FIRST AID FOR THE

USMLE STEP 1

A STUDENT TO 2004 STUDENT GUIDE

FIRST AID FOR THE

USMLE STEP 1

A STUDENT TO 2004 STUDENT GUIDE

VIKAS BHUSHAN, MD
University of California, San Francisco, Class of 1991
Diagnostic Radiologist

TAO LE, MD
University of California, San Francisco, Class of 1996
Johns Hopkins University, Fellow in Allergy and Immunology

JOSHUA KLEIN, PhD
Yale University School of Medicine, Class of 2005

ANIL SHIVARAM, MD
Yale University School of Medicine, Class of 2003
Mt. Auburn Hospital, Intern

Boston   Burr Ridge, IL   Dubuque, IA   Madison, WI   New York   San Francisco   St. Louis
Bangkok   Bogotá   Caracas   Kuala Lumpur   Lisbon   London   Madrid   Mexico City
Milan   Montreal   New Delhi   Santiago   Seoul   Singapore   Sydney   Taipei   Toronto

The McGraw·Hill Companies

First Aid for the USMLE Step 1 2004: A Student to Student Guide
International Edition 2004

Previous editions copyright © 2003, 2002, 2001, 2000 by The McGraw-Hill Companies, Inc.;
copyright © 1991 through 1999 by Appleton & Lange.
First edition copyright © 1990, 1989 by Vikas Bhushan, Jeffrey Hansen, and Edward Hon.
Portions of the material in Section 1 are copyright © 2000 by The Federation of State Medical Boards of the United States, Inc., and the National Board of Medical Examiners.

10 09 08 07 06 05 04 03 02 01
20 09 08 07 06 05 04
CTF   BJE

ISBN 007-142948-4

Notice

Medicine is an ever-changing science. As new research and clinical experience broaden our knowledge, changes in treatment and drug therapy are required. The authors and the publisher of this work have checked with sources believed to be reliable in their efforts to provide information that is complete and generally in accord with the standards accepted at the time of publication. However, in view of the possibility of human error or changes in medical sciences, neither the authors nor the publisher nor any other party who has been involved in the preparation or publication of this work warrants that the information contained herein is in every respect accurate or complete, and they disclaim all responsibility for any errors or omissions or for the results obtained from use of the information contained in this work. Readers are encouraged to confirm the information contained herein with other sources. For example and in particular, readers are advised to check the product information sheet included in the package of each drug they plan to administer to be certain that the information contained in this work is accurate and that changes have not been made in the recommended dose or in the contraindications for administration. The recommendation is of particular importance in connection with new or infrequently used drugs.

When ordering this title, use ISBN 007-123710-0

Printed in Singapore

To the contributors to this and future editions, who took time to share their knowledge, insight, and humor for the benefit of students.

&

To our families, friends, and loved ones, who endured and assisted in the task of assembling this guide.

Contributors

ROHIT CHANDWANI
Yale University,
Class of 2005

JORGE GALVEZ
Yale University,
Class of 2005

ZACHARY GOLDBERGER
Yale University,
Class of 2004

DOUGLAS JACOBSON
Yale University,
Class of 2005

BRIAN NAHED
Yale University,
Class of 2004

ALI OZTURK
Yale University,
Class of 2005

MATTHEW WHITLEY
Yale University,
Class of 2004

ALIREZA KHAZAEIZADEH, MD
Associate Professor of Biochemistry
St. Luke's University School of Medicine

BAHAR SEDARATI, MD
Associate Professor of Pathology
St. Luke's University School of Medicine

Associate Contributors

FADI ABU SHAHIN, MD
Northwestern University
   Resident in Obstetrics and Gynecology

MAE SHEIKH-ALI, MD
Drexel University College of Medicine
Resident in Internal Medicine

Faculty Reviewers

LINDA COSTANZO, PhD
Professor of Physiology
Medical College of Virginia
Virginia Commonwealth University

STUART FLYNN, MD
Professor of Pathology
Yale University School of Medicine

WILLIAM GANONG, MD
Lange Professor of Physiology Emeritus
University of California, San Francisco

BERTRAM KATZUNG, MD, PhD
Professor of Pharmacology
University of California, San Francisco

WARREN LEVINSON, MD, PhD
Professor of Microbiology and Immunology
University of California, San Francisco

WILLIAM STEWART, PhD
Associate Professor of Surgery
Yale University School of Medicine

Contents

Preface to the 2004 Edition

With the 2004 edition of *First Aid for the USMLE Step 1*, we continue our commitment to providing students with the most useful and up-to-date preparation guide for the USMLE Step 1. This edition represents a thorough revision in many ways and includes:

- A revised and updated exam preparation guide for the USMLE Step 1. Includes detailed analysis as well as study and test-taking strategies for the computer-based testing (CBT) format.
- Revisions and new material based on student experience with the 2003 administrations of the computerized USMLE Step 1.
- Expanded USMLE advice for international medical graduates, osteopathic medical students, podiatry students, and students with disabilities.
- An updated collection of over 140 high-yield glossy photos similar to those appearing on the USMLE Step 1 exam.
- More than 900 frequently tested facts and useful mnemonics, including hundreds of new or revised entries with many new diagrams and illustrations.
- An updated listing of more than 100 high-yield clinical vignette topics that highlight key areas of basic science and clinical material recently emphasized on the USMLE Step 1.
- An in-depth guide to hundreds of recommended basic science review and sample examination books, based on a nationwide survey of randomly selected third-year medical students.

The 2004 edition would not have been possible without the help of the hundreds of students and faculty members who contributed their feedback and suggestions. We invite students and faculty to continue sharing their thoughts and ideas to help us improve *First Aid for the USMLE Step 1*. (See How to Contribute, p. xv, and User Survey, p. xxiii.)

Los Angeles   Vikas Bhushan
Baltimore   Tao Le
New Haven   Joshua Klein
Boston   Anil Shivaram

November 2003

Foreword

The purpose of *First Aid for the USMLE Step 1: A Student-to-Student Guide* is to help medical students and international medical graduates review the basic medical sciences and prepare for the United States Medical Licensing Examination Step 1 (USMLE Step 1). Preparing for this examination can be a stressful, difficult, and costly task. This book helps students make the most of their limited time, money, and energy. As is often the case in medical school, we found that the best advice a student can receive is from other medical students. We also recognized that certain basic science topics and details are "popular" and appear frequently on examinations. With this in mind, *First Aid for the USMLE Step 1* was started in 1989.

As we studied for the NBME Part I, we examined and evaluated scores of review books and thousands of sample questions. We kept track of useful study strategies, frequently tested facts, and helpful mnemonics through a simple computer database. The printed database was first distributed to the medical school class of 1992 at the University of California, San Francisco (UCSF). The next year, a revised edition was self-published under the name *High-Yield Basic Science Boards Review: A Student-to-Student Guide*. This guide was distributed to the UCSF class of 1993 and to numerous faculty and medical students at various institutions.

The title reflects the potential value of this book as the "first" one to get before buying others, and the fact that boards examinations are stressful and unpleasant experiences that students may "aid" each other in overcoming. We feel that this study guide provides a unique and pragmatic approach to the USMLE Step 1 and that it contains useful components not found in current boards review material. *First Aid for the USMLE Step 1* has three major sections:

Section I: Guide to Efficient Exam Preparation is a compilation of general student advice and study strategies for taking the computerized USMLE Step 1.

Section II: Database of High-Yield Facts contains short descriptions of frequently tested facts and concepts as well as mnemonics, diagrams, and high-quality photo illustrations to facilitate learning. It includes a unique summary of subject-by-subject examination emphases as estimated by students who have recently taken the examination.

Section III: Database of Basic Science Review Books is designed to save students time and money by identifying high-quality, reasonably priced review and sample examination books and software. The comments and ratings are based on our analyses and on an annual nationwide random sampling of third-year medical students.

First Aid for the USMLE Step 1 is not designed to be a comprehensive text or the sole study source for the USMLE Step 1; it is meant as a guide to one's preparation for the USMLE Step 1. The material in this book has been written to strengthen one's familiarity with a large number of topics in a short, fact-based review. The authors do not advocate blindly memorizing the lists of facts, and we hope medical students realize that memorization cannot replace an understanding of the concepts that underlie these key points.

Entries in *First Aid for the USMLE Step 1* originated from hundreds of students, international medical graduates, and faculty members, who synthesized the facts, notes, and mnemonics from a variety of text-books, review books, lecture notes, and personal notes. We regret the inability to reference each individual fact or mnemonic owing to the diverse and often anecdotal sources. Although the material has been reviewed by faculty members and medical students, errors and omissions are inevitable. We urge readers to identify errors and suggest improvements. We regret that some students may find certain mnemonics trivializing or offensive. The mnemonics are meant solely as optional devices for learning.

The authors and McGraw-Hill intend to continue updating *First Aid for the USMLE Step 1* so that the book grows in quality and scope and continues to reflect the material covered on the USMLE Step 1. If you have any study strategies, high-yield facts with mnemonics, or book reviews for the next edition, please use the forms included to submit your contributions. (See How to Contribute, p. xv.) Any student or faculty member who submits material subsequently used in the next edition of *First Aid for the USMLE Step 1* will receive personal acknowledgment in the next edition and a $10 gift certificate per complete entry.

Good luck in your studies!

Acknowledgments

This has been a collaborative project from the start. We gratefully acknowledge the thoughtful comments, corrections, and advice of the many hundreds of medical students, international medical graduates, and faculty who have supported the authors in the continuing development of *First Aid for the USMLE Step 1*.

Thanks to Noam Maitless for the original book design, as well as Evenson Design Group, Ashley Pound, and Elizabeth Sanders for design revisions.

For support and encouragement throughout the process, we are grateful to Thao Pham and Jonathan Kirsch, Esq.

Thanks to our publisher, McGraw-Hill, for the valuable assistance of their staff. For enthusiasm, support, and commitment for this ongoing and ever-challenging project, thanks to our editor, Catherine Johnson. Thanks to Selina Bush for organizing and supporting the project. For editorial support, an enormous thanks to Andrea Fellows. A special thanks to Rainbow Graphics for remarkable production work.

Thanks to Kristopher Jones, Kristina Panizzi, and Peter Anderson of the Department of Pathology, University of Alabama at Birmingham, for use of images from the Pathology Education Instructional Resource Digital Library (http://peir.net). Special thanks to Dr. Raoul Fresco for his generous contributions to the glossy photo section.

For submitting contributions and corrections for the 2004 edition, we thank Aimee Chung, Sina Dadfarmay, Abdulla Fakhro, Michael Galuska, Jessie Glasser, Chivonne Harrigal, Peter Johnson, Geoffrey Lam, Anthony Migura, Linh Nguyen, Amay Parikh, and Haider Saeed.

For submitting book reviews, we thank Ingrid Abashamleh, Heba Abdulla, Jim Alexander, Beth Augustine, Justin Blasberg, Michelle Brand, Calandrella Casciano, Nicole Castonguay, Esther J. Cheung, Eugene Choo, Jonathan Christopher, Raisa Chyorny, Heidi Dambach, Malinda Danforth, Dana Dumitru, Raman Singh Dusan, Daniel Feldman, Celia Garner, Julia Gloeckler, David Goldberg, Jaime Terner Goodman, Gregory B. Gullung, Jessica Hoots, Michael V. Huppmann, Barbara Huynh, Roland M. Jermyn, Jennifer Jocson, Reza John Karimi, Melissa Keca, Rachel Kerford, Sajid Khan, Christi A. Kidd, James Knight, Robert Koval, Melissa Krebs, Carey Kucirek, Shilpa Kumbhani, Melissa Kurkjian, Ashwini Lakshmanan, Katie Laures, Jacqueline K. Le, Phuoc Le, Grace Lee, Monica Lee, Robert Lee, Diana Leu, Joseph Levison, Heather Liu, Sarah Macleish, Karla Maguire, Miranda McCann, Cheryl McGary, Paul Meier, Amie Y. Miklavic, Arun Mohan, Jacquelyn Nohl, Harry W. Ou, Jay Pahade, Ben Peake, Judy Peters, Yelena Podorozhansky, Paul Polyar, Jennifer Poon, Zainab Rashid, Jennifer Rasmussen, Susan Rhee, Alison Rudy, David Spence, Greg Stancel, Kalyan Tatineny, Pamela Traisak, Svetlana Volokh, Amy E. Williams, Joanna Wu, Andrew Zinkel, and Anna Zou.

Finally, thanks to Ted Hon, one of the founding authors of this book, for his vision in developing this guide on the computer, and to Chirag Amin for his enormous contributions as an editor and author over many editions.

Los Angeles   Vikas Bhushan
Baltimore   Tao Le
New Haven   Joshua Klein
Boston   Anil Shivaram

How to Use This Book

Medical students who have used previous editions of this guide have given us feedback on how best to make use of the book.

It is recommended that you begin using this book as early as possible when learning the basic medical sciences. You can use Section III to select first-year course review books and Internet resources and then use those books for review while taking your medical school classes.

Use different parts of the book at different stages in your preparation for the USMLE Step 1. Before you begin to study for the USMLE Step 1, we suggest that you read Section I: Guide to Efficient Exam Preparation and Section III: Database of Basic Science Review Resources. **If you are an international medical graduate student, an osteopathic medical student, a podiatry student, or a student with a disability,** refer to the appropriate Section I supplement for additional advice. Devise a study plan and decide what resources to buy. We strongly recommend that you invest in at least one or two top-rated review books in each subject. *First Aid* is not a comprehensive review book, and it is not a panacea that can compensate for not studying during the first two years of medical school. Scanning Section II will give you an initial idea of the diverse range of topics covered on the USMLE Step 1.

As you study each discipline, **use the corresponding high-yield-fact section in *First Aid for the USMLE Step 1* as a means of consolidating the material and testing yourself** to see if you have covered some of the frequently tested items. Work with the book to integrate important facts into your fund of knowledge. Using *First Aid for the USMLE Step 1* as a review can serve as both a self-test of your knowledge and a repetition of important facts to learn. High-yield topics and vignettes are abstracted from recent exams to help guide your preparation.

Return to Section II frequently during your preparation and fill your short-term memory with remaining high-yield facts a few days before the USMLE Step 1. The book can serve as a useful way of retaining key associations and keeping high-yield facts fresh in your memory just prior to the examination.

Reviewing the book immediately after the exam is probably the best way to **help us improve the book in the next edition.** Decide what was truly high and low yield and **send in the contribution forms or your entire annotated book.**

First Aid Checklist for the USMLE Step 1

This is an example of how you might use the information in Section I to prepare for the USMLE Step 1. Refer to corresponding topics in Section I for more details.

Years Prior

☐ Select top-rated review books as study guides for first-year medical school courses.

Months Prior

☐ Review computer test format and registration information.
☐ Register six months in advance. Carefully verify name and address printed on scheduling permit. Call Prometric for test date ASAP.
☐ Define goals for the USMLE Step 1 (e.g., comfortably pass, beat the mean, ace the test).
☐ Set up a realistic timeline for study. Cover less crammable subjects first. Review subject-by-subject emphasis and clinical vignette format.
☐ Simulate the USMLE Step 1 to pinpoint strengths and weaknesses in knowledge and test-taking skills.
☐ Evaluate and choose study methods and materials (e.g., review books, practice tests, software).
☐ Ask advice from those who have recently taken the USMLE Step 1.

Weeks Prior

☐ Simulate the USMLE Step 1 again. Assess how close you are to your goal.
☐ Pinpoint remaining weaknesses. Stay healthy (exercise, sleep).
☐ Verify information on admission ticket (e.g., location, date).

One Week Prior

☐ Remember comfort measures (loose clothing, earplugs, etc.).
☐ Work out test site logistics such as location, transportation, parking, and lunch.
☐ Call Prometric and confirm your exam appointment.

One Day Prior

☐ Relax.
☐ Light review of short-term material if necessary. Skim high-yield facts.
☐ Get a good night's sleep.
☐ Make sure the name printed on your photo ID appears EXACTLY the same as the name printed on your scheduling permit. You will not be allowed to take the exam unless the names match EXACTLY.

Day of Exam

☐ Relax. Eat breakfast. Minimize bathroom breaks during exam by avoiding excessive morning caffeine.
☐ Analyze and make adjustments in test-taking technique. You are allowed to review notes/study material during breaks on exam day.

After the Exam

☐ Celebrate, regardless.
☐ Please fill out the contribution forms and receive $10 gift certificates. See p. xv for details.

Guide to Efficient Exam Preparation

INTRODUCTION

Relax.

This section is intended to make your exam preparation easier, not harder. Our goal is to reduce your level of stress and help you make the most of your study effort by helping you understand more about the United States Medical Licensing Examination, Step 1 (USMLE Step 1)—especially what the new computer-based testing (CBT) is likely to mean to you. As a medical student, you are no doubt familiar with taking standardized examinations and quickly absorbing large amounts of material. When you first confront the USMLE Step 1, however, you may find it easy to become sidetracked and not achieve your goal of studying with maximum effectiveness. Common mistakes that students make when studying for the boards include the following:

- "Stressing out" owing to an inadequate understanding of the new computer-based format
- Not understanding how scoring is performed or what your score means
- Starting *First Aid* too late
- Starting to study too late
- Using inefficient or inappropriate study methods
- Buying the wrong books or buying more books than you can ever use
- Buying only one publisher's review series for all subjects
- Not using practice examinations to maximum benefit
- Not using review books along with your classes
- Not analyzing and improving your test-taking strategies
- Getting bogged down by reviewing difficult topics excessively
- Studying material that is rarely tested on the USMLE Step 1
- Failing to master certain high-yield subjects owing to overconfidence
- Using *First Aid* as your sole study resource

In this section, we offer advice to help you avoid these pitfalls and be more productive in your studies. To begin, it is important for you to understand what the examination involves.

USMLE STEP 1—THE CBT BASICS

The USMLE assesses a physician's ability to apply knowledge, concepts, and principles that are important in health and disease and that constitute the basis of safe and effective patient care.[2]

Some degree of concern about your performance on the USMLE Step 1 examination is both expected and appropriate. All too often, however, medical students become unnecessarily anxious about the examination. It is therefore important to understand precisely what the USMLE Step 1 involves. As you become familiar with Step 1, you can translate your anxiety into more efficient preparation.

The USMLE Step 1 is the first of three examinations that you must pass in order to become a licensed physician in the United States.[1] The USMLE is a joint endeavor of the National Board of Medical Examiners (NBME) and the Federation of State Medical Boards (FSMB). In previous years, the examination was strictly organized around seven traditional disciplines: anatomy, behavioral science, biochemistry, microbiology, pathology, pharmacology, and physiology. In June 1991, the NBME began administering the "new" NBME Part I examination, which offered a more integrated and multidisciplinary format coupled with more clinically oriented questions.

In 1992, the USMLE replaced both the Federation Licensing Examination (FLEX) and the certifying examinations of the NBME.[3] The USMLE now serves as the single examination system for United States medical students and international medical graduates (IMGs) seeking medical licensure in the United States.

How Is the CBT Structured?

In 1999, the traditional two-day paper-and-pencil exam gave way to an eight-hour computer-based test. The exam, administered by Prometric, Inc®, a subsidiary of Thomson Learning™, is now offered year-round at hundreds of sites around the world.

The CBT format of Step 1 is simply a computerized version of the former paper exam.

The CBT Step 1 exam consists of seven question "blocks" of 50 questions each (Figure 1) for a total of 350 questions, timed at 60 minutes per block. A short 11-question survey follows the last question block. The computer begins the survey with a prompt to proceed to the next block of questions. Don't be fooled! "Block 8" is the NBME survey.

These blocks were designed to reduce eyestrain and fatigue during the exam. Once an examinee finishes a particular block, he or she must click on a screen icon to continue to the next block. Examinees will **not** be able to go back and change answers to questions from any previously completed block. Changing answers, however, is allowed **within** a block of questions as long as time permits.

Don't be fooled! After the last question block comes the NBME survey ("Block 8").

Prometric test centers offer Step 1 on a year-round basis, except for the first two weeks in January. The exam is given every day except Sunday at most centers. Some schools administer the exam on their own campuses.

FIGURE 1. Schematic of CBT Exam.

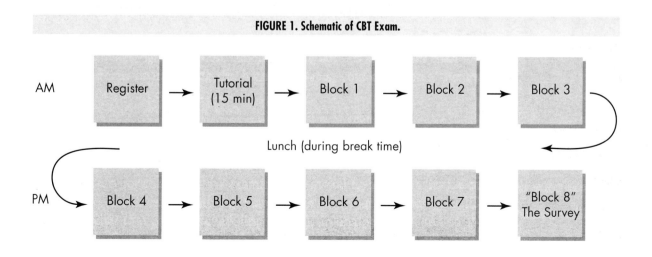

What Is the CBT Like?

Skip the tutorial and add

15 minutes to your break

time!

Because of the unique environment of the CBT, it's important that you be familiar ahead of time with what your test-day conditions will be like. Familiarizing yourself with the testing interface before the exam can add 15 minutes to your break time! This is because a 15-minute tutorial, offered on exam day, may be skipped if you are already familiar with the exam procedures and the testing interface (see description of CD-ROM below). The 15 minutes is added to your allotted break time (should you choose to skip the tutorial).

For security reasons, examinees are not allowed to bring any personal electronic equipment into the testing area. This includes digital watches, watches with computer communication and/or memory capability, cellular telephones, and electronic paging devices. Food and beverages are also prohibited. The testing centers are monitored by audio and video surveillance equipment.

The typical question screen (Figure 2) has a question followed by a number of choices on which an examinee can click, together with a number of navigational buttons at the bottom. There is also a button that allows the examinee to mark the question for review. There is a countdown timer in the upper right-hand corner of the screen as well. If the question happens to be longer than the screen (very rare), a scroll bar appears on the right, allowing the examinee to see the rest of the question. Regardless of whether the examinee clicks on an answer or leaves it blank, he or she must click the "Next" button to advance to the next question.

Some questions contain figures or color illustrations (Figure 3). These are typically situated to the right of the question. Although the contrast and bright-

FIGURE 2. Typical Question Screen.

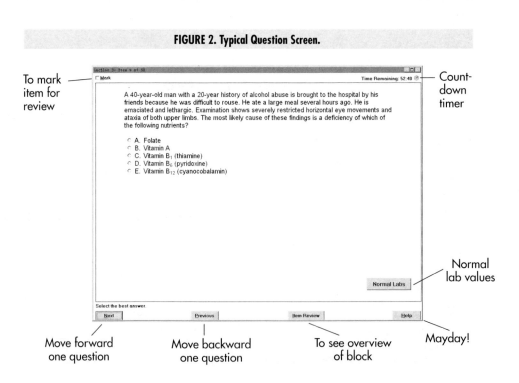

To mark item for review

Count-down timer

Normal lab values

Move forward one question

Move backward one question

To see overview of block

Mayday!

FIGURE 3. Question Screen with Illustration.

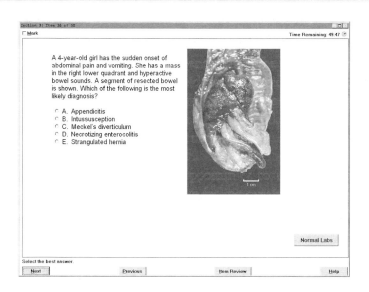

Test illustrations include:

- *Gross photos*

- *Histology slides*

- *Radiographs*

- *EMs*

- *Line drawings*

ness of the screen can be adjusted, there are no other ways to manipulate the picture (e.g., no zooming or panning).

The examinee can call up a window displaying normal lab values (Figure 4). However, if he or she does not press "Tile" on the normal-values screen, the normal-values window may obscure the question. The examinee may have to scroll down searching for the needed laboratory values.

Clicking "Item Review" at the bottom of the screen brings up a screen showing an overview of the block (Figure 5). This screen allows the examinee to pinpoint questions marked for review as well as unanswered questions. This

FIGURE 4. Lab-Values Screen—Floating and Tiled.

Floating lab values   Tile function   Tiled lab values

FIGURE 5. Item Review Screen.

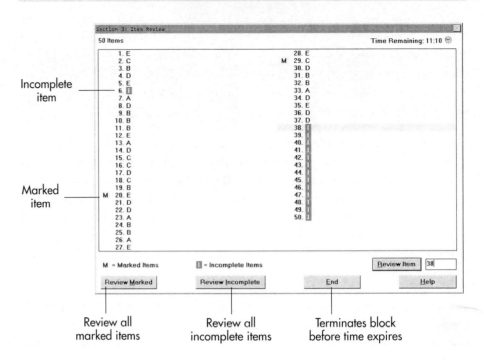

Incomplete item

Marked item

M = Marked Items   ☐ = Incomplete Items

Review Marked   Review Incomplete   End   Help

Review all marked items   Review all incomplete items   Terminates block before time expires

also serves as a quick way of navigating to any question in the block—even unmarked completed questions.

What Does the CBT Format Mean to Me?

The significance of the CBT to you depends on the requirements of your school and your level of computer knowledge. If you hate computers and freak out whenever you see one, you might want to face your fears as soon as possible. Spend some time playing with a Windows-based system and pointing and clicking icons or buttons with a mouse. These are the absolute basics, and you won't want to waste valuable exam time figuring them out on test day. Your test taking will proceed by pointing and clicking, essentially without the use of the keyboard. The free CD is an excellent way to become familiar with the test interface.

For those who feel they would benefit, the USMLE offers an opportunity to take a simulated test, or "CBT Practice Session at a Prometric center." Students are eligible to take the three-and-one-half-hour practice session after they have received their fluorescent orange scheduling permit (see below).

The same USMLE Step 1 sample test items (150 questions) available on the CD or USMLE Web site, www.usmle.org, are used at these sessions. *No new items will be presented.* The session is divided into three one-hour blocks of 50 test items each and costs about $42. The student receives a printed percent-correct score after completing the session. No explanations of questions are provided.

You may register for a practice session online at www.usmle.org.

How Do I Register to Take the Exam?

Starting with the 2001 USMLE application cycle, registration packets with printed materials are no longer provided to medical schools. Your medical school should have a supply of the 2004 CD, which contains electronic files of all of the printed materials, such as the *2004 USMLE Bulletin of Information*. Step 1 or Step 2 applications, which are not on the CD, may be printed from the USMLE Web site.

The preliminary registration process for the USMLE Step 1 is essentially unchanged, which is to say that students are required to complete registration forms and send exam fees to the NBME. The application allows applicants to select one of 12 overlapping three-month blocks in which to be tested (e.g., April–May–June, June–July–August). The application includes a photo ID form that must be certified by an official at your medical school to verify your enrollment. After the NBME processes your application, it will send you a fluorescent orange slip of paper called a scheduling permit.

The scheduling permit you receive from the NBME will contain your USMLE identification number, the eligibility period in which you may take the exam, and two unique numbers. One of these is known as your "scheduling number." You must have this number to make your exam appointment with Prometric. The other number is known as the "candidate identification number," or CIN. Examinees must enter their CINs at the Prometric workstation to access their exams. Prometric has no access to the codes. **Do not lose your permit!** You will not be allowed to take the boards unless you present this permit along with an unexpired, government-issued photo identification with your signature (such as a driver's license or passport). Make sure the name on your photo ID exactly matches the name appearing on your scheduling permit.

Once you receive your scheduling permit, you may call the Prometric toll-free number to arrange a time to take the exam. Although requests for taking the exam may be completed more than six months before the test date, examinees will not receive their scheduling permits earlier than six months before the eligibility period. The eligibility period is the three-month period you have chosen to take the exam. Most medical students choose the April–June or June–August period. Because exams are scheduled on a "first-come, first-served" basis, it is recommended that you telephone Prometric as soon as you have received your permit. After you've scheduled your exam, it's a good idea to confirm your exam appointment with Prometric at least one week prior to your test date. Prometric does not provide written confirmation of exam date, time, or location. Be sure to read the *2004 USMLE Bulletin of Information* for further details.

What if I Need to Reschedule the Exam?

You can change your date and/or center by contacting Prometric at 1-800-MED-EXAM (1-800-633-3926) or www.prometric.com. Make sure to have your CIN when rescheduling. If you are rescheduling by phone, you must

Test scheduling is on a "first-come, first-served" basis. It's important to call and schedule an exam date as soon as you receive your scheduling permit.

Testing centers are closed on major holidays and during the first two weeks of January.

Register six months in advance for seating and scheduling preference.

speak with a Prometric representative; leaving a voice-mail message will not suffice. To avoid a rescheduling fee, you will need to request a change before noon EST at least five business days before your appointment. Please note that your rescheduled test date must fall within your assigned three-month eligibility period.

When Should I Register for the Exam?

Although there are no deadlines for registering for Step 1, you should plan to register at least six months ahead of your desired test date. This will guarantee that you will get either your test center of choice or one within a 50-mile radius of your first choice. For most U.S. medical students, the desired testing window is in June, since most medical school curricula for the second year end in May or June. Thus, U.S. medical students should plan to register before January for a June test date. The timing of the exam is more flexible for IMGs, as it is related only to when they finish exam preparation.

Choose your three-month eligibility period wisely. If you need to reschedule outside your initial three-month period, you must submit a new application along with another application fee.

Where Can I Take the Exam?

Your testing location is arranged with Prometric when you call for your test date (after you receive your scheduling permit). For a list of Prometric locations nearest you, visit www.prometric.com.

How Long Will I Have to Wait Before I Get My Scores?

The USMLE reports scores three to six weeks after the examinee's test date. Scores are always released on a Wednesday. During peak times, score reports may take up to six weeks. Official information concerning the time required for score reporting is posted on the USMLE Web site.

What Did Other Students Like/Dislike About the CBT Format?

Feedback from students about the CBT format has been overwhelmingly positive. Students note that the testing environment was not as stressful as imagined and add that they enjoyed the test's point-and-click simplicity. "It's nice to be able to work at your own pace and take breaks whenever you want," commented one student.

Beware of the awkward lab-values screen, background noise, variable image quality, and eyestrain.

Of the complaints expressed, students were most concerned with image quality, eyestrain, temperature extremes (heat/cold), and background noise at the Prometric center. Students noted that the quality of some images made it difficult to answer certain questions and that they would like to be able to enlarge images. Eyestrain seemed to affect other test takers; taking a short break usually afforded relief. In addition, some students noted that the clicking of mice and keyboard chatter by other students bothered them. Earplugs helped but didn't completely block all such sounds.

What About Time?

Time is of special interest on the CBT exam. Here's a breakdown of the exam schedule:

15 minutes	Tutorial (skip if familiar)
7 hours	60-minute question blocks
45 minutes	Break time (includes time for lunch)

The computer will keep track of how much time has elapsed. However, the computer will show you only how much time you have remaining in a given block. Therefore, it is up to you to determine if you are pacing yourself properly (at a rate of approximately one question per 72 seconds).

The computer will **not** warn you if you are spending more than your allotted time for a break. Taking long breaks between question blocks or for lunch may result in your not being able to take breaks later. You should budget your time so that you can take a short break when you need it and have time to eat.

You must be especially careful not to spend too much time in between blocks (you should keep track of how much time elapses from when you finish a block of questions to when you start the next block). After you finish one question block, you'll need to click the mouse when you are ready to proceed to the next block of questions.

Forty-five minutes is the minimum break time for the day. You can gain extra break time (but not time for the question blocks) by skipping the tutorial or by finishing a block ahead of the allotted time.

For security reasons, digital watches are not allowed. This means that only analog watches are permitted. You should therefore get used to timing yourself with an analog watch so that you know exactly how much time you have left. Some analog watches come with a bevel that helps keep track of 60-minute periods. This may be useful for keeping track of break time.

If I Freak Out and Leave, What Happens to My Score?

Your scheduling permit shows a CIN that you will enter onto your computer screen to start your exam. Entering the CIN is the same as breaking the seal on a test book, and you are considered to have started the exam. However, no score will be reported if you do not complete the exam. In fact, if you leave at any time from the start of the test to the last block, no score will be reported. The fact that you started but did not complete the exam, however, will appear on your USMLE score transcript.

Be careful to watch the clock on your break time.

Gain extra break time by skipping the tutorial or finishing a block early.

If you have one unanswered question remaining during any block, the computer will allow you to answer it before you are closed out of the block. (Note: This will use up some of your break time.)

The exam ends when all blocks have been completed or their time has expired. As you leave the testing center, you receive a printed test-completion notice to document your completion of the exam.

To receive an official score, you must finish the entire exam. This means that you must start and either finish or run out of time for each block of the exam. Again, if you do not complete all blocks, your exam is documented as an incomplete attempt, and no score is reported.

What Types of Questions Are Asked?

Nearly three-fourths of the 2003 Step 1 questions began with a description of a patient.

Although numerous changes had to be made for the CBT format, the question types are the same as in previous years.

One-best-answer items have been the most commonly used multiple-choice format. Test takers report that every question was of this format. Most questions consist of a clinical scenario or a direct question followed by a list of five or more options. You are required to select the one best answer among the options. A number of options may be partially correct, in which case you must select the option that best answers the question or completes the statement. Additionally, keep in mind that experimental questions may appear on the exam (see Difficult Questions, p. 28).

How Is the Test Scored?

The mean Step 1 score for U.S. medical students rose from 200 in 1991 to 215 in 2000.

Each Step 1 examinee receives a score report that has the examinee's pass/fail status, two test scores, and a graphic depiction of the examinee's performance by discipline and organ system or subject area (Figures 6A and 6B). The actual organ system profiles reported may depend on the statistical characteristics of a given administration of the examination.

For 1999, the NBME provided two overall test scores based on the total number of items answered correctly on the examination (Figure 7). The first score, the three-digit score, was reported as a scaled score in which the mean was 215 and the standard deviation was 20. The second score scale, the two-digit score, defines 75 as the minimum passing score (equivalent to a score of 179 on the first scale). A score of 82 is equivalent to a score of 200 on the first score scale. To avoid confusion, we refer to scores using the three-digit scale with a mean of 215 and a standard deviation of 20.

Passing the CBT Step 1 is estimated to correspond to answering 60 to 70% of the questions correctly.

Starting in 2001, a score of 182 or higher is required to pass Step 1. Passing the CBT Step 1 is estimated to correspond to answering 60 to 70% of questions correctly. In 2001, the pass rates for first-time test takers from accredited U.S. and Canadian medical schools were 93% and 91%, respectively (Table 1). These statistics prove it—you're much more likely to pass than fail. Although the NMBE may adjust the minimum passing score at any time, no further adjustment is expected for several years.

FIGURE 6A. Sample Score Report—Front Page.

UNITED STATES MEDICAL LICENSING EXAMINATION™

USMLE Step 1 is administered to students and graduates of U.S. and Canadian medical schools by the
NATIONAL BOARD OF MEDICAL EXAMINERS® (NBME®)
3750 Market Street, Philadelphia, Pennsylvania 19104-3190.
Telephone: (215) 590-9700

STEP 1 SCORE REPORT

Schmoe, Joe T	USMLE ID: 1-234-567-8
Anytown, CA 12345	Test Date: June 2002

The USMLE is a single examination program for all applicants for medical licensure in the United States; it replaces the Federation Licensing Examination (FLEX) and the certifying examinations of the National Board of Medical Examiners (NBME Parts I, II and III). The program consists of three Steps designed to assess an examinee's understanding of and ability to apply concepts and principles that are important in health and disease and that constitute the basis of safe and effective patient care. Step 1 is designed to assess whether an examinee understands and can apply key concepts of the basic biomedical sciences, with an emphasis on principles and mechanisms of health, disease and modes of therapy. The inclusion of **Step 1** in the USMLE sequence is intended to ensure mastery of not only the basic medical sciences undergirding the safe and competent practice of medicine in the present, but also the scientific principles required for maintenance of competence through lifelong learning. Results of the examination are reported to medical licensing authorities in the United States and its territories for use in granting an initial license to practice medicine. The two numeric scores shown below are equivalent; each state or territory may use either score in making licensing decisions. These scores represent your results for the administration of Step 1 on the test date shown above.

PASS	This result is based on the minimum passing score set by USMLE for Step 1. Individual licensing authorities may accept the USMLE-recommended pass/fail result or may establish a different passing score for their own jurisdictions.
215	This score is determined by your overall performance on Step 1. For recent administrations, the mean and standard deviation for first-time examinees from U.S. and Canadian medical schools are approximately 215 and 20, respectively, with most scores falling between 175 and 255. A score of 179 is set by USMLE to pass Step 1. The standard error of measurement (SEM)‡ for this scale is four points.
85	This score is also determined by your overall performance on the examination. A score of 82 on this scale is equivalent to a score of 200 on the scale described above. A score of 75 on this scale, which is equivalent to a score of 182 on the scale described above, is set by USMLE to pass Step 1. The SEM‡ for this scale is one point.

‡Your score is influenced both by your general understanding of the basic biomedical sciences and the specific set of items selected for this Step 1 examination. The SEM provides an estimate of the range within which your scores might be expected to vary by chance if you were tested repeatedly using similar tests.

121JP452

NOTE: Original score report has copy-resistant watermark.

According to the USMLE, medical schools receive a listing of total scores and pass/fail results plus group summaries by discipline and organ system. Students can withhold their scores from their medical school if they wish. Official USMLE transcripts, which can be sent on request to residency programs, include only total scores, not performance profiles.

Consult the USMLE Web site or your medical school for the most current and accurate information regarding the examination.

What Does My Score Mean?

For students, the most important point with the Step 1 score is passing versus failing. Passing essentially means, "Hey, you're on your way to becoming a fully licensed doc."

11

FIGURE 6B. Sample Score Report—Back Page.

INFORMATION PROVIDED FOR EXAMINEE USE ONLY

The Performance Profile below is provided solely for the benefit of the examinee.
These profiles are developed as assessment tools for examinees only and will not be reported or verified to any third party.

USMLE STEP 1 PERFORMANCE PROFILES

	Lower Performance	Borderline Performance	Higher Performance
Behavioral Sciences			xxxxxxxxxxxxxxx
Biochemistry			xxxxxxxxxxx
Cardiovascular System			xxxxxxxxxxxxxx *
Gastrointestinal System			xxxxxxxxxxxxxxx
General Principles of Health & Disease			xxxxxxxxx
Genetics			xxxxxxxxxxxxxx
Gross Anatomy & Embryology			xxxxxxxxxxxxx *
Hematopoietic & Lymphoreticular Systems		xxxxxxxxxxxxxx	
Histology & Cell Biology		xxxxxxxxxxxxxxxx	
Microbiology & Immunology			xxxxxxxxxx
Musculoskeletal, Skin & Connective Tissue		xxxxxxxxxxxxxx	
Nervous System/Special Senses			xxxxxxxxxx
Pathology			xxxxxxxxxx
Pharmacology			xxxxxxxxx
Physiology			xxxxxxxxx
Renal/Urinary System			xxxxxxxxxxxxxxx
Reproductive & Endocrine Systems			xxxxxxxxxxxxx
Respiratory System		xxxxxxxxxxxxxxxx	

The above Performance Profile is provided to aid in self-assessment. The shaded area defines a borderline level of performance for each content area; borderline performance is comparable to a HIGH FAIL/LOW PASS on the total test.

Performance bands indicate areas of relative strength and weakness. Some bands are wider than others. The width of a performance band reflects the precision of measurement: narrower bands indicate greater precision. An asterisk indicates that your performance band extends beyond the displayed portion of the scale. Small differences in the location of bands should not be over interpreted. If two bands overlap, the performance in the associated areas should not be interpreted as significantly different.

This profile should not be compared to those from other Step 1 administrations.

Additional information concerning the topics covered in each content area can be found in the *USMLE Step 1 General Instructions, Content Description and Sample Items.*

452JP121

Beyond that, the main point of having a quantitative score is to give you a sense of how you've done aside from the fact that you've passed the exam. The two-digit or three-digit score gauges how you have done with respect to the content on the exam.

Since the content of the exam is what drives the score, the profile of the exam is what remains relatively constant over the years. That is to say that each exam profile includes a certain number of "very hard" questions along with "medium" and "easy" ones. The questions vary, but the profile of the exam doesn't change much. This ensures that someone who scored 200 on the boards yesterday achieved a level of knowledge similar to that of the person who scored 200 four years ago.

FIGURE 7. Scoring Scales for the USMLE Step 1.

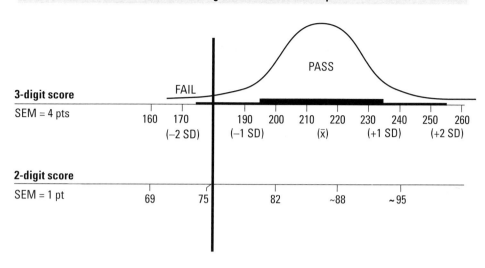

TABLE 1. Passing Rates for the 2001–2002 USMLE Step 1.[a]

	2001		2002	
	No. Tested	Passing (%)	No. Tested	Passing (%)
NBME-registered examinees (U.S./Canadian) Allopathic students				
First-time takers	16,368	91	16,420	92
Repeaters	2012	58	2,085	59
Allopathic total	**18,380**	**88**	**18,505**	**88**
Osteopathic students First-time takers	723	72	892	70
Repeaters	51	31	57	32
Osteopathic total	**774**	**69**	**949**	**67**
Total (U.S./Canadian)	**19,154**	**87**	**19,454**	**87**
FMG examinees (ECFMG[b] registrants) First-time takers	9,835	66	11,821	64
Repeaters	4,259	35	5,298	36
FMG total	**14,094**	**56**	**17,119**	**55**
Total Step 1 examinees	**33,248**	**74**	**36,573**	**72**

[a]Reflects the most current data available at the time of publishing.
[b]Educational Commission for Foreign Medical Graduates.

13

Official NBME/USMLE Resources

We strongly encourage students to use the free materials provided by the testing agencies (see p. 32) and to study in detail the following NBME publications, all of which are available on CD-ROM or at the USMLE Web site www.usmle.org:

- *USMLE Step 1 2004 Computer-based Content and Sample Test Questions* (information given free to all examinees)
- *2004 USMLE Bulletin of Information* (information given free to all examinees)

The *USMLE Step 1 2004 Computer-based Content and Sample Test Questions* contains approximately 150 questions that are similar in format and content to the questions on the actual USMLE Step 1. This practice test offers one of the best methods for assessing your test-taking skills. However, it does not contain enough questions to simulate the full length of the examination, and its content represents a limited sampling of the basic science material that may be covered on Step 1. Most students felt that the questions on the actual 2003 exam were more challenging than those contained in these questions. Others report encountering a few near-duplicates of these questions on the actual Step 1. Presumably, these are "experimental" questions, but who knows! Bottom line: Know these questions!

The extremely detailed *Step 1 Content Outline* provided by the USMLE has not proved useful for students studying for the exam. The USMLE even states that ". . . the content outline is not intended as a guide for curriculum development or as a study guide."[4] We concur with this assessment.

The *2004 USMLE Bulletin of Information* is found on the CD-ROM. This publication contains detailed procedural and policy information regarding the CBT, including descriptions of all three Steps, scoring of the exams, reporting of scores to medical schools and residency programs, procedures for score rechecks and other inquiries, policies for irregular behavior, and test dates.

Starting in 2003, the NBME unveiled the Comprehensive Basic Science Self-Assessment (CBSSA), which tests users on topics covered during basic science courses in a format similar to the USMLE Step 1 examination. The Web-based information provided via the CBSSA is intended for use as a study tool and not as an indicator of Step 1 performance. However, students who prepared for the examination using this Web-based tool found the format and content highly indicative of questions tested for the Step 1 examination. The CBSSA exists in two forms: a standard-paced and a self-paced format, both of which consist of four sections of 50 questions (a total of 200 multiple-choice items). The standard-paced format allows the user up to one hour to complete each section, reflecting the time limits of the actual exam. The self-paced format, however, places no time limit on answering the multiple-choice questions. Keep in mind that this bank of questions is available only over the Web. The NBME requires that users log on, register, and start within 30 days of registration. Once the assessment has begun, users are required to complete the sections within 20 days. Upon completion of the questions, the CBSSA will provide the user with a performance profile, indicating relative strengths and weaknesses, similar to the report profile for the USMLE Step 1 exam. However, please keep in mind that this self-assessment does not provide the user with a list of correct answers. Feedback from the self-assessment is entirely in the format of a performance profile and nothing more. The NBME charges $45 for this service, which is payable by credit card or money order. For more information regarding the CBSSA, please visit the NBME's Web site at www.nbme.org and click on the link for "NBME Web-based Self-Assessment Service."

DEFINING YOUR GOAL

It is useful to define your own personal performance goal when approaching the USMLE Step 1. Your style and intensity of preparation can then be matched to your goal. Your goal may depend on your school's requirements, your specialty choice, your grades to date, and your personal assessment of the test's importance.

Comfortably Pass

As mentioned earlier, the USMLE Step 1 is the first of three standardized examinations that you must pass in order to become a licensed physician in the United States. Also, at many medical schools, passing the USMLE Step 1 is required before you can continue with your clinical training. The NBME, however, feels that medical schools should not use Step 1 as the sole determinant of advancement to the third year.[5] If you are headed for a "noncompetitive" residency program and you have consulted advisers and fourth-year medical students in your area of interest, you may feel comfortable with this approach. Obviously, however, aiming for a score of 182 is a risky way to "comfortably pass" the exam.

Fourth-year medical students have the best feel for how Step 1 scores factor into the residency application process.

Beat the Mean

Although the NBME warns against the misuse of examination scores to evaluate student qualifications for residency positions, some residency program directors continue to use Step 1 scores to screen applicants. Thus, many students feel it is important to score higher than the national average.

Internship and residency programs vary greatly in their policy toward requesting scores. Some simply request your pass/fail status, whereas others ask for your total score. Some programs have even been known to request a photocopy of your score report to determine how well you performed on individual sections; however, this is unusual. It is unclear how continuing changes in USMLE Step 1 examination and score reporting will affect the application process for residency programs. The best sources of bottom-line information are fourth-year medical students who have recently completed the residency application process.

Some medical students may wish to "beat the mean" for their own personal satisfaction. For these students, there may be a psychological advantage to scoring higher than the national average.

Ace the Exam

Some competitive residency programs use Step 1 scores in their selection process.

Certain highly competitive residency programs, such as those in otolaryngology and orthopedic surgery, have acknowledged their use of Step 1 scores in the selection process. In such residency programs, greater emphasis may be placed on attaining a high score, so students who wish to enter these programs may wish to consider aiming for a very high score on the USMLE Step 1. However, use of the USMLE scores for residency selection has been criticized because neither Step 1 nor Step 2 was designed for this purpose.[6] In addition, only a subset of the basic science facts and concepts that are tested is important to functioning well on the wards. Alternatively, some students may wish to score well in order to feel a sense of mastery. High scores are particularly important for IMGs applying in all specialties.

TIMELINE FOR STUDY

Time management is key. Customize your schedule to your goals and available time following any final exams.

Make a Schedule

After you have defined your goals, map out a study schedule that is consistent with your objectives, your vacation time, and the difficulty of your ongoing coursework (Figure 8). Determine whether you want to spread out your study time or concentrate it into 14-hour study days in the final weeks. Then factor in your own history in preparing for standardized examinations (e.g., SAT, MCAT).

FIGURE 8. Typical Timeline for the USMLE Step 1.

There are three basic study patterns:
The compulsive (months— ace exam).
The crammer (weeks— just pass).
The IMG (months— variable).

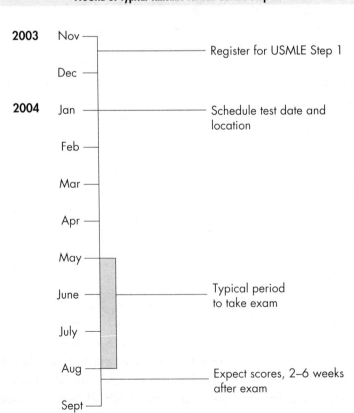

2003	Nov	Register for USMLE Step 1
	Dec	
2004	Jan	Schedule test date and location
	Feb	
	Mar	
	Apr	
	May	
	June	Typical period to take exam
	July	
	Aug	Expect scores, 2–6 weeks after exam
	Sept	

Another important consideration is when you will study each subject. Some subjects lend themselves to cramming, whereas others demand a substantial long-term commitment. The "crammable" subjects for Step 1 are those for which concise yet relatively complete review books are available. (See Section III for highly rated review and sample examination books.) Behavioral science and physiology are two subjects with concise review books. Three subjects with longer but quite complete review books are microbiology, pharmacology, and biochemistry. Thus, these subjects could be covered toward the end of your schedule, whereas other subjects (anatomy and pathology) require a longer time commitment and could be studied earlier. An increasing number of students report using a "systems-based" approach (e.g., GI, renal, cardiovascular) to integrate the material across basic science subjects.

"Crammable" subjects should be covered later and less crammable subjects earlier.

Practically speaking, spending a given amount of time on a crammable or high-yield subject (particularly in the last few days before the test) generally produces more correct answers on the examination than spending the same amount of time on a low-yield subject. Student opinion indicates that knowing the crammable subjects extremely well probably results in a higher overall score than knowing all subjects moderately well.

Allow time in your study schedule for getting sidetracked by personal emergencies.

If you are having difficulty deciding when to start your test preparation, you may find the reverse-calendar approach helpful. Start with the day of the test and plan backward, setting deadlines for objectives to be met. Where the planning ends on your calendar defines a possible starting point.

Make your schedule realistic, and set achievable goals. Many students make the mistake of studying at a level of detail that requires too much time for a comprehensive review—reading *Gray's Anatomy* in a couple of days is not a realistic goal! Revise your schedule regularly based on your actual progress. Be careful not to lose focus. Beware of feelings of inadequacy when comparing study schedules and progress with your peers. **Avoid students who stress you out.** Focus on a few top-rated books that suit your learning style—not on some obscure books your friends may pass down to you. Do not set yourself up for frustration. Accept the fact that you cannot learn it all. Maintain your sanity throughout the process.

Avoid burnout. Maintain proper diet, exercise, and sleep habits.

You will need time for uninterrupted and focused study. Plan your personal affairs to minimize crisis situations near the date of the test. Allot an adequate number of breaks in your study schedule to avoid burnout. Maintain a healthy lifestyle with proper diet, exercise, and sleep.

Year(s) Prior

The USMLE asserts that the best preparation for the USMLE Step 1 resides in "broadly based learning that establishes a strong general foundation of understanding of concepts and principles in basic sciences."[6] We agree. Although you may be tempted to rely solely on cramming in the weeks and months before the test, you should not have to do so. The knowledge you gained during your first two years of medical school and even during your

Don't let the exam take over your life.

undergraduate years should provide the groundwork on which to base your test preparation. The preponderance of your boards preparation should thus involve resurrecting dormant information that you have stored away during the basic science years.

Some ways to help resurrect and integrate this information are as follows:

Buy review books early (first year) and use while studying for courses.

- Tutor first-year students during your second year.
- Review related first-year material in your second year. For example, review first-year cardiac physiology and histology while learning second-year cardiac pathology.
- At the end of each medical school course, compile and organize key tables, charts, and mnemonics into a "Step 1" binder. Then, when it comes time to study, you will have a head start with familiar high-yield material.
- Attend all "Introduction to Clinical Medicine" and "problem-based learning" classes and reviews to gain experience with clinical vignettes.
- Spend time using computer-based medical education software.

We also recommend that you buy highly rated review books early in your first year of medical school and use them as you study throughout the two years. When Step 1 comes along, the books will be familiar and personalized to the way in which you learn. It is risky and intimidating to use unfamiliar review books in the final two or three weeks.

Review first-year material in parallel with related second-year topics.

You should talk with third- and fourth-year medical students to familiarize yourself with strengths and weaknesses in your school's curriculum. Identify subject areas in which you excel or with which you have difficulty. If you have any doubts concerning your reading speed, consider a speed-reading course. Content typically learned in the second year receives more coverage on Step 1 than do first-year topics owing to the emphasis placed on integration of basic science information across many courses.[7] Be aware of your school's testing format, and determine whether you have adequate exposure to multiple-choice and matching questions in the form of clinical vignettes.

Months Prior

Simulate the USMLE Step 1 under "real" conditions before beginning your studies.

Review test dates and the application procedure. In 2003, the testing for the USMLE Step 1 continues on a year-round basis (Table 2). Choose the most appropriate Prometric testing site for optimal performance. Many U.S. students simply take the exam at the closest site along with all their classmates. By contrast, a few students report a preference for traveling to more distant sites in the interest of privacy. Judge for yourself whether you find familiarity reassuring or stressful. If you have any disabilities or "special circumstances," contact the NBME as early as possible to discuss test accommodations (see p. 62, First Aid for the Student with a Disability).

TABLE 2. 2004 USMLE Exams.

Step	Focus	No. of Questions/ No. of Blocks	Test Schedule Length of CBT Exam	Passing Score
Step 1	Basic mechanisms and principles	350/7	One day (eight hours)	182
Step 2	Clinical diagnosis and disease pathogenesis	400/8	One day (nine hours)	174
Step 3	Clinical management	500/10	Two days (16 hours)	182

Before you begin to study earnestly, simulate the USMLE Step 1 under "real" conditions (even down to the earplugs if you plan to use them during the real exam) to pinpoint strengths and weaknesses in your knowledge and test-taking skills. Be sure that you are well informed about the examination and that you have planned your strategy for studying. Consider what study methods you will use, the study materials you will need, and how you will obtain your materials. Some review books and software may not be available at your local bookstore, and you may have to order ahead of time to get copies (see the list of publisher contacts at the end of Section III). Plan ahead. Get advice from third- and fourth-year medical students who have recently taken the USMLE Step 1. There might be strengths and weaknesses in your school's curriculum that you should take into account in deciding where to focus your efforts. You might also choose to share books, notes, and study hints with classmates. That is how this book began.

Three Weeks Prior

Two to four weeks before the examination is a good time to resimulate the USMLE Step 1. You may want to do this earlier depending on the progress of your review, but do not do it later, when there will be little time to remedy defects in your knowledge or test-taking skills. Make use of remaining good-quality sample USMLE test questions, and try to simulate the computerized test conditions so that you get a fair assessment of your test performance. Recognize, too, that time pressure is increasing as more and more questions are framed as clinical vignettes. Most sample exam questions are shorter than the real thing. Focus on reviewing the high-yield facts, your own notes, picture books, and very short review books.

In the final two weeks, focus on review and endurance. Avoid unfamiliar material. Stay confident!

One Week Prior

Make sure you have your CIN (found on your scheduling permit) and other items necessary for the day of the examination, including a driver's license or other photo identification with signature (make sure your name on your ID *exactly* matches that on your scheduling permit), an analog watch, and possibly earplugs. Confirm the Prometric testing center location and test time.

Confirm your testing date at least one week in advance.

Work out how you will get to the testing center and what parking and traffic problems you might encounter. Visit the testing site (if possible) to get a better idea of the testing conditions. Determine what you will do for lunch. Make sure you have everything you need to ensure that you will be comfortable and alert at the test site. Prometric will provide earplugs on request. Assess your pre-exam living and sleeping arrangements. Take aggressive measures to ensure an environment fit for concentration and sufficient sleep. If you must travel a long distance to the test site, consider arriving the day before and staying overnight with a friend or at a nearby hotel (make early hotel reservations).

One Day Prior

Ensure that you will be comfortable and alert. You must be able to think, not just regurgitate.

Try your best to relax and rest the night before the test. Double-check your admissions and test-taking materials as well as comfort measures as discussed earlier so you do not have to deal with such details the morning of the exam. Do not study any new material. If you feel compelled to study, then quickly review short-term-memory material (e.g., Section II: Database of High-Yield Facts) before going to sleep (the brain does a lot of information processing at night). However, do not quiz yourself, as you may risk becoming flustered and confused. Remember that regardless of how hard you studied, you cannot know everything. There will be things on the exam that you have never even seen before, so do not panic. Do not underestimate your abilities.

No notes, books, calculators, pagers, recording devices, or digital watches are allowed in the testing area.

Many students report difficulty sleeping the night prior to the exam. This is often exacerbated by going to bed much earlier than usual. Do whatever it takes to ensure a good night's sleep (e.g., massage, exercise, warm milk). Do not change your daily routine prior to the exam. Exam day is not the day for a caffeine-withdrawal headache.

Morning of the Exam

Wake up at your regular time and eat a normal breakfast. Drink coffee, tea, or soda in moderation, or you may end up wasting exam time on bathroom breaks. Make sure you have your scheduling permit admission ticket, test-taking materials, and comfort measures as discussed earlier. Wear loose, comfortable clothing. Plan for a variable temperature in the testing center. Remember that you will arrive early in the morning, when it may be cool, and that you will not leave until late in the afternoon, when it may be warmer.

Arrive at the testing center 30 minutes before your scheduled exam time. If you arrive more than half an hour late you will not be allowed to take the test.

Arrive at the test site 30 minutes before the time designated on the admission ticket; however, do not come too early, as this may increase your anxiety. The proctor should give you a blue, laminated USMLE information sheet to read, which explains important things such as the use of break time. Seating may be assigned, but ask to be reseated if necessary; you need to be seated in an area that will allow you to remain comfortable and to concentrate. Get to know your testing station, especially if you have never been in a Prometric testing center before. Adjust your chair and the monitor. Test the mouse, keyboard, lamp, dry markers, and whiteboard to make sure everything is functioning properly before the exam starts. Listen to your proctors regarding any changes in instructions or testing procedures that may apply to your test site.

Remember that it is natural (and even beneficial) to be a little nervous. Focus on being mentally clear and alert. Avoid panic. Avoid panic. Avoid panic. When you are asked to begin the exam, take a deep breath, focus on the screen, and then begin. Keep an eye on the timer. Take advantage of breaks between blocks to stretch and relax for a moment.

The break for lunch is an excellent opportunity to relax, reorganize your thoughts, and regain composure if you are feeling overly stressed or panicked. Some students use the break to discuss questions with classmates or to look up information. Some even recommend reviewing theme topics during lunch. However, do what feels comfortable, as time will be short. If you decide to review the morning session, do not dwell on perceived mistakes.

Some students recommend reviewing certain "theme" topics that tend to recur throughout the exam.

After the Test

Have fun and relax regardless of how you may feel. Taking the test is an achievement in itself. Remember, you are much more likely to have passed than not. Enjoy the free time you have before your clerkships. Expect to experience some "reentry" phenomena as you try to regain a real life. Once you have recovered sufficiently from the test (or from partying), we invite you to send us your feedback, corrections, and suggestions for entries, facts, mnemonics, strategies, book ratings, and the like (see p. xv, How to Contribute). Sharing your experience benefits fellow medical students and IMGs.

IF YOU THINK YOU FAILED

After the test, many examinees feel that they have failed, and most are at the very least unsure of their pass/fail status. There are several sensible steps you can take to plan for the future in the event that you do not achieve a passing score. First, save and organize all your study materials, including review books, practice tests, and notes. If you studied from borrowed materials, make sure you have immediate access to them. Review your school's policy regarding requirements for graduation and promotion to the third year. About one-half of the medical schools accredited by the Liaison Committee on Medical Education (LCME) require passing Step 1 for promotion to the third year, and two-thirds require passing Step 1 as a requirement for graduation.[7] Familiarize yourself with the reapplication procedures for Step 1, including application deadlines and upcoming test dates. The CBT format allows an examinee who has failed the exam to retake it no earlier than the first day of the month after 60 days have elapsed since the last test date. Examinees will, however, be allowed to take the exam no more than three times within a 12-month period should they repeatedly fail.

If you pass Step 1, you are not allowed to retake the exam in an attempt to raise your score.

TABLE 3. Pass Rates for USMLE Step 1 Repeaters 1999.[8]

Initial Score	% Pass
176–178	83
173–175	74
170–172	71
165–169	64
160–164	54
150–159	31
< 150	0
Overall	**67**

The performance profiles on the back of the USMLE Step 1 score report provide valuable feedback concerning your relative strengths and weaknesses (see Figure 6B). Study the performance profiles closely. Set up a study timeline to strengthen gaps in your knowledge as well as to maintain and improve what you already know. Do not neglect high-yield subjects. It is normal to feel somewhat anxious about retaking the test. If anxiety becomes a problem, however, seek appropriate counseling.

Fifty-two percent of the NBME-registered first-time takers who failed the June 1998 Step 1 repeated the exam in October 1998. The overall pass rate for that group in October was 60%. Eighty-five percent of those scoring near the old pass/fail mark of 176 (173–176) in June 1998 passed in October. However, 1999 pass rates varied widely depending on initial score (see Table 3, which reflects the most current data available at time of publishing).

Although the NBME allows an unlimited number of attempts to pass Step 1, both the NBME and the FSMB recommend that licensing authorities allow a minimum of three and a maximum of six attempts for each Step examination.[8] Again, review your school's policy regarding retakes.

IF YOU-FAILED

Even if you came out of the exam room feeling that you failed, seeing that failing grade can be traumatic, and it is natural to feel upset. Different people react in different ways: For some it is a stimulus to buckle down and study harder; for others it may "take the wind out of their sails" for a few days; and for still others it may lead to a reassessment of individual goals and abilities. In some instances, however, failure may trigger weeks or months of sadness, feelings of hopelessness, social withdrawal, and inability to concentrate—in other words, true clinical depression.

Near the failure threshold, each three-digit scale point is equivalent to about 1.5 questions answered correctly.[9]

If you think you are depressed, seek help. Depression is a common yet potentially disabling, and at times even fatal, illness. Depression is also very treatable, so you must use the same resources that you plan to offer your patients. In other words, you must seek treatment, whether from a school counselor, a psychiatrist, or a psychologist. Do not "treat" yourself with alcohol, illicit drugs, or anything else; you need the same skilled help that anyone else with this problem warrants.

As Table 3 shows, the majority of people who fail Step 1 the first time pass on their second attempt, especially if they were near the passing threshold. If you repeatedly fail the exam despite maximum preparation, you may need to reevaluate your goals. Seek testing and career counseling early.

STUDY METHODS

It is important to have a set of study methods for preparing for the USMLE Step 1. There is too much material to justify a studying plan that is built on random reading and memorization. Experiment with different ways of studying. You do not know how effective something might be until you try it. This is best done months before the test to determine what works and what you enjoy. Possible study options include:

- Studying review material in groups
- Creating personal mnemonics, diagrams, and tables
- Using *First Aid* as a framework on which to add notes
- Taking practice computer as well as pencil-and-paper tests (see Section III for reviews)
- Attending faculty review sessions
- Making or sharing flash cards
- Reviewing old syllabi and notes
- Making cassette tapes of review material to study during commuting time
- Playing Trivial Pursuit–style games with facts and questions
- Getting away from home for an extended period to avoid distractions and to immerse yourself in studying

Study Groups

A good study group has many advantages. It can relieve stress, organize your time, and allow people with different strengths to exchange information. Study groups also allow you to pool resources and spend less money on review books and sample tests.

There are, however, potential problems associated with study groups. Above all, it is difficult to study with people who have different goals and study paces. Avoid large, unwieldy groups. Otherwise, studying can be inefficient and time-consuming. Avoid study groups that tend to socialize more than study.

Balance individual and group study.

If you choose not to belong to a study group, it may be a good idea to find a support group or a study partner simply to keep pace with and share study ideas. It is beneficial to get different perspectives from other students in evaluating what is and is not important to learn. Do not become intimidated or discouraged by interactions with a few overly compulsive students; everyone studies and learns differently.

Mnemonics and Memorizing

Cramming is a viable way of memorizing short-term information just before a test, but after one or two days you will find that much of that knowledge has dissipated. For that reason, cramming and memorization by repetition ("brute force") in the weeks before the exam are not ideal techniques for long-term

Developing good mnemonics takes time and work. Quiz yourself periodically. Do not simply reread highlighted material.

memorization of the overwhelming body of information covered in Step 1. Mnemonics are memory aids that work by linking isolated facts or abstract ideas to acronyms, pictures, patterns, rhymes, and stories—information that the mind tends to store well.[10] The best mnemonics are your own, and developing them takes work. The first step to creating a mnemonic is understanding the information to be memorized. Play around with the information and look for unique features that help you remember it. In addition, make the mnemonic as colorful, humorous, or outlandish as you can; such mnemonics are the most memorable. Effective mnemonics should link the topic with the facts in as specific and unambiguous a manner as possible. In memorizing the mnemonic, engage as many senses as possible by repeating the fact aloud or by writing or acting it out. Keep the information fresh by quizzing yourself periodically with flash cards, in study groups, and so on. Do not make the common mistake of simply rereading highlighted review material. The material may start to look familiar, but that does not mean you will be able to remember it in another context during the exam. Strive to gain an understanding rather than rote memorization.

Review Sessions

Faculty review sessions can also be helpful. Review sessions that are geared specifically toward the USMLE Step 1 tend to be more helpful than general review sessions. By contrast, open "question and answer" sessions tend to be inefficient and not worth the time. Focus on reviews given by faculty who are knowledgeable in the content and testing format of the USMLE Step 1.

Commercial Courses

Commercial preparation courses can be helpful for some students, but they are expensive and require significant time commitment. They are often effective in organizing study material for students preparing for Step 1 who feel overwhelmed by the sheer volume of material. Note, however, that multiple-week courses may be quite intense and may thus leave limited time for independent study. Note also that some commercial courses are designed for first-time test takers while others focus on students who are repeating the examination. Still other courses focus on IMGs, who must take all three Steps in a limited time period. See Section III for summarized data and excerpted information from several commercial review courses.

STUDY MATERIALS

Quality and Cost Considerations

Although an ever-increasing number of review books and software are now available on the market, the quality of such material is highly variable. Some common problems are as follows:

- Certain review books are too detailed for review in a reasonable amount of time or cover subtopics that are not emphasized on the exam (e.g., a 400-page histology book).
- Many sample question books were originally written years ago and have not been adequately updated to reflect trends on the revised USMLE Step 1.
- Many sample question books use poorly written questions or contain factual errors in their explanations.
- Explanations for sample questions range from nonexistent to overly detailed.
- The available review software is of highly variable quality, may be difficult to install, and may be fraught with bugs.

In 2003, many students felt that even the top-rated sample exams did not accurately reflect the clinical focus of the actual exam.

Basic Science Review Books

Most review books are the products of considerable effort by experienced educators. There are, however, many such books, so you must choose which ones to buy on the basis of their relative merits. Although recommendations from other medical students are useful, many students simply recommend whatever books they used without having compared them to other books on the same subject. Do not waste time with outdated "hand-me-down" review books. Some students blindly advocate one publisher's series without considering the broad range of quality encountered within most series. Weigh different opinions against each other, read the reviews and ratings in Section III of this guide, examine the books closely in the bookstore, and choose review books carefully. You are investing not only money but also your limited study time. Do not worry about finding the "perfect" book, as many subjects simply do not have one, and different students prefer different styles.

If a given review book is not working for you, stop using it no matter how highly rated it may be or how much it costs.

There are two types of review books: books that are stand-alone titles and books that are part of a series. The books in a series generally have the same style, and you must decide if that style works for you. However, a given style is not optimal for every subject. For example, charts and diagrams may be the best approach for physiology and biochemistry, whereas tables and outlines may be preferable for microbiology.

You should also find out which books are up to date. Some new editions represent major improvements, whereas others contain only cursory changes. Take into consideration how a book reflects the format of the USMLE Step 1. Some of the books reviewed in Section III have not been updated adequately to reflect the clinical emphasis and question format of the current USMLE Step 1. Books that emphasize obscure facts and minute details tend to be less helpful for the current USMLE Step 1 because there are now fewer "picky" questions and more problem-solving questions.

Many students regret not having used the same books for medical school exam review and Step 1 review.

Practice Tests

Taking practice tests provides valuable information about potential strengths and weaknesses in your fund of knowledge and test-taking skills. Some students use practice examinations simply as a means of breaking up the monotony of studying and adding variety to their study schedule, whereas other students study almost solely from practice tests. There is, moreover, a wide range of quality in available practice material, and finding good practice exams is likely to become even more complicated with the advent of the computerized Step 1. Your best preview of the computerized exam can be found in the practice exams on the USMLE CD-ROM. Some students also recommend using computerized test simulation programs such as Kaplan's Qbank (see Section III for reviews). In addition, students report that many current practice-exam books have questions that are, on average, shorter and less clinically oriented than the current USMLE Step 1. Many Step 1 questions demand fast reading skills and application of basic science facts in a problem-solving format. Approach sample examinations and simulation software critically, and do not waste time with low-quality questions until you have exhausted better sources.

After taking a practice test, try to identify concepts and areas of weakness, not just the facts that you missed. Do not panic if you miss a lot of questions on a practice examination; instead, use the experience you have gained to motivate your study and prioritize those areas in which you need the most work. Use quality practice examinations to improve your test-taking skills. Analyze your ability to pace yourself so that you have enough time to complete each block of 50 questions comfortably. Practice examinations are also a good means of training yourself to concentrate for long periods of time under appropriate time pressure. Consider taking practice tests with a friend or in a small group to increase motivation while simulating more accurately the format and schedule of the real examination. Analyze the pattern of your responses to questions to determine if you have made systematic errors in answering questions. Common mistakes are reading too much into the question, second-guessing your initial impression, and misinterpreting the question.

Clinical Review Books

Keep your eye out for more clinically oriented review books; purchase them early and begin to use them. A number of students are turning to Step 2 books, pathophysiology books, and case-based reviews to prepare for the clinical vignettes. Examples of such books include:

- *Blueprint* clinical series (Blackwell Science)
- *PreTest Physical Diagnosis* (McGraw-Hill)
- *Washington Manual* (Lippincott Williams & Wilkins)
- Various USMLE Step 2 review books

Texts, Syllabi, and Notes

Limit your use of texts and syllabi for Step 1 review. Many textbooks are too detailed for high-yield review and include material that is generally not tested on the USMLE Step 1 (e.g., drug dosages, complex chemical structures). Syllabi, although familiar, are inconsistent and frequently reflect the emphasis of individual faculty, which often does not correspond to that of the USMLE Step 1. Syllabi also tend to be less organized and to contain fewer diagrams and study questions than do top-rated review books. In our opinion, they are often a waste of time for the faculty to write and suboptimal for the student to read (when compared with the best review books). Make sure that your instructors are aware of the best books, and supplement your classes with case-based problem-solving curricula that reflect the current exam format. Your class notes have the advantage of presenting material in the way you learned it but suffer from the same disadvantages as syllabi.

When using texts or notes, engage in active learning by making tables, diagrams, new mnemonics, and conceptual associations whenever possible. Supplement unclear material with reference to other appropriate textbooks. Keep a good medical dictionary at hand to sort out definitions.

GENERAL STUDY STRATEGIES

The USMLE Step 1 was created according to an integrated outline that organizes basic science material in a multidisciplinary approach. Broad-based knowledge is now more important than it was in the exams of prior years. The exam is designed to test basic science material and its application to clinical situations. A little over half of the questions include clinical vignettes, although some are brief. Some useful studying guidelines are as follows:

- Be familiar with the CBT tutorial. This will give you 15 minutes of extra break time.
- Use computerized practice tests in addition to paper exams.
- Consider doing a simulated test at a Prometric center.
- Practice taking 50 questions in one-hour bursts.
- Be familiar with the Windows environment.
- Consider scheduling a light rotation for your first clinical block in case you get a test date later than you expected.

Familiarize yourself with the commonly tested normal laboratory values.

In spite of the change in the organization of the subject matter, the detailed Step 1 content outline provided by the USMLE has not proved useful for students. We feel that it is still best to approach the material along the lines of the seven traditional disciplines. In Section II, we provide suggestions on how to approach the material within each subject.

Practice questions that include case histories or descriptive vignettes are critical in preparing for the clinical slant of the USMLE Step 1. The normal lab values provided on the computerized test are difficult to use and access. For quick reference, see the table of high-yield laboratory values on the inside back cover.

Practice questions that include case histories or descriptive vignettes are critical for Step 1 preparation.

TEST-TAKING STRATEGIES

Your test performance will be influenced by both your fund of knowledge and your test-taking skills. You can increase your performance by considering each of these factors. Test-taking skills and strategies should be developed and perfected well in advance of the test date so that you can concentrate on the test itself. We suggest that you try the following strategies to see if they might work for you.

Practice and perfect test-taking skills and strategies well before the test date.

Pacing

You have seven hours to complete 350 questions. Note that each one-hour block contains 50 questions. This works out to about 72 seconds per question. NBME officials note that time was not an issue for most takers of the CBT field test. However, pacing errors have in the past been detrimental to the performance of even highly prepared examinees. The bottom line is to keep one eye on the clock at all times! If you find yourself running out of time, fill in all remaining blanks with C or B or your favorite letter, but also click on the "mark" button for each so that you can come back to them from the item review screen.

Dealing with Each Question

Time management is an important skill for exam success.

There are several established techniques for efficiently approaching multiple-choice questions; see what works for you. One technique begins with identifying each question as easy, workable, or impossible. Your goal should be to answer all easy questions, work out all workable questions in a reasonable amount of time, and make quick and intelligent guesses on all impossible questions. Most students read the stem, think of the answer, and turn immediately to the choices. A second technique is to first skim the answer choices and the last sentence of the question and then read through the passage quickly, extracting only relevant information to answer the question. Try a variety of techniques on practice exams and see what works best for you.

In general, when you eliminate an incorrect choice on a question, avoid rereading it unnecessarily. Move on. If you are unsure about a choice, mark it for later review. When you think you have determined the best answer, click on it and move on.

Difficult Questions

Do not dwell excessively on questions that you are on the verge of "figuring out." Make your best guess and move on.

Questions on the USMLE Step 1 require varying amounts of time to answer. Some problem-solving questions take longer than simple, fact-recall questions. Because of the exam's clinical emphasis, you may find that many of the questions appear workable but take more time than is available to you. It can be tempting to dwell on such a question for an excessive amount of time because you feel you are on the verge of "figuring it out," but resist this temptation and budget your time. Answer the question with your best guess, mark it for review, and come back to it if you have time after you have completed the rest of the questions in the block. This will keep you from inadvertently leaving any questions blank in your efforts to "beat the clock." Remember to save a few minutes at the end to make sure that all questions have been answered.

Inevitably, there will be some questions about which you will not have a clue (i.e., impossible questions). Do not be disturbed by these questions. Guess, mark them for later review, and move on. As a medical student, you are used to scoring well on standardized examinations (otherwise you would not be in medical school), so the USMLE Step 1 may be your first experience with facing lots of questions for which you do not know the answer. Prepare yourself for this. After narrowing down the answers as best you can, have a plan for guessing so that you do not waste time. Remember that you are not expected to know all the answers.

Another reason for not dwelling too long on any one question is that certain questions may be **experimental** or may be **incorrectly phrased.** Moreover, not all questions are scored. Some questions serve as "embedded pretest items" that do not count toward your overall score.[10] In fact, anywhere from 10 to 20% of exam questions have been designated as experimental on past exams.

Remember that some questions may be experimental.

Students have also noted several errors in past USMLE Step 1 examinations. The lesson here is that you should not waste too much time with ambiguous or "flawed" questions. The reason you are having difficulty with a question may lie in the question itself, not with you!

Guessing

There is **no penalty** for wrong answers. Thus, no test block should be left with unanswered questions. A hunch is probably better than a random guess. If you have to guess, we suggest selecting an answer you recognize over one that is totally unfamiliar. Go where the money is! If you have studied the subject and do not recognize a particular answer, then it is more likely a distractor than a correct answer.

Changing Your Answer

The conventional wisdom regarding "reconsidering" answers is not to change answers that you have already marked unless there is a convincing and logical reason to do so—in other words, go with your first hunch. You can test this strategy for yourself by keeping a running total of the questions on which you seriously considered changing your answer when taking practice exams. Experience eventually tells you how strongly to trust your first hunches. Remember, with the CBT format you can go back and change answers only within the question block you're working on. Once you move to the next block, you cannot return to questions in the previous block.

Fourth-Quarter Effect (Avoiding Burnout)

Do not terminate the block too early. Carefully review your answers if possible.

Pacing and endurance are important. Practice helps develop both. Fewer and fewer examinees are leaving the examination session early. Use any extra time you might have at the end of each block to return to marked questions or to recheck your answers; you cannot add the extra time to any remaining blocks of questions or to your break time. Do not be too casual in your review or you may overlook serious mistakes. A few students report that near the end of a section they suddenly remember facts that help answer questions they had guessed on earlier.

Remember your goals, and keep in mind the effort you have devoted to studying compared with the small additional effort you will need to maintain focus and concentration throughout the examination.

Never give up. If you begin to feel frustrated, try taking a 30-second breather. Look away from the screen, breathe deeply, and slowly count to ten. Hopefully, you can return to the exam refreshed and clear. Every point you earn is to your advantage. The difference between passing and an average score is far fewer questions than you might think—about 25% of students who failed past exams were within 15 questions of passing.

CLINICAL VIGNETTE STRATEGIES

In recent years, the USMLE Step 1 has become increasingly clinically oriented. Students polled from 2003 exams report that nearly 80% of the questions were presented as clinical vignettes. This change mirrors the trend in medical education toward introducing students to clinical problem solving during the basic science years. The increasing clinical emphasis on Step 1 may be challenging to those students who attend schools with a more traditional curriculum.

The first step toward approaching the clinical vignette is not to panic. The same basic science concepts are often being tested in the guise of a clinical vignette.

What Is a Clinical Vignette?

Be prepared to read fast and think on your feet!

A clinical vignette is a short (usually paragraph-long) description of a patient, including demographics, presenting symptoms, signs, and other information concerning the patient. Sometimes this paragraph is followed by a brief listing of important physical findings and/or laboratory results. The task of assimilating all this information and answering the associated question in the span of one minute can be intimidating. Be prepared to read fast and think on your feet. Remember that the question is often indirectly asking something you already know.

Here are two examples of vignettes that appear complex but actually ask relatively straightforward questions.

Vignette #1

A 38-year-old African-American woman visits her physician. She explains that she has been experiencing palpitations, shortness of breath, and syncopal episodes for several months. In addition to a constant feeling of impending doom, she also has episodes of dizziness without nausea or vomiting. Her sleep pattern is normal. The physician's first course of action should be to:

A) provide psychotherapy
B) treat the patient with benzodiazepines
C) perform a physical examination
D) refer the patient to a psychiatrist
E) teach the patient self-hypnosis

Answer: C. Regardless of whether a psychiatric or organic disorder is present, a history and physical examination should always be performed during the first visit. As the history is summarized in the vignette, the physical exam would be the first course of action before considering any of the other answer choices.

Vignette #2

J.B. is a seven-year-old white male who complains of a chronic, persistent cough. The cough is often elicited by physical activity or cold exposure. His mother says that she had an uncomplicated, full-term pregnancy and that the child has been healthy except for one episode of pneumonia when he was five years old. She also notes that his appetite is variable and that he frequently has light-colored and foul-smelling stool. On physical exam, his weight was 20.5 kg (25th percentile) and his height was 119.5 cm (25th percentile). His physician orders a sweat chloride test (Cook-Gibson method) and receives the following results:

Right arm	103 mEq/L
Left arm	108 mEq/L
Normal	< 70 mEq/L

What is the mode of inheritance of this disorder?

A) autosomal dominant
B) autosomal recessive
C) mitochondrial
D) X-linked recessive
E) Y-linked

Answer: B.

Strategy

Remember that the Step 1 vignettes usually describe diseases or disorders in their most classic presentation. Look for buzzwords or cardinal signs (e.g., malar rash for SLE or nuchal rigidity for meningitis) in the narrative history. Be aware, however, that the question may contain classic signs and symptoms instead of mere buzzwords. Sometimes the data from labs and the physical exam will help

Step 1 vignettes usually describe diseases or disorders in their most classic presentation.

you confirm or reject possible diagnoses, thereby helping you rule answer choices in or out. In some cases, they will be a dead giveaway for the diagnosis.

Making a diagnosis from the history and data is often not the final answer. Not infrequently, the diagnosis is divulged at the end of the vignette, after you have just struggled through the narrative to come up with a diagnosis of your own. The question instead asks about a related aspect of the diagnosed disease.

One strategy that many students suggest is to skim the questions and answer choices before reading a vignette, especially if the vignette is lengthy. This focuses your attention on the relevant information and reduces the time spent on that vignette. Sometimes you may not need much of the information in the vignette to answer the question.

Sometimes making a diagnosis is not necessary at all.

For vignette #2, consider the following approach:

- Take a look at the question and answer choices first. We see that a diagnosis of some inherited disease will likely have to be made to answer this question.
- As in many vignettes, the first sentence presents the patient's age, sex, and race. This information can help direct your diagnosis. For the case above, you are looking for a genetic disease in a young white male, which may already tip you off to cystic fibrosis. If you are looking for an inherited anemia, sickle cell disease would be more likely for an African-American patient. If, by contrast, the patient were Asian or Mediterranean, then thalassemia might be more likely.
- Next, look for the chief complaint, in this case "chronic, persistent cough."
- Even if the diagnosis of cystic fibrosis is not apparent at this point, fear not! The vignette further describes other classic symptoms of the disease (e.g., fat malabsorption due to pancreatic insufficiency, growth retardation, elevated sweat chloride levels).
- Instead of asking for the diagnosis, the question asks its mode of inheritance. Questions such as this require the test taker to go beyond the first stage in the reasoning process. These "two-step questions" are appearing with increasing frequency on the Step 1 exam.

"Two-step questions" are appearing with increasing frequency on the Step 1 exam.

TESTING AGENCIES

National Board of Medical Examiners (NBME)
Department of Licensing Examination Services
3750 Market Street
Philadelphia, PA 19104-3102
(215) 590-9500
Fax: (215) 590-9457
E-mail: webmail@nbme.org
www.nbme.org

Educational Commission for Foreign Medical Graduates (ECFMG)
3624 Market Street, Fourth Floor
Philadelphia, PA 19104-2685
(215) 386-5900 or (215) 375-1913
Toll free within North America: (800) 500-8249
Fax: (215) 386-9196
E-mail: info@ecfmg.org
www.ecfmg.org

Federation of State Medical Boards (FSMB)
P.O. Box 619850
Dallas, TX 75261-9850
(817) 868-4000
Fax: (817) 868-4099
E-mail: usmle@fsmb.org
www.fsmb.org

USMLE Secretariat
3750 Market Street
Philadelphia, PA 19104-3190
(215) 590-9700
E-mail: webmail@nbme.org
www.usmle.org

REFERENCES

1. Bidese, Catherine M., *U.S. Medical Licensure Statistics and Current Licensure Requirements 1995*, Chicago, American Medical Association, 1995.

2. National Board of Medical Examiners, *2002 USMLE Bulletin of Information*, Philadelphia, 2001.

3. National Board of Medical Examiners, *Bulletin of Information and Description of National Board Examinations, 1991*, Philadelphia, 1990.

4. Federation of State Medical Boards and National Board of Medical Examiners, *USMLE: 1993 Step 1 General Instructions, Content Outline, and Sample Items*, Philadelphia, 1992.

5. Swanson, David B., Case, Susan M., Melnick, Donald E., et al., "Impact of the USMLE Step 1 on Teaching and Learning of the Basic Biomedical Sciences," *Academic Medicine*, September Supplement 1992, Vol. 67, No. 9, pp. 553–556.

6. Case, Susan M., and Swanson, David B., "Validity of NBME Part I and Part II Scores for Selection of Residents in Orthopaedic Surgery, Dermatology, and Preventive Medicine," *Academic Medicine*, February Supplement 1993, Vol. 68, No. 2, pp. S51–S56.

7. "Report on 1995 Examinations," *National Board Examiner*, Winter 1997, Vol. 44, No. 1, pp. 1–4.

8. "Report on 1996 Examinations," op. cit.

9. O'Donnell, M. J., Obenshain, S. Scott, and Erdmann, James B., "I: Background Essential to the Proper Use of Results of Step 1 and Step 2 of the USMLE," *Academic Medicine*, October 1993, Vol. 68, No. 10, pp. 734–739.

10. Robinson, Adam, *What Smart Students Know*, New York, Crown Publishers, 1993.

Special Situations

"International medical graduate" (IMG) is the term now used to describe any student or graduate of a non–U.S., non–Canadian, non–Puerto Rican medical school, regardless of whether he or she is a U.S. citizen. The old term "foreign medical graduate" (FMG) was replaced because it was misleading when applied to U.S. citizens attending medical schools outside the United States.

The IMG's Steps to Licensure in the United States

If you are an IMG, you must go through the following steps (not necessarily in this order) to become licensed to practice in the United States. You must complete these steps even if you are already a practicing physician and have completed a residency program in your own country.

- Complete the basic sciences program of your medical school (equivalent to the first two years of U.S. medical school).
- Take the USMLE Step 1. You can do this while still in school or after graduating, but in either case your medical school must certify that you completed the basic sciences part of your school's curriculum before taking the USMLE Step 1.
- Complete the clinical clerkship program of your medical school (equivalent to the third and fourth years of U.S. medical school).
- Take the USMLE Step 2. If you are still in medical school, your school must certify that you are within one year of graduating for you to be allowed to take Step 2.
- Take the Test of English as a Foreign Language (TOEFL), recognized by the Educational Commission for Foreign Medical Graduates (ECFMG).
- Take the Clinical Skills Assessment (CSA).
- Graduate with your medical degree.
- Then, send the ECFMG a copy of your degree and transcript, which they will verify with your medical school.
- Obtain an ECFMG certificate. To do this, candidates must accomplish the following:
    - —Graduate from a medical school that is listed in the International Medical Education Directory (IMED). The list can be accessed at www.ecfmg.org.
    - —Pass Step 1 and Step 2 within a seven-year period.
    - —Pass the TOEFL.
    - —Pass the CSA.
    - —Have medical credentials verified by the ECFMG.
- The standard certificate is usually sent two weeks after all the above requirements have been fulfilled. You must have a valid certificate before entering an accredited residency program, although you may begin the application process before you receive your certification.
- Apply for residency positions in your field of interest, either directly or through the Electronic Residency Application Service (ERAS) and the National Residency Matching Program ("the Match"). To be entered

More detailed information can be found in the 2004 edition of the ECFMG Information Booklet, available at www.ecfmg.org/pubshome. html.

Applicants may apply online for the TOEFL at www.toefl.org

Applicants may apply online for the USMLE Step 1 or Step 2, for the ECFMG Clinical Skills Assessment, or to request an extension of the USMLE eligibility period at http://iwa.ecfmg.org.

into the Match, you need to have passed all the examinations necessary for ECFMG certification (i.e., Step 1, Step 2, the CSA, and the TOEFL) by a certain deadline (January 31, 2004, for the 2004 Match). If you do not pass these exams by the deadline, you will be withdrawn from the Match.

- Obtain a visa that will allow you to enter and work in the United States if you are not already a U.S. citizen or a green-card holder (permanent resident).

- If required for IMGs by the state in which your residency is located, obtain an educational/training/limited medical license. Your residency program may assist you with this application. Note that medical licensing is the prerogative of each individual state, not of the federal government, and that states vary with respect to their laws about licensing (although all 50 states recognize the USMLE).

- In order to begin your residency program, make sure your TOEFL and CSA scores are valid. A passing TOEFL score is valid for two years, and a passing CSA score is valid for three years. If more time has elapsed, you must revalidate your scores by passing a subsequent TOEFL or CSA exam.

- Take the USMLE Step 3 during your residency, and then obtain a full medical license. Once you have a license in any state, you are permitted to practice in federal institutions such as VA hospitals and Indian Health Service facilities in any state. This can open the door to "moonlighting" opportunities and possibilities for an H1B visa application. For details on individual state rules, write to the licensing board in the state in question or contact the FSMB.

- Complete your residency and then take the appropriate specialty board exams in order to become board certified (e.g., in internal medicine or surgery). If you already have a specialty certification in your home country (e.g., in surgery or cardiology), some specialty boards may grant you six months' or one year's credit toward your total residency time.

- Currently, many residency programs are accepting applications through ERAS. For more information, see *First Aid for the Match* or contact:

ECFMG/ERAS Program
P.O. Box 11746
Philadelphia, PA 19101-1746
(215) 386-5900
Fax: (215) 222-5641
e-mail: eras_support@ecfmg.org
www.ecfmg.org/eras

The USMLE and the IMG

The USMLE is a series of standardized exams that gives IMGs a level playing field. It is the same exam series taken by U.S. graduates even though it is administered by the ECFMG rather than by the NBME. This means that passing marks for IMGs for both Step 1 and Step 2 are determined by a statistical process that is based on the scores of U.S. medical students. For example, to pass Step 1, you will probably have to score higher than the bottom 8 to 10% of U.S. and Canadian graduates.

Timing of the USMLE

For an IMG, the timing of a complete application is critical. It is extremely important that you send in your application early if you are to garner the maximum number of interview calls. A rough guide would be to complete all exam requirements by August of the year in which you wish to apply. This would translate into sending both your score sheets and your ECFMG certificate with your application.

In terms of USMLE exam order, arguments can be made for taking the Step 1 or the Step 2 exam first. For example, you may consider taking the Step 2 exam first if you have just graduated from medical school and the clinical topics are still fresh in your mind. However, keep in mind that there is a large overlap between Step 1 and Step 2 topics in areas such as pharmacology, pathophysiology, and biostatistics. You might therefore consider taking the Step 1 and Step 2 exams close together to take advantage of this overlap in your test preparation.

USMLE Step 1 and the IMG

What Is the USMLE Step 1? It is a computerized test of the basic medical sciences consisting of 350 multiple-choice questions.

Significance of the Test. Step 1 is required for the ECFMG certificate as well as for registration for the CSA. Since most U.S. graduates apply to residency with their Step 1 scores only, it may be the only objective tool available with which to compare IMGs with U.S. graduates.

Official Web Sites. www.usmle.org/step1 and www.ecfmg.org/usmle.

Eligibility. Both students and graduates from medical schools that are listed in IMED are eligible to take the test. Students must have completed at least two years of medical school by the beginning of the eligibility period selected.

Eligibility Period. A three-month period of your choice.

Fee. The fee for Step 1 is $660 plus an international test delivery surcharge (if you choose a testing region other than the United States or Canada).

Retaking the Exam. In the event that you failed the test, you can reapply and select an eligibility period that begins at least 60 days after the last attempt. You cannot take the same Step more than three times in any 12-month period. You cannot retake the exam if you passed.

Statistics. In 2001, only 66% of ECFMG candidates passed Step 1 on their first attempt, compared with 91% of U.S. and Canadian medical students and graduates. Of note, 1994–1995 data showed that USFMGs (U.S. citizens attending non-U.S. medical schools) performed 0.4 SD lower than IMGs (non-U.S. citizens attending non-U.S. medical schools). Although their overall scores were lower, USFMGs performed better than IMGs on behavioral sciences. In general, students from non-U.S. medical schools perform worst in behavioral science and biochemistry (1.9 and 1.5 SDs below U.S. students) and comparatively better in gross anatomy and pathology (0.7 and 0.9 SD below U.S. students). Although derived from data collected in 1994–1995, these data may help you focus your studying efforts.

Tips. Although few if any students feel totally prepared to take Step 1, IMGs in particular require serious study and preparation to reach their full potential on this exam. It is also imperative that IMGs do their best on Step 1, as a poor score on Step 1 is a distinct disadvantage in applying for most residencies. Remember that if you pass Step 1, you cannot retake it to try to improve your score. Your goal should thus be to beat the mean, because you can then confidently assert that you have done better than average for U.S. students. Good Step 1 scores will lend credibility to your residency application.

Commercial Review Courses. Do commercial review courses help improve your scores? Reports vary, and such courses can be expensive. Many IMGs decide to try the USMLE on their own and then consider a review course only if they fail. Just keep in mind that many states require that you pass the USMLE within three attempts. (For more information on review courses, see Section III.)

USMLE Step 2 and the IMG

What Is the USMLE Step 2? It is a computerized test of the clinical sciences consisting of 370 multiple-choice questions.

Significance of the Test. Step 2 is required for the ECFMG certificate. It reflects the level of clinical knowledge of the applicant.

Official Web Sites. www.usmle.org/step2 and www.ecfmg.org/usmle.

Eligibility. Students and graduates from medical schools that are listed in IMED are eligible to take Step 2. Students must be within 12 months of graduation by the beginning of the eligibility period selected.

Eligibility Period. A three-month period of your choice.

Fee. The fee for Step 2 is $660 plus an international test delivery surcharge (if you choose a testing region other than the United States or Canada).

Retaking the Exam. In the event that you fail Step 2, you can reapply and select an eligibility period that begins at least 60 days after the last attempt. You cannot take the same Step more than three times in any 12-month period. You cannot retake the exam if you passed.

Statistics. In 2000–2001, 75% of ECFMG candidates passed Step 2 on their first attempt, compared with 95% of U.S. and Canadian candidates.

Tips. Because this is a clinical sciences exam, cultural and geographic considerations play a greater role than is the case with Step 1. For example, if your medical education gave you ample exposure to malaria, brucellosis, and malnutrition but little to alcohol withdrawal, child abuse, and cholesterol screening, you must work to familiarize yourself with topics that are more heavily emphasized in U.S. medicine. You must also have a basic understanding of the legal and social aspects of U.S. medicine, because you will be asked questions about communicating with and advising patients.

The English Language Test

What Is the TOEFL? The TOEFL is a computer-based or paper-based test of the English language that evaluates grammar, structure, reading, listening, and writing. Topics include proper use of grammar and vocabulary, proper evaluation of sentence structure, comprehension of reading texts, comprehension of audio dialogues, and writing a brief essay.

Significance of the Test. The TOEFL is required for the ECFMG certificate and for registration for the CSA.

Official Web Sites. www.toefl.org and www.ecfmg.org/elpt/index.html.

Scoring. The minimum passing score accepted by the ECFMG is 550 with the paper-based test or 213 with the computer-based test. Test results are valid for two years.

Clinical Skills Assessment

What Is the CSA? The CSA is a test of clinical and communication skills administered as a one-day, eight-hour exam. It includes 10 to 12 encounters with standardized patients (15 minutes each, with 10 minutes to write a note after each encounter). Test results are valid for three years.

Topics Covered by This Exam. The CSA tests the ability to communicate in English as well as interpersonal skills, data-gathering skills, the ability to perform a physical exam, and the ability to formulate a brief note, a differential diagnosis, and a list of diagnostic tests. The areas that are covered in the exam are:

- Internal medicine
- Surgery
- Obstetrics and gynecology
- Pediatrics
- Psychiatry
- Family medicine

Significance of the Test. The CSA is required for the ECFMG certificate.

Official Web Site. www.ecfmg.org/csa.

Eligibility. Both medical school students and graduates must have passed the USMLE Step 1 and TOEFL exams. Students should be within 12 months of graduation from medical school.

Fee. The fee for the CSA is $1200.

Scheduling. You must schedule your CSA within **four months** of the date indicated on your notification of registration. You must take the CSA within 12 months of the date indicated on your notification of registration.

Retaking the Exam. If you fail the CSA, the period of time you must wait before retaking it depends on the total number of times you have failed.

- If you have failed the CSA **one** time, you must wait at least **three months** from the date of your most recent CSA fail before retaking it.
- If you have failed the CSA **two** times, you must wait at least **six months** from the date of your most recent CSA fail before retaking it.
- If you have failed the CSA **three or more** times, you must wait at least **one year** from the date of your most recent CSA fail before retaking it.

Test Site Locations. The CSA is currently administered at the following locations:

ECFMG CSA Center—Philadelphia
3624 Market Street, Third Floor
Philadelphia, PA 19104-2685

ECFMG CSA Center—Atlanta
Two Crown Center
1745 Phoenix Boulevard, Suite 500
Atlanta, GA 30349-5585

For more information about the CSA, please refer to *First Aid for the CSA,* which will be available in 2004.

USMLE Step 3 and the IMG

What Is the USMLE Step 3? It is a computerized test in clinical medicine consisting of multiple-choice questions and computer-based case simulations (CCS).

Significance of the Test. Taking Step 3 before residency is critical if an IMG is seeking an H1B visa and is a bonus that can be added to the application for residency. Step 3 is also required to obtain a full medical license in the United States and can be taken during residency for this purpose.

Official Web Site. www.usmle.org/step3.

Fee. The fee for Step 3 is $590 (the total application fee can vary among states).

Eligibility. Most states require that applicants have completed one, two, or three years of postgraduate training (residency) prior to applying for Step 3 and permanent state licensure. The exceptions are the 11 states mentioned below, which allow IMGs to take Step 3 at the beginning of or even before residency. So if you don't fulfill the prerequisites to take Step 3 in your state of choice, simply use the name of one of the 11 states in your Step 3 application. You can take the exam in any state you choose regardless of the state that you mentioned on your application. Once you pass Step 3, it will be recognized by all states. Basic eligibility requirements for the USMLE Step 3 are as follows:

- Obtaining an MD or DO degree (or its equivalent) by the application deadline.
- Obtaining an ECFMG certificate if you are a graduate of a foreign medical school or are successfully completing a "fifth pathway" program (at a date no later than the application deadline).
- Meeting the requirements imposed by the individual state licensing authority to which you are applying to take Step 3. Please refer to www.fsmb.org for more information.

The following states do not have postgraduate training as an eligibility requirement to apply for Step 3:

- Arkansas
- California
- Connecticut
- Florida
- Louisiana
- Maryland
- Nebraska*
- New York
- South Dakota
- Texas
- Utah*
- Washington
- West Virginia

* Requires that IMGs obtain a "valid indefinite" ECFMG certificate.

Step 3 applications can be found online at www.fsmb.org and must be submitted to the FSMB.

Residencies and the IMG

It is becoming increasingly difficult for IMGs to obtain residencies in the United States given the rising concern about an oversupply of physicians in the United States. Official bodies such as the Council on Graduate Medical

Education (COGME) have recommended that the total number of residency slots be reduced from the current 144% of the number of U.S. graduates to 110%. Furthermore, changes in immigration law are likely to make it much harder for noncitizens or legal residents of the United States to remain in the country after completing a residency.

In the residency Match, the number of U.S.-citizen IMG applications has been stable for the last few years, while the percentage accepted has slowly increased. For non-U.S.-citizen IMGs, applications fell from 7977 in 1999 to 4556 in 2002, while the percentage accepted significantly increased (see Table 4). This decrease in the total number of IMGs applying for the Match may be attributed to several factors:

- A decrease in the CSA passing rate to 80%.
- Increased difficulty obtaining a U.S. visa.
- Increased expenses associated with the USMLE exams, the CSA, ERAS, and travel to the United States.
- An increase in the number of IMGs who are withdrawing from the Match to sign a separate "pre-Match" contract with programs. This was to be eliminated in the 2004 Match through a new policy adopted by the NRMP stating that "beginning with the 2004 Match, all sponsoring institutions participating in the NRMP Main Match must register and attempt to fill all their positions in the Match except for those specialties or programs participating in other national matching programs." However, the implementation of this policy has been postponed. For more information, refer to www.nrmp.org.

Visa Options for the IMG

If you are living outside the United States, you will need to apply for a visa that will allow you lawful entry into the United States in order to take the CSA and/or do your interviews for residency. A B1 or B2 visitor visa may be issued by the U.S. consulate in your country. Citizens of some countries may have to undergo an additional security check that could take up to six

TABLE 4. IMGs in the Match.			
Applicants	2000	2001	2002
U.S.-citizen IMGs	2169	1999	2029
% U.S. citizens accepted	51	52	54
Non-U.S.-citizen IMGs	7287	5116	4556
% non-U.S. citizens accepted	38	45	51
U.S. graduates (non-IMGs)	14,358	14,455	14,336
% U.S. graduates accepted	94	94	94

months. Upon entry to the United States, either the B1 or, more commonly, the B2 will be issued on your I-94. Both visas allow you a limited period to stay in the United States (two to six months) in order to take the exam. If the given period is not sufficient, you may apply for an extension before the expiration of your I-94.

Documents that are recommended to facilitate this process include:

- The CSA admission permit and a letter from the ECFMG (which explains why the applicant must enter the United States)
- Your medical diploma
- Transcripts from your medical school
- Your USMLE score sheets
- A sponsor letter or affidavit of support stating that you (if you are sponsoring yourself) or your sponsor will bear the expense of your trip and that you have sufficient funds to meet that expense
- An alien status affidavit

Individuals from certain countries may be allowed to enter the United States for up to 90 days without a visa under the Visa Waiver Program. See www.immigration.gov.

As an IMG, you need a visa to work or train in the United States unless you are a U.S. citizen or a permanent resident (i.e., hold a green card). Two types of visas enable you to accept a residency appointment in the United States: J1 and H1B. Most sponsoring residency programs (SRPs) prefer a J1 visa. Above all, this is because SRPs are authorized by the Department of Homeland Security (DHS)—which in 2003 took the place of the U.S. Immigration and Naturalization Service—to issue a Form DS-2019 (which replaced Form IAP-66 as of September 1, 2002) directly to an IMG. By contrast, SRPs must complete considerable paperwork, including an application to the Immigration and Labor Department, to apply to the DHS for an H1B visa on behalf of an IMG.

The J1 Visa

Also known as the Exchange Visitor Program, the J1 visa was introduced to give IMGs in diverse specialties the chance to use their training experience in the United States to improve conditions in their home countries. As mentioned above, the DHS authorizes most SRPs to issue Form DS-2019 in the same manner that I-20s are issued to regular international students in the United States.

To enable an SRP to issue a DS-2019, you must obtain a certificate from the ECFMG indicating that you are eligible to participate in a residency program in the United States. First, however, you must ask the Ministry of Health in your country to issue a statement indicating that your country needs physicians with the skills you propose to acquire from a U.S. residency program. This statement, which must bear the seal of your country's government and must be signed by a duly designated government official, is intended to satisfy the U.S. Secretary of Health and Human Services (HHS) that there is such a need. The Health Ministry in your country should send this statement to the ECFMG (or they may allow you to mail it to the ECFMG).

How can you find out if the government of your country will issue such a statement? In many countries, the Ministry of Health maintains a list of medical specialties in which there is a need for further training abroad. You can also consult seniors in your medical school. A word of caution: If you are applying for a residency in internal medicine and internists are not in short supply in your country, it may help to indicate an intention to pursue a subspecialty after completing your residency training.

The text of your statement of need should read as follows:

> Name of applicant for visa: _____. There currently exists in _____ (your country) a need for qualified medical practitioners in the specialty of _____. (Name of applicant for visa) has filed a written assurance with the government of this country that he/she will return to _____ (your country) upon completion of training in the United States and intends to enter the practice of medicine in the specialty for which training is being sought.
>
> Stamp (or seal and signature) of issuing official of named country. Dated _____

To facilitate the issuing of such a statement by the Ministry of Health in your country, you should submit a certified copy of the agreement or a contract from your SRP in the United States. The agreement or contract must be signed by you and the residency program official responsible for the training.

Armed with Form DS-2019, you should then go to the U.S. consulate closest to the residential address indicated in your passport. As for other nonimmigrant visas, you must show that you have a genuine nonimmigrant intent to return to your home country. You must also show that all your expenses will be paid.

When you enter the United States, bring your Form DS-2019 along with your visa. You are usually admitted to the United States for the length of the JI program, designated as "D/S," or duration of status. The duration of your program is indicated on the DS-2019.

In the wake of the terrorist attacks of September 11, 2001, a number of new regulations have been introduced to improve the monitoring of exchange visitors during their time in the United States. As of January 30, 2003, all SRPs and students are required to register with the Student and Exchange Visitor Program (SEVP) via the Student and Exchange Visitor Information System (SEVIS). SEVIS allows the DHS to maintain up-to-date information (e.g., enrollment status, current address) on exchange visitors. As of January 30, 2002, SEVIS Form DS-2019 will be used for visa applications, admission, and change of status. Non-SEVIS forms such as Form IAP-66 issued prior to January 30, 2003, will not be accepted after August 1, 2003. Procedural details for this new legislation are still being hammered out, so contact your SRP or check the DHS Web site (www.immigration.gov) for the most current information.

Duration of Participation. The duration of a resident's participation in a program of graduate medical education or training is limited to the time normally required to complete such a program. If you would like to get an idea of the typical training time for the various medical subspecialties, you may consult the *Directory of Medical Specialties*, published by Marquis Who's Who for the American Board of Medical Specialties. The authority charged with determining the duration of time required by an individual IMG is the State Department. The maximum amount of time for participation in a training program is ordinarily limited to seven years unless the IMG has demonstrated to the satisfaction of the ECFMG and the State Department that his or her home country has an exceptional need for the specialty in which he or she will receive further training. An extension of stay may be granted in the event that an IMG needs to repeat a year of clinical medical training or needs time for training or education to take an exam required for board certification.

Requirements After Entry into the United States. Each year, all IMGs participating in a residency program on a J1 visa must furnish the Attorney General of the United States with an affidavit (Form I-644) attesting that they are in good standing in the program of graduate medical education or training in which they are participating and that they will return to their home countries upon completion of the education or training for which they came to the United States.

Restrictions Under the J1 Visa. No later than two years after the date of entry into the United States, an IMG participating in a residency program on a J1 visa is allowed one opportunity to change his or her designated program of graduate medical education or training if his or her director approves that change.

The J1 visa includes a condition called the "two-year foreign residence requirement." The relevant section of the Immigration and Nationality Act states:

> Any exchange visitor physician coming to the United States on or after January 10, 1977, for the purpose of receiving graduate medical education or training is automatically subject to the two-year home-country physical presence requirement of section 212(e) of the Immigration and Nationality Act, as amended. Such physicians are not eligible to be considered for section 212(e) waivers on the basis of "No Objection" statements issued by their governments.

The law thus requires that a J1 visa holder, upon completion of the training program, leave the United States and reside in his or her home country for a period of at least two years. Currently, there is pressure from the American Medical Association (AMA) to extend this period to five years.

An IMG on a J1 visa is ordinarily not allowed to change from a J1 to most other types of visas or (in most cases) to change from J1 to permanent residence while in the United States until he or she has fulfilled the "foreign residence requirement." The purpose of the foreign residence requirement is to ensure that an IMG uses the training he or she obtained in the United States for the benefit of his or her home country. The U.S. government may, however, waive the two-year foreign residence requirement under the following circumstances:

- If you as an IMG can prove that returning to your country would result in "exceptional hardship" to you or to members of your immediate family who are U.S. citizens or permanent residents;
- If you as an IMG can demonstrate a "well-founded fear of persecution" due to race, religion, or political opinions if forced to return to your country;
- If you obtain a "no objection" statement from your government; or
- If you are sponsored by an "interested governmental agency" or a designated state Department of Health in the United States.

Applying for a J1 Visa Waiver. IMGs who have sought a waiver on the basis of the last alternative have found it beneficial to approach the following potentially "interested government agencies":

- **The Department of Health and Human Services.** As of 2003, HHS has expanded its role in reviewing J1 waiver applications. HHS's considerations for a waiver have classically been as follows: (1) the program or activity in which the IMG is engaged is "of high priority and of national or international significance in an area of interest" to HHS; (2) the IMG must be an "integral" part of the program or activity "so that the loss of his/her services would necessitate discontinuance of the program or a major phase of it"; and (3) the IMG "must possess outstanding qualifications, training, and experience well beyond the usually expected accomplishments at the graduate, postgraduate, and residency levels and must clearly demonstrate the capability to make original and significant contributions to the program." Under these criteria, HHS waivers are granted to physicians working in high-level biomedical research.

  New rules will also allow HHS to review J1 waiver applications from community health centers, rural hospitals, and other health care providers. In the past, the U.S. Department of Agriculture (USDA) served as the interested federal government agency that reviewed waiver applications to allow foreign doctors to serve in rural underserved communities outside Appalachia, while the Appalachian Regional Commission (ARC) played that role for Appalachian communities. The USDA is no longer handling applications for J1 waivers. HHS will now review waiver applications for primary care practitioners and psychiatrists who have completed residency training within one year of application to practice in designated Health Professional Shortage Areas (HPSAs), Medically Underserved Areas and Populations (MUA/Ps), and Mental Health Professional Shortage Areas (MHPSAs). HHS waiver applications should be mailed to Joyce E. Jones, Executive Secretary, Exchange Visitor Waiver Review Board, Room 639-H, Hubert H. Humphrey Building, Department of Health and Human Services, 200 Independence Avenue, S.W., Washington, D.C. 20201; phone (202)-690-6174; fax (202)-690-7127.

- **The Veterans Administration.** With more than 170 health care facilities located in various parts of the United States, the VA is a major employer of physicians in this country. In addition, many VA hospitals are affiliated with university medical centers. The VA sponsors IMGs working in research, patient care (regardless of specialty), and teaching. The waiver applicant may engage in teaching and research in conjunction with clinical duties. The VA's latest guidelines (issued on June 22, 1994) provide that it will act as an interested government agency only when the loss of an IMG's services would necessitate the discontinuance of a program or a major phase of it and when recruitment efforts have failed to locate a U.S. physician to fill the position.

  The procedure for obtaining a VA sponsorship for a J1 waiver is as follows: (1) the IMG should deal directly with the Human Resources Department at the local VA facility; and (2) the facility must request that the VA's chief medical director sponsor the IMG for a waiver. The waiver request should include the following documentation: (1) a letter from the director of the local facility describing the program, the IMG's immigration status, the health care needs of the facility, and the facility's recruitment efforts; (2) recruitment efforts, including copies of all job advertisements run within the preceding year; and (3) copies of the IMG's licenses, test results, board certifications, IAP-66 or SEVIS DS-2019 forms, and the like. The VA contact person in Washington, D.C., should be contacted by the local medical facility rather than by IMGs or their attorneys.

- **The Appalachian Regional Commission.** ARC sponsors physicians in certain places in the eastern and southern United States—namely, in Alabama, Georgia, Kentucky, Maryland, Mississippi, New York, North Carolina, Ohio, Pennsylvania, South Carolina, Tennessee, Virginia, and West Virginia. Since 1992, ARC has sponsored approximately 200 primary care IMGs annually in counties within its jurisdiction that have been designated as HPSAs by HHS.

  In accordance with its February 1994 revision of its J1 waiver policies, ARC requires that waiver requests initially be submitted to the ARC contact person in the state of intended employment. Contact information for each state can be found on the ARC Web site (www.arc.gov). If the state concurs, a letter from the state's governor recommending the waiver must be addressed to Anne B. Pope, the new federal cochairman of ARC. The waiver request should include the following: (1) a letter from the facility to Ms. Pope stating the proposed dates of employment, the IMG's medical specialty, the address of the practice location, an assertion that the IMG will practice primary care for at least 40 hours per week in the HPSA, and details as to why the facility needs the services of the IMG; (2) a J1 Visa Data Sheet; (3) the ARC federal cochairman's J1 Visa Waiver Policy and the J1 Visa Waiver Policy Affidavit and Agreement with the notarized signature of the IMG; (4) a contract of at least three years' duration; (5) evidence of the IMG's qualifications, including a résumé, medical diplomas and licenses, and IAP-66 or SEVIS DS-2019 forms; and (6) evidence of unsuccessful attempts to recruit qualified U.S. physicians within the preceding six months. Copies of advertisements, copies of résumés received, and reasons for rejection must also be included. The ARC will not sponsor IMGs who have been out of status for six months or longer.

Requests for ARC waivers are then processed in Washington, D.C. (ARC, 1666 Connecticut Avenue, N.W., Washington, D.C. 20235). ARC is usually able to forward a letter confirming that a waiver has been recommended to the United States Information Agency (USIA) to the requesting facility or attorney within 30 days of the request.

- **The Department of Agriculture.** At the time of publication, the USDA is no longer sponsoring J1 waivers. The scope of the HHS J1 waiver program has been expanded to fill the gap.

- **State Departments of Public Health.** There is no application form for a state-sponsored J1 waiver. However, USIA regulations specify that an application must include the following documents: (1) a letter from the state Department of Public Health identifying the physician and specifying that it would be in the public interest to grant him or her a J1 waiver; (2) an employment contract that is valid for a minimum of three years and that states the name and address of the facility that will employ the physician and the geographic areas in which he or she will practice medicine; (3) evidence that these geographic areas are located within HPSAs; (4) a statement by the physician agreeing to the contractual requirements; (5) copies of all IAP-66 or SEVIS DS-2019 forms; and (6) a completed USIA Data Sheet. Applications are numbered in the order in which they are received, since only 30 physicians per year may be granted waivers in a particular state under the Conrad State 30 program. Individual states may choose to participate or not to participate in this program. At the time of publication, nonparticipating states included Idaho, Oklahoma, and Wyoming, while Texas had suspended its J1 waiver program pending new legislation.

The H1B Visa

Since 1991, the law has allowed medical residency programs to sponsor foreign-born medical residents for H1B visas. There are no restrictions on changing the H1B visa to any other kind of visa, including permanent resident status (green card), through employer sponsorship or through close relatives who are U.S. citizens or permanent residents. The overall ceiling for the number of H1B visas issued to professionals in all categories was increased to 195,000 for the years 2002–2003. This ceiling is scheduled to revert to 65,000 visas in 2004. It is advisable for SRPs to apply for H1B visas as soon as possible in the official year (beginning October 1) when the new quota officially opens up.

According to the Web site www.immihelp.com, as of October 17, 2000, the following beneficiaries of approved H1B petitions are exempt from the H1B annual cap:

- Beneficiaries who are in J1 nonimmigrant status in order to receive graduate medical education or training, and who have obtained a waiver of the two-year home residency requirement
- Beneficiaries who are employed at, or who have received an offer of employment at, an institution of higher education or a related or affiliated nonprofit entity
- Beneficiaries who are employed by, or who have received an offer of employment from, a nonprofit research organization
- Beneficiaries who are employed by, or who have received an offer of employment from, a governmental research organization
- Beneficiaries who are currently maintaining, or who have held within the last six years, H1B status, and are ineligible for another full six-year stay as an H1B
- Beneficiaries who have been counted once toward the numerical limit and are the beneficiary of multiple petitions

H1B visas are intended for "professionals" in a "specialty occupation." This means that an IMG intending to pursue a residency program in the United States with an H1B visa needs to clear all three USMLE Steps before becoming eligible for the H1B. The ECFMG administers Steps 1 and 2, whereas Step 3 is conducted by the individual states. You will need to contact the FSMB or the medical board of the state where you intend to take Step 3 for details (see p. 41, USMLE Step 3 and the IMG).

H1B Application. An application for an H1B visa is filed not by the IMG but rather by his or her employment sponsor—in your case, by the SRP in the United States. If an SRP is willing to do so, you will be told about it at the time of your interview for the residency program.

Before filing an H1B application with the DHS, an SRP must file an application with the U.S. Department of Labor affirming that the SRP will pay at least the normal salary for your job that a U.S. professional would earn. After receiving approval from the Labor Department, your SRP should be ready to file the H1B application with the DHS. The SRP's supporting letter is the most important part of the H1B application package; it must describe the job duties to make it clear that the physician is needed in a "specialty occupation" (resident) under the prevalent legal definition of that term.

Most SRPs prefer to issue a SEVIS Form DS-2019 for a J1 visa rather than file papers for an H1B visa because of the burden of paperwork and the attorney costs involved in securing approval of an H1B visa application. Even so, a sizable number of SRPs are willing to go through the trouble, particularly if an IMG is an excellent candidate or if the SRP concerned finds it difficult to fill all the available residency slots (although this is becoming rarer with continuing cuts in residency slots). If an SRP is unwilling to file for an H1B visa because of attorney costs, you could suggest that you would be willing to bear the burden of such costs. The entire process of getting an H1B visa can take anywhere from 10 to 20 weeks.

H1B Premium Processing Service. According to the Web site www.myvisa.com, the DHS offers the opportunity to obtain processing of an H1B visa application within 15 calendar days. Within 15 days of receiving Form I-907, the DHS will mail you a notice of approval, request for evidence, intent to deny, or notice of investigation for fraud or misrepresentation. If the notice requires the submission of additional evidence or indicates an intent to deny, a new 15-day period will begin upon delivery to the DHS of a complete response to the request for evidence or notice of intent to deny. The fee for this service is $1000. With this service, the total time needed to obtain an H1B visa has become significantly shorter than that required for the J1.

Although an H1B visa can be stamped by any U.S. consulate abroad, it is advisable that you have it stamped at the U.S. consulate where you first applied for a visitor visa to travel to the United States for interviews.

A Final Word

IMGs should also be aware of a new program called the National Security Entry-Exit Registration System, which aims to tighten up homeland security by keeping closer tabs on nonimmigrants residing in or entering the United States on temporary visas.

Male citizens or nationals of specific countries who are already residing in the United States may be required to report to a designated DHS office for registration, which includes being fingerprinted, photographed, and interviewed under oath. The official list of countries includes Bangladesh, Egypt, Indonesia, Jordan, Kuwait, Pakistan, Saudi Arabia, Afghanistan, Algeria, Bahrain, Eritrea, Lebanon, Morocco, North Korea, Oman, Qatar, Somalia, Tunisia, the United Arab Emirates, Yemen, Iran, Iraq, Libya, Sudan, and Syria. Different registration deadlines and criteria have been assigned to citizens of the above-mentioned countries, so please refer to the DHS Web site for details (www. immigration.gov).

If you are entering the United States, you may be registered at the port of entry if you are (1) a citizen or national of Iran, Iraq, Libya, Sudan, or Syria; (2) a nonimmigrant who has been designated by the State Department; or (3) any other nonimmigrant identified by immigration officers at airports, seaports, and land ports of entry in accordance with new regulation 8 CFR 264.1(f)(2). If you will be staying in the United States for more than 30 days, you will then be required to register in person at a DHS district office within 30 days for an interview and will be required to reregister annually.

Once you are registered, certain special procedures will apply. If you leave the United States for any reason, you must appear in person before a DHS inspecting officer at a preapproved airport, seaport, or land port and leave the United States from that port on the same day. If you change your address, employment, or school, you must report to the DHS in writing within ten days using Form AR-11 SR. If any of these regulations are not followed, you may be considered out of status and subject to arrest, detention, fines, and/or removal from the United States, and any further application for immigration may be affected.

For the most up-to-date information regarding policies and procedures, please consult www.immigration.gov.

Summary

Despite some significant obstacles, a number of viable methods are available to IMGs who seek visas to pursue a residency program or eventually practice medicine in the United States. There is no doubt that the best alternative for an IMG is to obtain an H1B visa to pursue a medical residency. However, in cases where an IMG joins a residency program with a J1 visa, there are some possibilities for obtaining waivers of the two-year foreign residency requirement, particularly for those who are willing to make a commitment to perform primary care medicine in medically underserved areas.

Resources for the IMG

- ECFMG
  3624 Market Street, Fourth Floor
  Philadelphia, PA 19104-2685
  (215) 386-5900 or (215) 375-1913
  Fax: (215) 386-9196
  www.ecfmg.org

  The ECFMG telephone number is answered only between 9:00 A.M. and 12:30 P.M. and between 1:30 P.M. and 5:00 P.M. Monday through Friday EST. The ECFMG often takes a long time to answer the phone, which is frequently busy at peak times of the year, and then gives you a long voice-mail message—so it is better to write or fax early than to rely on a last-minute phone call. Do not contact the NBME, as all IMG exam matters are conducted by the ECFMG. The ECFMG also publishes an information booklet on ECFMG certification and the USMLE program, which gives details on the dates and locations of forthcoming USMLE, CSA, and English tests for IMGs together with application forms. It is free of charge and is also available from the public affairs offices of U.S. embassies and consulates worldwide as well as from Overseas Educational Advisory Centers. You may order single copies of the handbook by calling (215) 386-5900, preferably on weekends or between 6 P.M. and 6 A.M. Philadelphia time, or by faxing to (215) 387-9963. Requests for multiple copies must be made by fax or mail on organizational letterhead. The full text of the booklet is also available on the ECFMG's Web site at www.ecfmg.org.

- Federation of State Medical Boards
  P.O. Box 619850
  Dallas, TX 75261-9850
  (817) 868-4000
  Fax: (817) 868-4099
  www.fsmb.org

The FSMB has a number of publications available, including *The Exchange, Section I*, which gives detailed information on examination and licensing requirements in all U.S. jurisdictions. The cost is $30. (Texas residents must add 8.25% state sales tax.) To obtain these publications, submit the online order form. Payment options include Visa or Master-Card. Alternatively, write to Federation Publications at the above address. All orders must be prepaid with a personal check drawn on a U.S. bank, a cashier's check, or a money order payable to the federation. Foreign orders must be accompanied by an international money order or the equivalent, payable in U.S. dollars through a U.S. bank or a U.S. affiliate of a foreign bank. For Step 3 inquiries, the telephone number is (817) 868-4041. You may e-mail the FSMB at usmle@fsmb.org or write to Examination Services at the address above.

- United States Information Agency
  301 4th Street, S.W.
  Washington, D.C. 20547
  (202) 619-6531
  www.ecfmg.com

This Web site summarizes the agency's policy regarding various program administration issues arising from the pursuit of graduate medical education or training in the United States by foreign medical graduates under the aegis of the Exchange Visitor Program.
- The Internet newsgroups misc.education.medical and bit.listserv.medforum can be valuable forums through which to exchange information on licensing exams, residency applications, and the like.

- Immigration information for IMGs is available from the sites of Siskind, Susser, Haas & Devine, a firm of attorneys specializing in immigration law: www.visalaw.com/IMG/resources.html.
- Another source of immigration information can be found on the Web site of the law offices of Carl Shusterman, a Los Angeles attorney specializing in medical immigration law: www.shusterman.com.
- The AMA has dedicated a portion of its Web site to information on IMG demographics, residencies, immigration (double-check that the information is up to date), and the like: www.ama-assn.org/ama/pub/category/17.html.
- International Medical Placement Ltd., a U.S. company specializing in recruiting foreign physicians to work in the United States, has a site at www.intlmedicalplacement.com.
- Two more useful Web sites are www.myvisa.com and www.immihelp.com.
- *First Aid for the International Medical Graduate*, 2nd ed., by Keshav Chander (2002; 313 pages; ISBN 0071385320), is an excellent resource written by a successful IMG. The book includes interviews with successful IMGs and students gearing up for the USMLE, complete "getting settled" information for new residents, and tips for dealing with possible social and cultural transition difficulties. The book provides useful advice on the U.S. curriculum, the health care delivery system, and ethical issues—and the differences IMGs should expect. Dr. Chander points out the weaknesses often found in IMG hopefuls and suggests ways to improve their performance on standardized tests as well as on academic and clinical evaluations. As a bonus, the guide contains information on how to get good fellowships after residency. The bottom line is that this is a reassuring guide that can help IMGs boost their confidence and proficiency. A great "first of its kind" that will empower IMGs with information that they need to succeed.

Other books that may be useful and of interest to IMGs are as follows:

- *International Medical Graduates in U.S. Hospitals: A Guide for Directors and Applicants*, by Faroque A. Khan and Lawrence G. Smith (1995; ISBN 094312641x).
- *Insider's Guide for the International Medical Graduate to Obtain a Medical Residency in the U.S.A.*, by Ahmad Hakemi (1999; ISBN 1929803001).

What Is the COMLEX Level 1?

In 1995, the National Board of Osteopathic Medicine Examiners (NBOME) introduced a new assessment tool called the Comprehensive Osteopathic Medical Licensing Examination, or COMLEX-USA. As with the former NBOME examination series, the COMLEX-USA is administered over three levels. In 1995, only Level 3 was administered, but by 1998 all three levels were implemented. The COMLEX-USA is now the only exam offered to osteopathic students. One goal of this changeover is to have all 50 states recognize this examination as equivalent to the USMLE. Currently, the COMLEX-USA exam sequence is accepted for licensure in all 50 states. Another stated goal of the COMLEX-USA Level 1 is to create a more primary care–oriented exam that integrates osteopathic principles into clinical situations.

To be eligible to take the COMLEX-USA Level 1, you must have satisfactorily completed at least one-half of your sophomore year in an American Osteopathic Association (AOA)–approved medical school. In addition, you must obtain verification that you are in good standing at your medical school via approval of your dean.

For all three levels of the COMLEX-USA, raw scores are converted to a percentile score and a score ranging from 5 to 800. For Levels 1 and 2, a score of 400 is required to pass; for Level 3, a score of 350 is needed. COMLEX-USA scores are usually mailed six to eight weeks after the test date. The mean score on the June 2002 exam was 500 with a standard deviation of 79.

If you pass a COMLEX-USA examination, you are not allowed to retake it to improve your grade. If you fail, there is no specific limit to the number of times you can retake it in order to pass. Level 2 and 3 exams must be passed in sequential order within seven years of passing Level 1. Table 5 lists the upcoming examination dates for all levels of the COMLEX-USA in 2004.

What Is the Structure of the COMLEX Level 1?

The COMLEX-USA Level 1 is a multiple-choice examination that is administered over two days. The exam consists of four booklets, each of which must

TABLE 5. Test Dates for COMLEX-USA Exams in 2004.

Level 1	June 8–9
	October 12–13
Level 2	January 13–14
	August 24–25
Level 3	June 15–16
	December 14–15

be completed in four hours. In the 2003 exam, each booklet contained 200 questions for a two-day total of 800 questions. Since the number of questions may change, the best way to determine the number of questions to expect is to consult the most recent *Examination Guidelines and Sample Exam* (you can download this material from the Web site).

The COMLEX-USA Level 1 questions consist of one-best-answer questions, clinical vignettes, and matching sets. In the 2003 exam, approximately 50 to 60% of the questions were one-best-answer, 20 to 45% were clinical vignettes, and 3 to 5% were matching sets. There were no answer choices such as "all the above," "none of the above," negatively phrased best-answer questions, or K-type questions.

Each test booklet had a similar format. The 2003 COMLEX-USA exam consisted of 120 multiple-choice questions and 80 clinical vignette questions per test booklet. All four test booklets had approximately ten matching questions. Each multiple-choice question was preceded by a one- to two-sentence case.

The 2003 exam included only black-and-white (no color) photos with an accompanying brief clinical description, along with questions asking for the diagnosis. For example, there were photos of an eye movement deficit, an illustration of radical immunodiffusion, x-rays of upper and lower extremities, lung images showing lobar pneumonia, a blood smear showing megaloblastic anemia, ECGs, and an EEG. All photos appeared in the fourth book of the exam.

What Is the Difference Between the USMLE and the COMLEX-USA?

Although the COMLEX-USA and the USMLE are similar in scope, content, and emphasis, some differences are worth noting. For example, the COMLEX-USA Level 1 tests osteopathic principles in addition to basic science materials but does not emphasize lab techniques. In addition, although both exams often require that you apply and integrate knowledge over several areas of basic science to answer a given question, many students who took both tests in 2003 reported that the questions differed somewhat in style. Students reported, for example, that USMLE questions generally required that the test taker reason and draw from the information given (often a two-step process), whereas those on the COMLEX-USA exam tended to be more straightforward. Furthermore, USMLE questions were on average found to be considerably longer than those on the COMLEX-USA.

Students also commented that the COMLEX-USA utilized "buzzwords," although limited in their use (e.g., "rose spots" in typhoid fever), whereas the USMLE avoided buzzwords in favor of descriptions of clinical findings or symptoms (e.g., rose-colored papules on the abdomen rather than rose spots). Finally, the 2003 USMLE had many more photographs than did the COMLEX-USA. In general, the overall impression was that the USMLE was a more "thought-provoking" exam, while the COMLEX-USA was more of a "knowledge-based" exam.

Who Should Take Both the USMLE and the COMLEX-USA?

Aside from facing the COMLEX-USA Level 1, you must decide if you will also take the USMLE Step 1. We recommend that you consider taking both the USMLE and the COMLEX-USA under the following circumstances:

- **If you are applying to allopathic residencies.** Although there is grow-ing acceptance of COMLEX-USA certification on the part of allo-pathic residencies, some allopathic programs prefer or even require pas-sage of the USMLE Step 1. These include many academic programs, programs in competitive specialties (e.g., orthopedics, ophthalmology, or dermatology), and programs in competitive geographic areas (such as California). Fourth-year doctor of osteopathy (DO) students who have already matched may be a good source of information about which pro-grams and specialties look for USMLE scores. It is also a good idea to contact program directors at the institutions you are interested in to ask about their policy regarding the COMLEX-USA versus the USMLE.
- **If you are unsure about your postgraduate training plans.** Successful passage of both the COMLEX-USA Level 1 and the USMLE Step 1 is certain to provide you with the greatest possible range of options when you are applying for internship and residency training.

The clinical coursework that some DO students receive during the summer of their third year (as opposed to their starting clerkships) is considered helpful in integrating basic science knowledge for the COMLEX-USA or the USMLE.

How Do I Prepare for the COMLEX-USA Level 1?

Student experience suggests that you should start studying for the COMLEX-USA four to six months before the test is given, as an early start will allow you to spend up to a month on each subject. The recommendations made in Section I regarding study and testing methods, strategies, and resources, as well as the books suggested in Section III for the USMLE Step 1, hold true for the COMLEX-USA as well.

Another important source of information is in the *Examination Guidelines and Sample Exam*, a booklet that discusses the breakdown of each subject while also providing sample questions. Many students, however, felt that this breakdown provided only a general guideline and was not representative of the level of difficulty of the actual COMLEX-USA. The sample questions did not provide examples of clinical vignettes, which made up approximately 25% of the exam. You will receive this publication with registration materials for the COMLEX-USA Level 1 exam, but you can also receive a copy and additional information by writing:

NBOME
8765 W. Higgins Road, Suite 200
Chicago, IL 60631-4101
(773) 714-0622
Fax: (773) 714-0631

or by visiting the NBOME Web page at www.nbome.org.

Level 1 Practice Items is a new feature offered by the NBOME. It contains about 200 COMLEX-USA Level 1 items and answers. It is important to note that items in this booklet have been used in previous exams. The booklet costs $15 and can be purchased via the NBOME Web site.

The 2003 COMLEX-USA exam consisted of 120 multiple-choice questions and 80 clinical vignette questions per test booklet. There were four test booklets, two of which had approximately ten matching questions. Each multiple-choice question accompanied a small case (about one to two sentences long).

In 2003, students reported an emphasis in certain areas. For example:

- There was an increased emphasis on lower limb anatomy.
- High-yield osteopathic manipulative technique (OMT) topics on the 2003 exam included basic craniosacral theory, sacral testing/diagnosis, lumbar mechanics, spinal motion and diagnosis, and an emphasis on the sympathetic and parasympathetic innervation of viscera.
- Specific topics were repeatedly tested on the exam. These included cardiovascular physiology and pathology, acid-base physiology, diabetes, benign prostatic hyperplasia, sexually transmitted diseases, measles, and rubella. Thyroid and adrenal function, neurology (head injury), specific drug treatments for bacterial infection, migraines/cluster headaches, and drug mechanisms also received heavy emphasis.
- Behavioral science questions were based on psychiatry.
- Since topics that were repeatedly tested appeared in all four booklets, students found it useful to review them in between the two test days. It is important to understand that the topics emphasized on the 2003 exam may not be stressed on the 2004 exam. However, some topics are heavily tested each year; it may be beneficial to have a solid foundation of the above-mentioned topics.

FIRST AID FOR THE PODIATRIC MEDICAL STUDENT

The National Board of Podiatric Medical Examiners (NBPME) tests are designed to assess whether a candidate possesses the knowledge required to practice as a minimally competent entry-level podiatrist. In all states that recognize them, the NBPME examinations are used as part of the licensing process governing the practice of podiatric medicine. Individual states use the examination scores differently; therefore, doctor of podiatric medicine (DPM) candidates should refer to the *NBPME Bulletin of Information: 2004 Examinations* (www.nbpme.info/PDFs/NBPME1Bull.pdf).

The NBPME Part I is generally taken after the completion of the second year of podiatric medical education. Unlike the USMLE Step 1, there is no behavioral science section. The exam does sample the seven basic science disciplines: general anatomy; lower extremity anatomy; biochemistry; physiology; medical microbiology and immunology; pathology; and pharmacology. Questions covering these content areas are interspersed throughout the test.

Candidates performing at extreme levels are passed or failed at 90 minutes.

Your NBPME Appointment

In early spring, your college registrar will have you fill out an application for the NBPME Part I. After your application and registration fees are received, you will be mailed the *NBPME Bulletin of Information: 2004 Examinations*. This bulletin gives you a list of Sylvan Learning Centers across the country that are administering the exam. You may then find the location nearest you and set up an appointment to take the exam. We suggest that you do this as soon as you receive your *NBPME Bulletin*, because reservation slots fill up quickly, especially in the home cities of the seven podiatric medical schools.

On the day of the exam, be sure to arrive at the testing center at least 30 minutes before your scheduled appointment. At that time, you will be registered, escorted to a computer terminal, and given a tutorial to acquaint you with the format of the examination. At the end of the examination, you will be asked to complete a survey regarding your computer-based testing experience.

Computer-Based Testing

The NBPME Part I is a Computerized Mastery Test (CMT) whose format is multiple choice. Each candidate is administered a base test of 90 questions. The maximum amount of time permitted for this base test is 90 minutes. Following the base test, candidates performing at either extreme (either high or low) are passed or failed immediately. By contrast, candidates with an intermediate level of performance are administered additional "testlets" (consisting of 15 questions each), permitting them additional opportunity to demonstrate minimal competence. The maximum time allowed for each additional testlet is 15 minutes. You should try your best on each question, marking any questions that you would like to review should time permit. There is no penalty for guessing. No more than 180 questions are administered to a candidate.

Interpreting Your Score

After you complete the NBPME Part I, a pass/fail decision is reported on the computer. You need a scaled score of at least 75 to pass. Eighty-five percent of first-time test takers pass the NBPME Part I. In computing the scaled score, the number of questions varies from candidate to candidate; however, this is taken into consideration along with the number of questions answered correctly. Approximately two weeks after the examination, you will receive your official score report by mail. Passing candidates receive a message of congratulations but no numerical score. Failing candidates receive a report with one score between 55 and 74 in addition to diagnostic messages intended to help identify strengths or weaknesses in particular content areas. If you fail the NBPME Part I, you must retake the entire examination at a later date. There is no limit to the number of times you can retake the exam.

Preparation for the NBPME Part I

Students suggest that you begin studying for the NBPME Part I at least three months prior to the test date. Each of the colleges of podiatric medicine conducts a series of board reviews. Ask a third-year student which review sessions are most informative. The suggestions made in Section I regarding study and testing methods for the USMLE Step 1 can be applied to the NBPME as well. This book should, however, be used as a supplement and not as the sole source of information.

Know everything about lower extremity anatomy.

Approximately 24% of the NBPME Part I focuses on lower extremity anatomy. In this area, students should rely on the notes and material that they received from their class. Remember, lower extremity anatomy is the podiatrist's specialty—so everything about it is important. Do not forget to study osteology. Keep your old tests and look through old lower extremity class exams, because each of the podiatric colleges submits questions from its own exams. This strategy will give you an understanding of the types of questions that may be asked.

The NBPME, like the USMLE, requires that you apply and integrate knowledge over several areas of basic science to answer the questions. Students report that many questions emphasize clinical presentations; however, the facts in this book are very useful in helping students recall the different diseases and organisms. DPM candidates should expand on the high-yield pharmacology section and study antifungal drugs and treatment protocols for *Pseudomonas*, candidiasis, erythrasma, and the like. The high-yield section focusing on pathology is very useful; however, additional emphasis on diabetes mellitus and all its secondary manifestations should not be overlooked. Students should also focus on classic podiatric dermatopathologies, gout, and arthritis.

A sample set of questions is found in the *NBPME Bulletin of Information: 2004 Examinations*. If you do not receive an *NBPME Bulletin* or if you have any questions regarding registration, fees, test centers, authorization forms, or score reports, please contact your college registrar or:

National Board of Podiatric Medical Examiners (NBPME)
P.O. Box 510
Bellefonte, PA 16823
(814) 357-0487
Fax: (814) 357-0581
E-mail: NBPMEOfc@aol.com

or visit the NBPME Web page at www.nbpme.info.

The USMLE provides accommodations for students with documented disabilities. The basis for such accommodations is the Americans with Disabilities Act (ADA) of 1990. The ADA defines a disability as "a significant limitation in one or more major life activities." This includes both "observable/physical" disabilities (e.g., blindness, hearing loss, narcolepsy) and "hidden/mental disabilities" (e.g., attention deficit hyperactivity disorder, chronic fatigue syndrome, learning disabilities).

To provide appropriate support, the administrators of the USMLE must be informed of both the nature and the severity of an examinee's disability. Such documentation is required for an examinee to receive testing accommodations. Accommodations include extra time on tests, low-stimulation environments, extra or extended breaks, and zoom text.

Who Can Apply for Accommodations?

Students or graduates of a school in the United States or Canada that is accredited by the LCME or the AOA may apply for test accommodations directly from the NBME. Requests are granted only if they meet the ADA definition of a disability. If you are a disabled student or a disabled graduate of a foreign medical school, you must contact the ECFMG (see below).

Who Is Not Eligible for Accommodations?

Individuals who do not meet the ADA definition of disabled are not eligible for test accommodations. Difficulties not eligible for test accommodations include test anxiety, slow reading without an identified underlying cognitive deficit, English as a second language, or learning difficulties that have not been diagnosed as a medically recognized disability.

Understanding the Need for Documentation

Although most learning-disabled medical students are all too familiar with the often exhausting process of providing documentation of their disability, you should realize that **applying for USMLE accommodation is different from these previous experiences.** This is because the NBME determines whether an individual is disabled solely on the basis of the guidelines set by the ADA.

Getting the Information

The first step in applying for USMLE special accommodations is to contact the NBME and obtain a guidelines and questionnaire booklet. This can be obtained by calling or writing to:

Testing Coordinator
Office of Test Accommodations
National Board of Medical Examiners
3750 Market Street
Philadelphia, PA 19104-3102
(215) 590-9500

Internet access to this information is also available at www.nbme.org. This information is also relevant for IMGs, since the information is the same as that sent by the ECFMG.

Foreign graduates should contact the ECFMG to obtain information on special accommodations by calling or writing to:

ECFMG
3624 Market Street, Fourth Floor
Philadelphia, PA 19104-2685
(215) 386-5900

When you get this information, take some time to read it carefully. The guidelines are clear and explicit about what you need to do to obtain accommodations.

NOTES

Database of High-Yield Facts

"There comes a time when for every addition of knowledge you forget something that you knew before. It is of the highest importance, therefore, not to have useless facts elbowing out the useful ones."
—Arthur Conan Doyle, A Study in Scarlet

"Never regard study as a duty, but as the enviable opportunity to learn."
—Albert Einstein

"Live as if you were to die tomorrow. Learn as if you were to live forever."
—Gandhi

Anatomy
Behavioral Science
Biochemistry
Microbiology
Pathology
Pharmacology
Physiology
Rapid Review

The 2004 edition of *First Aid for the USMLE Step 1* contains a revised and expanded database of basic science material that student authors and faculty have identified as high yield for board reviews. The facts are loosely organized according to the seven traditional basic medical science disciplines (anatomy, behavioral science, biochemistry, microbiology, pathology, pharmacology, and physiology). Each discipline is then divided into smaller subsections of related facts. Individual facts are generally presented in a three-column format, with the **Title** of the fact in the first column, the **Description** of the fact in the second column, and the **Mnemonic** or **Special Note** in the third column. Some facts do not have a mnemonic and are presented in a two-column format. Others are presented in list or tabular form in order to emphasize key associations.

The database structure is useful for reviewing material already learned. This section is not ideal for learning complex or highly conceptual material for the first time. At the beginning of each basic science section we list supplementary high-yield clinical vignettes and topics that have appeared on recent exams in order to help focus your review.

The Database of High-Yield Facts is not comprehensive. Use it to complement your core study material and not as your primary study source. The facts and notes have been condensed and edited to emphasize the essential material, and as a result each entry is "incomplete." Work with the material, add your own notes and mnemonics, and recognize that not all memory techniques work for all students.

We update Section II annually to keep current with new trends in boards content as well as to expand our database of high-yield information. However, we must note that inevitably many other very high yield entries and topics are not yet included in our database.

We actively encourage medical students and faculty to submit entries and mnemonics so that we may enhance the database for future students. We also solicit recommendations of alternate tools for study that may be useful in preparing for the examination, such as diagrams, charts, and computer-based tutorials (see How to Contribute, p. xv).

Disclaimer

The entries in this section reflect student opinions of what is high yield. Owing to the diverse sources of material, no attempt has been made to trace or reference the origins of entries individually. We have regarded mnemonics as essentially in the public domain. All errors and omissions will gladly be corrected if brought to the attention of the authors, either through the publisher or directly by e-mail.

Anatomy

*"Dispel from your mind the thought that an understanding of the human body
in every aspect of its structure can be given in words ..."*
—Leonardo da Vinci

Several topics fall under this heading, including embryology, gross anatomy, histology, and neuroanatomy. Do not memorize all the small details; however, do not ignore anatomy altogether. Review what you have already learned and what you wish you had learned. Many questions require two steps. The first step is to identify a structure on anatomic cross section, electron micrograph, or photomicrograph. The second step may require an understanding of the clinical significance of the structure.

When studying, stress clinically important material. For example, be familiar with gross anatomy related to specific diseases (e.g., Pancoast's tumor, Horner's syndrome), traumatic injuries (e.g., fractures, sensory and motor nerve deficits), procedures (e.g., lumbar puncture), and common surgeries (e.g., cholecystectomy). There are also many questions on the exam involving x-rays, CT scans, and neuro MRI scans. Many students suggest browsing through a general radiology atlas, pathology atlas, and histology atlas. Focus on learning basic anatomy at key levels in the body (e.g., sagittal brain MRI; axial CT of midthorax, abdomen, and pelvis). Basic neuroanatomy (especially pathways, blood supply, and functional anatomy) also has good yield. Use this as an opportunity to learn associated neuropathology and neurophysiology. Basic embryology (especially congenital malformations) is worth reviewing.

**High-Yield Clinical
  Vignettes**
Cell Type
Embryology
Gross Anatomy
Histology
Neuroanatomy

These abstracted case vignettes are designed to demonstrate the thought processes necessary to answer multistep clinical reasoning questions.

Vignette	Question	Answer
■ Baby vomits milk when fed and has a gastric air bubble.	What kind of fistula is present?	Blind esophagus with lower segment of esophagus attached to trachea.
■ 20-year-old dancer reports ↓ plantar flexion and ↓ sensation over the back of her thigh, calf, and lateral half of her foot.	What spinal nerve is involved?	Tibial (L4 to S3).
■ Patient presents with ↓ pain and temperature sensation over the lateral aspects of both arms.	What is the lesion?	Syringomyelia.
■ Penlight in patient's right eye produces bilateral pupillary constriction. When moved to the left eye, there is paradoxical bilateral pupillary dilatation.	What is the defect?	Atrophy of the left optic nerve.
■ Patient describes ↓ prick sensation on the lateral aspect of her leg and foot.	A deficit in what muscular action can also be expected?	Dorsiflexion and eversion of foot (common peroneal nerve).
■ Elderly woman presents with arthritis and tingling over the lateral digits of her right hand.	What is the diagnosis?	Carpal tunnel syndrome, median nerve compression.
■ Woman involved in a motor vehicle accident cannot turn her head to the left and has right shoulder droop.	What structure is damaged?	Right CN XI (runs through jugular foramen with CN IX and X), innervating sternocleidomastoid and trapezius muscles.
■ Man presents with one wild, flailing arm.	Where is the lesion?	Contralateral subthalamic nucleus (hemiballismus).
■ Pregnant woman in 3rd trimester has normal blood pressure when standing and sitting. When supine, blood pressure drops to 90/50.	What is the diagnosis?	Compression of the IVC.
■ Soccer player who was kicked in the leg suffered a damaged medial meniscus.	What else is likely to have been damaged?	Anterior cruciate ligament (remember the "unhappy triad").

Vignette	Question	Answer
■ Gymnast dislocates her shoulder anteriorly.	What nerve is most likely to have been damaged?	Axillary nerve (C5, C6).
■ Patient with cortical lesion does not know that he has a disease.	Where is the lesion?	Right parietal lobe.
■ Child presents with cleft lip.	Which embryologic process failed?	Fusion of maxillary and medial nasal processes.
■ Patient cannot protrude tongue toward left side and has a right-sided spastic paralysis.	Where is the lesion?	Left medulla, CN XII.
■ Teen falls while rollerblading and hurts his elbow. He can't feel the medial part of his palm.	Which nerve and what injury?	Ulnar nerve due to broken medial condyle.
■ 24-year-old male develops testicular cancer.	Metastatic spread occurs by what route?	Para-aortic lymph nodes (recall descent of testes during development).
■ Field hockey player presents to the ER after falling on her arm during practice. X-ray shows midshaft break of the humerus.	Which nerve and which artery are most likely damaged?	Radial nerve and deep brachial artery, which run together.
■ Patient cannot blink his right eye or seal his lips and has mild ptosis on the right side.	What is the diagnosis, and which nerve is affected?	Bell's palsy; CN VII.
■ Patient complains of pain, numbness, and a tingling sensation. On exam, she has wasting of the thenar eminence.	What is the diagnosis, and what nerve is often affected?	Carpal tunnel syndrome; median nerve.

HIGH-YIELD FACTS

Anatomy

HIGH-YIELD FACTS

Anatomy

Blood cell differentiation

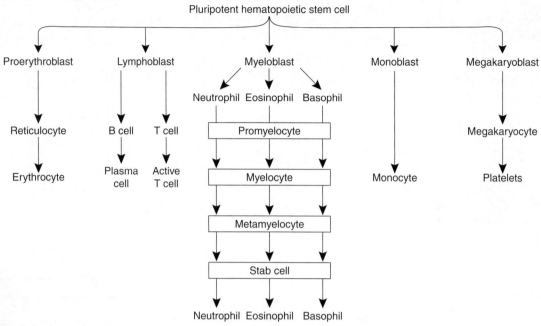

Pluripotent hematopoietic stem cell

Proerythroblast → Reticulocyte → Erythrocyte

Lymphoblast → B cell → Plasma cell

Lymphoblast → T cell → Active T cell

Myeloblast → Neutrophil, Eosinophil, Basophil

Promyelocyte

Myelocyte

Metamyelocyte

Stab cell

Neutrophil Eosinophil Basophil

Monoblast → Monocyte

Megakaryoblast → Megakaryocyte → Platelets

Erythrocyte	Anucleate, biconcave → large surface area: volume ratio → easy gas exchange (O_2 and CO_2). Source of energy—glucose (90% anaerobically degraded to lactate, 10% by HMP shunt). Survival time—120 days. Membrane contains the chloride-bicarbonate antiport important in the "physiologic chloride shift," which allows the RBC to transport CO_2 from the periphery to the lungs for elimination.	*Eryth* = red; *cyte* = cell. Erythrocytosis = polycythemia = ↑ number of red cells. Anisocytosis = varying sizes. Poikilocytosis = varying shapes. Reticulocyte = baby erythrocyte.

 (Erythrocyte image)

Leukocyte	Types: granulocytes (basophils, eosinophils, neutrophils) and mononuclear cells (lymphocytes, monocytes). Responsible for defense against infections. Normally 4000–10,000 per microliter.	*Leuk* = white; *cyte* = cell.

Basophil	Mediates allergic reaction. < 1% of all leukocytes. Bilobate nucleus. Densely basophilic granules containing heparin (anticoagulant), histamine (vasodilator) and other vasoactive amines, and SRS-A.	*Basophilic*—staining readily with *basic* stains.

  (Basophil images)

Mast cell	Mediates allergic reaction. Degranulation—release of histamine, heparin, and eosinophil chemotactic factors. Can bind IgE to membrane. Mast cells resemble basophils structurally and functionally but are not the same cell type.	Involved in type I hypersensitivity reactions. Cromolyn sodium prevents mast cell degranulation (used to treat asthma).

 (Mast cell images)

Eosinophil

1–6% of all leukocytes. Bilobate nucleus. Packed with large eosinophilic granules of uniform size. Defends against helminthic and protozoan infections (major basic protein). Highly phagocytic for antigen-antibody complexes.

Produces histaminase and arylsulfatase.

Eosin = a dye; *philic* = loving.

Causes of eosinophilia =
NAACP:
  Neoplastic
  Asthma
  Allergic processes
  Collagen vascular
    diseases
  Parasites

Neutrophil

Acute inflammatory response cell. 40–75% WBCs. Phagocytic. Multilobed nucleus. Large, spherical, azurophilic 1° granules (called lysosomes) contain hydrolytic enzymes, lysozyme, myeloperoxidase, and lactoferrin.

Hypersegmented polys are seen in vitamin B_{12}/ folate deficiency.

Monocyte

2–10% of leukocytes. Large. Kidney-shaped nucleus. Extensive "frosted glass" cytoplasm. Differentiates into macrophages in tissues.

Mono = one, single; *cyte* = cell.

Lymphocyte

Small. Round, densely staining nucleus. Small amount of pale cytoplasm. B lymphocytes produce antibodies. T lymphocytes manifest the cellular immune response as well as regulate B lymphocytes and macrophages.

B lymphocyte

CD19

CD20

Part of humoral immune response. Arises from stem cells in bone marrow. Matures in marrow. Migrates to peripheral lymphoid tissue (follicles of lymph nodes, white pulp of spleen, unencapsulated lymphoid tissue). When antigen is encountered, B cells differentiate into plasma cells and produce antibodies. Has memory. Can function as antigen-presenting cell (APC) via MHC II.

B = **B**one marrow.

Plasma cell

Off-center nucleus, clock-face chromatin distribution, abundant RER and well-developed Golgi apparatus. B cells differentiate into plasma cells, which can produce large amounts of antibody specific to a particular antigen.

Multiple myeloma is a plasma cell neoplasm.

HIGH-YIELD FACTS

Anatomy

T lymphocyte

Mediates cellular immune response. Originates from stem cells in the bone marrow, but matures in the thymus. T cells differentiate into cytotoxic T cells (MHC I, CD8), helper T cells (MHC II, CD4), suppressor T cells, and delayed hypersensitivity T cells.

T is for **Thymus**. **CD** is for **Cluster of Differentiation**. **MHC × CD = 8** (e.g., MHC 2 × CD4 = 8).

Macrophage

Phagocytizes bacteria, cell debris, and senescent red cells and scavenges damaged cells and tissues. Long life in tissues. Macrophages differentiate from circulating blood monocytes. Activated by γ-interferon. Can function as APC via MHC II.

Macro = large; *phage* = eater.

Airway cells

Ciliated cells extend to the respiratory bronchioles; goblet cells extend only to the terminal bronchioles. Type I cells (97% of alveolar surfaces) line the alveoli. Type II cells (3%) secrete pulmonary surfactant (dipalmitoylphosphatidylcholine), which ↓ the alveolar surface tension. Also serve as precursors to type I cells and other type II cells.

Mucus secretions are swept out of the lungs toward the mouth by ciliated cells. A lecithin-to-sphingomyelin ratio of > 2.0 in amniotic fluid is indicative of fetal lung maturity.

Microglia

CNS phagocytes. Mesodermal origin. Not readily discernible in Nissl stains. Have small irregular nuclei and relatively little cytoplasm. In response to tissue damage, transform into large ameboid phagocytic cells.

HIV-infected microglia fuse to form multinucleated giant cells in the CNS.

Oligodendroglia

Function to myelinate multiple CNS axons. In Nissl stains, they appear as small nuclei with dark chromatin and little cytoplasm. Predominant type of glial cell in white matter.

These cells are destroyed in multiple sclerosis.

Schwann cells

Each Schwann cell functions to myelinate only 1 PNS axon. Schwann cells promote axonal regeneration.

Acoustic neuroma is an example of a schwannoma. Location commonly associated with internal acoustic meatus (CN VII, VIII).

Gas exchange barrier

Surfactant
(constitutive secretion)

Macrophage

Type II
epithelial cell

Lamellar bodies

Alveolar
space

CO_2

Type I
epithelial cell

O_2

Air-blood
barrier

Tight junction
(continuous endothelium)

Capillary
lumen

Type II
pneumocytes
produce surfactant
and serve as progenitors
for type I and type II
cells.

ANATOMY—EMBRYOLOGY

Fetal landmarks

Day 0	Fertilization by sperm, initiating embryogenesis.
Within week 1	Implantation (as a blastocyst).
Within week 2	Bilaminar disk.
Within week 3	Gastrulation.
	Primitive streak, notochord, and neural plate begin to form.
Weeks 3–8	Neural tube formed.
	Organogenesis.
	Extremely susceptible to teratogens.
Week 4	Heart begins to beat.
	Upper and lower limb buds begin to form.
Week 10	Genitalia have male/female characteristics.

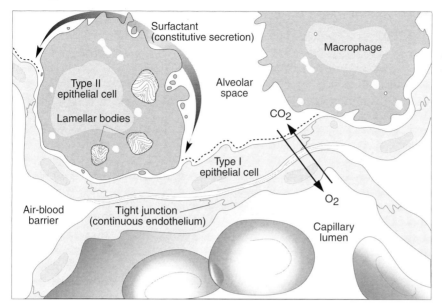

Day 2
Zygote

Day 3

Morula

Day 5
Blastocyst

Day 0
Fertilization

Endometrium

Day 6
Implantation

Uterine
wall

Neural plate

Day 18

Notochord

Neural crest

Neural tube

Neural
crest
cells

Day 21

Teratogens

Most susceptible in 3rd–8th weeks (organogenesis) of pregnancy.

Examples	Effects on fetus
ACE inhibitors	Renal damage
Cocaine	Abnormal fetal development and fetal addiction
DES	Vaginal clear cell adenocarcinoma
Iodide	Congenital goiter or hypothyroidism
13-*cis*-retinoic acid	Extremely high risk for birth defects
Thalidomide	Limb defects ("flipper" limbs)
Warfarin, x-rays	Multiple anomalies

Fetal infections can also cause congenital malformations. (Other medications contraindicated in pregnancy are shown in the pharmacology section.)

Umbilical cord

Contains 2 umbilical arteries, which return deoxygenated blood from the fetus, and 1 umbilical vein, which supplies oxygenated blood from the placenta to the fetus.

Single umbilical artery is associated with congenital and chromosomal anomalies.

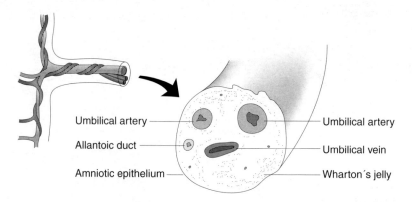

Umbilical artery — Umbilical artery
Allantoic duct — Umbilical vein
Amniotic epithelium — Wharton's jelly

Embryologic derivatives

Ectoderm

Surface ectoderm	Adenohypophysis, lens of eye, epithelial linings, epidermis.
Neuroectoderm	Neurohypophysis, CNS neurons, oligodendrocytes, astrocytes, pineal gland.
Neural crest	ANS, dorsal root ganglia, melanocytes, chromaffin cells of adrenal medulla, enterochromaffin cells, pia, celiac ganglion, Schwann cells, odontoblasts, parafollicular (C) cells of thyroid, laryngeal cartilage.

Mesoderm — Dura connective tissue, muscle, bone, cardiovascular structures, lymphatics, blood, urogenital structures, and serous linings of body cavities (e.g., peritoneal), spleen, adrenal cortex.

Endoderm — Gut tube epithelium and derivatives (e.g., lungs, liver, pancreas, thymus, thyroid, parathyroid).

Notochord — Induces ectoderm to form neuroectoderm (neural plate). Its postnatal derivative is the nucleus pulposus of the intervertebral disk.

Early development

Rule of 2's for 2nd week	2 germ layers (bilaminar disk): epiblast, hypoblast. 2 cavities: amniotic cavity, yolk sac. 2 components to placenta: cytotrophoblast, syncytiotrophoblast.	The epiblast (precursor to ectoderm) invaginates to form primitive streak. Cells from the primitive streak give rise to both intraembryonic mesoderm and endoderm.
Rule of 3's for 3rd week	3 germ layers (gastrula): ectoderm, mesoderm, endoderm.	

Fetal erythropoiesis

Fetal erythropoiesis occurs in:
1. **Y**olk sac (3–8 wk)
2. **L**iver (6–30 wk)
3. **S**pleen (9–28 wk)
4. **B**one marrow (28 wk onward)

Young **L**iver **S**ynthesizes **B**lood.

Heart embryology

Embryonic structure	Gives rise to
Truncus arteriosus	Ascending aorta and pulmonary trunk
Bulbus cordis	Smooth parts of left and right ventricle
Primitive ventricle	Trabeculated parts of left and right ventricle
Primitive atria	Trabeculated left and right atrium
Left horn of sinus venosus (SV)	Coronary sinus
Right horn of SV	Smooth part of right atrium
Right common cardinal vein and right anterior cardinal vein	SVC

Twinning

Monozygotic

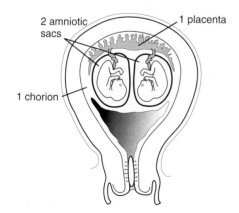

1 zygote splits evenly to develop 2 amniotic sacs with a single common chorion and placenta.

Dizygotic (fraternal) or monozygotic

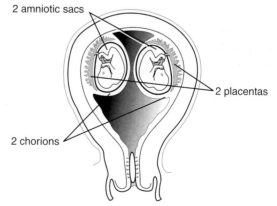

Dizygotes develop individual placentas, chorions, and amniotic sacs.

Monozygotes develop 2 placentas (separate/fused), chorions, and amniotic sacs.

Fetal circulation

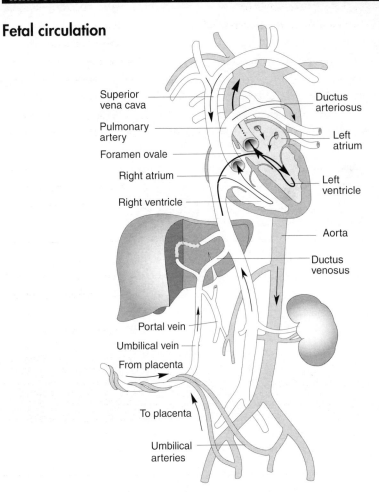

Superior vena cava	Ductus arteriosus
Pulmonary artery	Left atrium
Foramen ovale	
Right atrium	Left ventricle
Right ventricle	
	Aorta
	Ductus venosus
Portal vein	
Umbilical vein	
From placenta	
To placenta	
Umbilical arteries	

Blood in umbilical vein is ≈ 80% saturated with O_2.

Most oxygenated blood reaching the heart via the IVC is diverted through the foramen ovale and pumped out the aorta to the head.

Deoxygenated blood from the SVC is expelled into the pulmonary artery and ductus arteriosus to the lower body of the fetus.

At birth, infant takes a breath; ↓ resistance in pulmonary vasculature causes ↑ left atrial pressure vs. right atrial pressure; foramen ovale closes; ↑ in O_2 leads to ↓ in prostaglandins, causing closure of ductus arteriosus.

Indomethacin closes the PDA. Prostaglandins keep a PDA open.

(Adapted, with permission, from Ganong WF. *Review of Medical Physiology*, 19th ed. Stamford, CT: Appleton & Lange, 1999:600.)

Fetal-postnatal derivatives

1. Umbilical vein—ligamentum teres hepatis
2. Umbilical arteries—**medial** umbilical ligaments
3. Ductus arteriosus—ligamentum arteriosum
4. Ductus venosus—ligamentum venosum
5. Foramen ovale—fossa ovalis
6. Allantois—urachus—**median** umbilical ligament
7. Notochord—nucleus pulposus

Urachal cyst or sinus is a remnant of the allantois (urine drainage from bladder).

Aortic arch derivatives

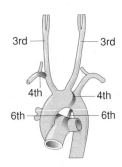

3rd — 3rd
4th — 4th
6th — 6th

1st—part of **MAX**illary artery.
2nd—**S**tapedial artery and hyoid artery.
3rd—common **C**arotid artery and proximal part of internal carotid artery.
4th—on left, aortic arch; on right, proximal part of right subclavian artery.
6th—proximal part of pulmonary arteries and (on left only) ductus arteriosus.

1st arch is **MAX**imal.
Second = **S**tapedial.
C is 3rd letter of alphabet.

4th arch (4 limbs) = systemic.

6th arch = pulmonary and the pulmonary-to-systemic shunt (ductus arteriosus).

HIGH-YIELD FACTS

Anatomy

Branchial apparatus	Branchial clefts are derived from ectoderm. Branchial arches are derived from mesoderm and neural crests. Branchial pouches are derived from endoderm.	**CAP** covers outside from inside (**C**lefts = ectoderm, **A**rches = mesoderm, **P**ouches = endoderm).
Branchial arch 1 derivatives	Meckel's cartilage: **M**andible, **M**alleus, incus, spheno**M**andibular ligament. Muscles: **M**uscles of **M**astication (temporalis, **M**asseter, lateral and **M**edial pterygoids), **M**ylohyoid, anterior belly of digastric, tensor tympani, tensor veli palatini. Nerve: CN V_3.	
Branchial arch 2 derivatives	Reichert's cartilage: **S**tapes, **S**tyloid process, lesser horn of hyoid, **S**tylohyoid ligament. Muscles: muscles of facial expression, **S**tapedius, **S**tylohyoid, posterior belly of digastric. Nerve: CN VII.	
Branchial arch 3 derivatives	Cartilage: greater horn of hyoid. Muscle: stylopharyngeus. Nerve: CN IX.	Think of pharynx: stylo**pharyngeus** innervated by glosso**pharyngeal** nerve.
Branchial arches 4 to 6 derivatives	Cartilages: thyroid, cricoid, arytenoids, corniculate, cuneiform. Muscles (4th arch): most pharyngeal constrictors, cricothyroid, levator veli palatini. Muscles (6th arch): all intrinsic muscles of larynx **except cricothyroid.** Nerve: 4th arch—CN X; 6th arch—CN X (recurrent laryngeal branch).	Arch 5 makes no major developmental contributions.
Branchial arch innervation	Arch 1 derivatives supplied by CN V_2 and V_3. Arch 2 derivatives supplied by CN VII. Arch 3 derivatives supplied by CN IX. Arch 4 and 6 derivatives supplied by CN X.	Primitive pharynx — CN V; Pharyngeal arches: 1st, 2nd — CN VII, 3rd — CN IX, 4th — CN X; Epicardial ridge; Primitive esophagus
Branchial cleft derivatives	1st cleft develops into external auditory meatus. 2nd through 4th clefts form temporary cervical sinuses, which are obliterated by proliferation of 2nd arch mesenchyme.	Persistent cervical sinus can lead to a branchial cyst in the neck.

Ear development

Bones	**Muscles**	**Miscellaneous**
Incus/malleus—1st arch	Tensor tympani (V_3)—1st arch	External auditory meatus—1st cleft
Stapes—2nd arch	Stapedius (VII)—2nd arch	Eardrum, eustachian tube—1st pharyngeal membrane

Branchial pouch derivatives	1st pouch develops into middle ear cavity, eustachian tube, mastoid air cells. 2nd pouch develops into epithelial lining of palatine tonsil. 3rd pouch (dorsal wings) develops into **inferior** parathyroids. 3rd pouch (ventral wings) develops into thymus. 4th pouch develops into **superior** parathyroids.	1st pouch contributes to endoderm-lined structures of ear. 3rd pouch contributes to 3 structures (thymus, left and right inferior parathyroids). Aberrant development of 3rd and 4th pouches → DiGeorge syndrome → leads to T-cell deficiency (thymic hypoplasia) and hypocalcemia (parathyroid glands).
Thymus	Site of T-cell maturation. Encapsulated. From epithelium of 3rd branchial pouches. Lymphocytes of mesenchymal origin. Cortex is dense with immature T cells; medulla is pale with mature T cells and epithelial reticular cells and contains Hassall's corpuscles. Positive and negative selection occurs at the corticomedullary junction.	Think of the **T**hymus as "finishing school" for **T** cells. They arrive immature and "dense" in the cortex; they are mature in the medulla.
Thyroid development	Thyroid diverticulum arises from floor of primitive pharynx, descends into neck. Connected to tongue by thyroglossal duct, which normally disappears but may persist as pyramidal lobe of thyroid. Foramen cecum is normal remnant of thyroglossal duct. Most common ectopic thyroid tissue site is the tongue.	
Tongue development 	1st branchial arch forms anterior $^2/_3$ (thus sensation via CN V_3, taste via CN VII). 3rd and 4th arches form posterior $^1/_3$ (thus sensation and taste mainly via CN IX, extreme posterior via CN X). Motor innervation is via CN XII.	Taste is CN VII, IX, X (solitary nucleus); pain is CN V_3, IX, X; motor is CN XII.
Cleft lip and cleft palate Cleft lip	Cleft lip—failure of fusion of the maxillary and medial nasal processes. Cleft palate—failure of fusion of the lateral palatine processes, the nasal septum, and/or the median palatine process.	 Cleft palate (partial)

Diaphragm embryology

Diaphragm is derived from:
1. **S**eptum transversum
2. **P**leuroperitoneal folds
3. **B**ody wall
4. **D**orsal mesentery of esophagus

Aorta
Pleuroperitoneal folds
Dorsal esophageal mesoderm
Foregut
Septum transversum
Body wall
Inferior vena cava

Several **P**arts **B**uild **D**iaphragm.
Diaphragm descends during development but maintains innervation from above C3–C5. "**C3, 4, 5** keeps the diaphragm alive."
Abdominal contents may herniate into the thorax due to incomplete development (hiatal hernia).

Bone formation

Intramembranous — Spontaneous bone formation without preexisting cartilage.

Endochondral — Ossification of cartilaginous molds. Long bones form by this type of ossification at 1° and 2° centers.

Meckel's diverticulum

Umbilicus
Meckel's diverticulum

Persistence of the vitelline duct or yolk stalk. May contain ectopic acid–secreting gastric mucosa and/or pancreatic tissue. Most common congenital anomaly of the GI tract. Can cause bleeding or obstruction near the terminal ileum. Contrast with omphalomesenteric cyst = cystic dilatation of vitelline duct.
Associated with intussusception and volvulus.

The five **2's:**
- **2** inches long.
- **2** feet from the ileocecal valve.
- **2%** of population.
- Commonly presents in first **2** years of life.
- May have **2** types of epithelia.

Pancreas and spleen embryology

Pancreas is derived from the foregut. Ventral pancreatic bud becomes pancreatic head, uncinate process (lower half of head), and main pancreatic duct. Dorsal pancreatic bud becomes everything else (body, tail, isthmus, and accessory pancreatic duct).
Spleen arises from dorsal mesentery but is supplied by artery of foregut.

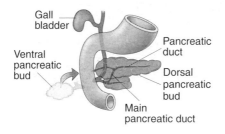

Gall bladder
Ventral pancreatic bud
Pancreatic duct
Dorsal pancreatic bud
Main pancreatic duct

Genital ducts

Mesonephric (wolffian) duct — Develops into **S**eminal vesicles, **E**pididymis, **E**jaculatory duct, and **D**uctus deferens.

Paramesonephric (müllerian) duct — Develops into fallopian tube, uterus, and part of vagina.

Müllerian inhibiting substance secreted by testes suppresses development of paramesonephric ducts in males.

SEED.

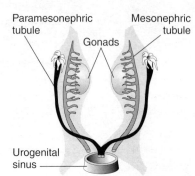

Bicornuate uterus

Results from incomplete fusion of the paramesonephric ducts. Associated with urinary tract abnormalities and infertility.

Male/female genital homologues

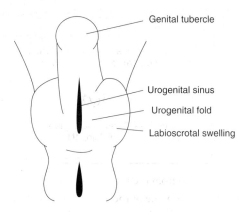

Male	Dihydrotestosterone		Estrogen	Female
Glans penis	←	Genital tubercle	→	Glans clitoris
Corpus spongiosum	←	Urogenital sinus	→	Vestibular bulbs
Bulbourethral glands (of Cowper)	←	Urogenital sinus	→	Greater vestibular glands (of Bartholin)
Prostate gland	←	Urogenital sinus	→	Urethral and paraurethral glands (of Skene)
Ventral shaft of penis (penile urethra)	←	Urogenital folds	→	Labia minora
Scrotum	←	Labioscrotal swelling	→	Labia majora

Congenital penile abnormalities

Hypospadias | Abnormal opening of penile urethra on inferior (ventral) side of penis due to failure of urethral folds to close. | Hypospadias is more common than epispadias. Fix hypospadias to prevent UTIs.

Epispadias | Abnormal opening of penile urethra on superior (dorsal) side of penis due to faulty positioning of genital tubercle. | Exstrophy of the bladder is associated with epispadias.

Sperm development

Spermatogenesis begins with spermatogonia (type A and type B). Full development takes 2 months. Spermatogenesis occurs in Seminiferous tubules. Type A forms both type A and type B spermatogonia.

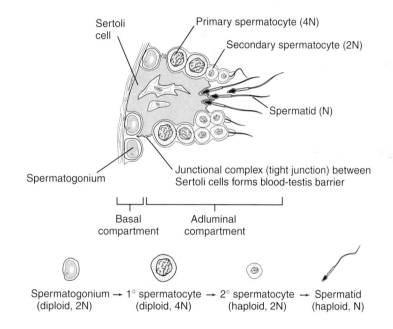

Derivation of sperm parts

Acrosome is derived from the Golgi apparatus and flagellum (tail) from one of the centrioles. Middle piece (neck) has Mitochondria. Sperm food supply is fructose.

Meiosis and ovulation

1° oocytes begin meiosis I during fetal life and complete meiosis I just prior to ovulation.

Meiosis I is arrested in prOphase for years until Ovulation.

Meiosis II is arrested in METaphase until fertilization.

An egg MET a sperm.

Amniotic fluid abnormalities

Polyhydramnios	> 1.5–2 L of amniotic fluid; associated with esophageal/duodenal atresia, causing inability to swallow amniotic fluid, and with anencephaly.
Oligohydramnios	< 0.5 L of amniotic fluid; associated with bilateral renal agenesis or posterior urethral valves (in males) and resultant inability to excrete urine.

Potter's syndrome

Bilateral renal agenesis → oligohydramnios → limb deformities, facial deformities, pulmonary hypoplasia. Caused by malformation of ureteric bud.

Babies with **P**otter's can't "**P**ee" in utero.

Horseshoe kidney

Inferior poles of both kidneys fuse. As they ascend from pelvis during fetal development, horseshoe kidneys get trapped under inferior mesenteric artery and remain low in the abdomen.

Aorta
Horseshoe kidney
Inferior mesenteric artery

ANATOMY—GROSS ANATOMY

Landmark dermatomes

C2 is a posterior half of a skull "cap."
C3 is a high turtleneck shirt.
C4 is a low-collar shirt.
T4 is at the nipple.
T7 is at the xiphoid process.
T10 is at the umbilicus (important for early appendicitis pain referral).
L1 is at the inguinal ligament.
L4 includes the kneecaps.
S2, S3, S4 erection and sensation of penile and anal zones.

Gallbladder pain referred to the right shoulder via the phrenic nerve.
T4 at the **teat pore.**

T10 at the belly but**TEN.**

L1 is **IL** (**I**nguinal **L**igament).
Down on **L4s (all fours).**
"**S2, 3, 4** keep the penis off the floor."

Rotator cuff muscles

Acromion **S**upraspinatus
Coracoid
Infra-spinatus
Biceps tendon
Teres minor
Sub-scapularis

Posterior   Anterior

Shoulder muscles that form the rotator cuff:
  Supraspinatus—helps deltoid abduct arm.
  Infraspinatus—laterally rotates arm.
  Teres minor—adducts and medially rotates arm.
  Subscapularis—medially rotates and adducts arm.

S I t S (small t is for teres minor).

Anatomy

HIGH-YIELD FACTS

| **Thenar-hypothenar muscles** | Thenar—**O**pponens pollicis, **A**bductor pollicis brevis, **F**lexor pollicis brevis. | Both groups perform the same functions: **O**ppose, **A**bduct, and **F**lex **(OAF).** |
| | Hypothenar—**O**pponens digiti minimi, **A**bductor digiti minimi, **F**lexor digiti minimi. | |

Thenar eminence
Hypothenar eminence

Unhappy triad/ knee injury	This common football injury (caused by clipping from the lateral side) consists of damage to medial collateral ligament (MCL), medial meniscus, and anterior cruciate ligament (ACL).	Positive anterior drawer sign indicates tearing of the ACL.
	PCL = posterior cruciate ligament. LCL = lateral collateral ligament.	Abnormal passive abduction indicates a torn MCL.
	"Anterior" and "posterior" in ACL and PCL refer to sites of **tibial** attachment.	

Lateral condyle
Medial condyle
ACL
PCL
LCL
MCL
Lateral meniscus
Medial meniscus

| **Recurrent laryngeal nerve** | Supplies all intrinsic muscles of the larynx **except the cricothyroid muscle.** Left recurrent laryngeal nerve wraps around the arch of the aorta and the ligamentum arteriosum. Right recurrent laryngeal nerve wraps around right subclavian artery. Damage results in hoarseness. Complication of thyroid surgery. | Branch of CN X. |

View from posterior

Esophageal muscle
Internal jugular vein
Left brachiocephalic vein
Thyroid gland
Right recurrent laryngeal nerve
Right subclavian artery and vein
Left recurrent laryngeal nerve
Arch of aorta
Trachea
Left vagus nerve (X)
Right vagus nerve (X)

Scalp and meninges: layers	Skin	SCALP–skull–DAP.
	Connective tissue	
	Aponeurosis	
	Loose connective tissue (vascular layer)	
	Pericranium (skull)	
	Dura mater, subdural (SD) space, **A**rachnoid, subarachnoid (SA) space, **P**ia mater, brain	

Meninges
D
SD
A
SA
P
Brain
CSF

Mastication muscles	3 muscles close jaw: **M**asseter, te**M**poralis, **M**edial pterygoid. 1 opens: lateral pterygoid. All are innervated by the trigeminal nerve (V_3).	**M**'s **M**unch. Lateral Lowers (when speaking of pterygoids with respect to jaw motion).
Muscles with glossus	All muscles with root *glossus* in their names (**except palatoglossus**, innervated by vagus nerve) are innervated by hypo*glossal* nerve.	*Palat:* vagus nerve. *Glossus:* hypo*glossal* nerve.
Muscles with palat	All muscles with root *palat* in their names (**except tensor veli palatini**, innervated by mandibular branch of CN V) are innervated by vagus nerve.	*Palat:* vagus nerve (except **TENS**or, who was too **TENSE**).
Carotid sheath	3 structures inside: 1. Internal jugular **V**ein (lateral) 2. Common carotid **A**rtery (medial) 3. Vagus **N**erve (posterior)	**VAN.**
Diaphragm structures	Structures perforating diaphragm: At T8: IVC. At T10: esophagus, vagus (2 trunks). At T12: aorta (red), thoracic duct (white), azygous vein (blue). Diaphragm is innervated by **C3, 4**, and **5** (phrenic nerve). Pain from the diaphragm can be referred to the shoulder.	**I 8 10 EGGs AT 12:** **I** = IVC @ **8**th vertebra; **EG** = Esopha**G**us; **G** = va**G**us @ **10**th vertebra; **A** = **A**orta, **A**zygous; **T** = **T**horacic duct @ **12**th vertebra. "**C3, 4, 5** keeps the diaphragm alive."

Central tendon
Inferior vena cava (T8)
Esophagus (T10)
Aorta (T12)
Rib
Vertebrae
Inferior view

Coronary artery anatomy

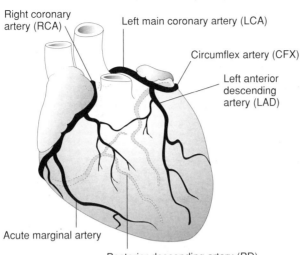

Right coronary artery (RCA)

Left main coronary artery (LCA)

Circumflex artery (CFX)

Left anterior descending artery (LAD)

Acute marginal artery

Posterior descending artery (PD)

(Adapted, with permission, from Ganong WF. *Review of Medical Physiology*, 19th ed. Stamford, CT: Appleton & Lange, 1999:592.)

In the majority of cases, the SA and AV nodes are supplied by the RCA. 80% of the time, the RCA supplies the inferior portion of the left ventricle via the PD artery (= right dominant).

Coronary artery occlusion occurs most commonly in the LAD, which supplies the anterior interventricular septum.

Coronary arteries fill during diastole.

The most posterior part of the heart is the left atrium; enlargement can cause dysphagia.

Bronchopulmonary segments

Each bronchopulmonary segment has a 3° (segmental) bronchus and 2 arteries (bronchial and pulmonary) in the center; veins and lymphatics drain along the borders.

Arteries run with Airways.

Lung relations

Right lung has 3 lobes; Left has 2 lobes and Lingula (homologue of right middle lobe). Right lung is more common site for inhaled foreign body owing to less acute angle of right main stem bronchus.

Instead of a middle lobe, the left lung has a space occupied by the heart. The relation of the pulmonary artery to the bronchus at each lung hilus is described by **RALS**— **R**ight **A**nterior; **L**eft **S**uperior.

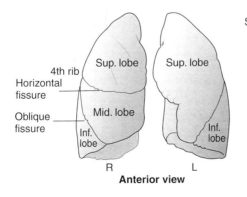

4th rib
Horizontal fissure
Oblique fissure
Sup. lobe
Sup. lobe
Mid. lobe
Inf. lobe
Inf. lobe
R
L
Anterior view

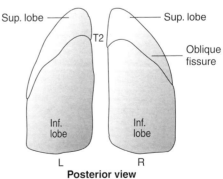

Sup. lobe
T2
Sup. lobe
Oblique fissure
Inf. lobe
Inf. lobe
L
R
Posterior view

HIGH-YIELD FACTS

Anatomy

Femoral triangle

Femoral sheath contains femoral artery, femoral vein, and femoral canal (containing deep inguinal lymph nodes). Femoral nerve lies outside femoral sheath.

Sartorius muscle
Femoral triangle
Inguinal ligament
Adductor longus muscle

Lateral to medial: **N–(AVEL)** = **N**erve–(**A**rtery–**V**ein–**E**mpty space–**L**ymphatics).

Femoral hernia is entrance of abdominal contents through the femoral canal.

The femoral triangle contains the femoral **V**ein, femoral **A**rtery, and femoral **N**erve.

Femoral hernia protrudes below and lateral to the pubic tubercle.

Abdominal hernias

Hernias are protrusions of peritoneum through an opening, usually sites of weakness.

Diaphragmatic hernia
: Abdominal structures enter the thorax; may occur in infants as a result of defective development of pleuroperitoneal membrane. Most commonly a hiatal hernia, in which stomach herniates upward through the esophageal hiatus of the diaphragm.

Direct hernia
: Protrudes through the inguinal (Hesselbach's) triangle. Direct hernia bulges directly through abdominal wall medial to inferior epigastric artery. Goes through the external inguinal ring only. Usually in older men.

Indirect hernia
: **IN**direct hernia goes through the internal (deep) inguinal ring and external (superficial) inguinal ring and **IN**to the scrotum. Indirect hernia enters internal inguinal ring lateral to inferior epigastric artery. **IN**direct hernias occur in **IN**fants owing to failure of processus vaginalis to close.

MDs don't **LI**e:
  Medial to inferior epigastric artery = **D**irect hernia.
  Lateral to inferior epigastric artery = **I**ndirect hernia.
Hesselbach's triangle:
  Inferior epigastric artery
  Lateral border of rectus abdominis
  Inguinal ligament

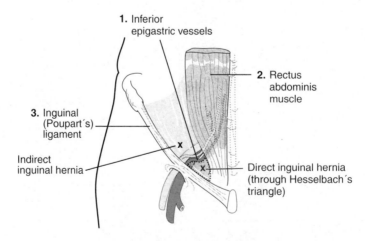

1. Inferior epigastric vessels
2. Rectus abdominis muscle
3. Inguinal (Poupart's) ligament
Indirect inguinal hernia
Direct inguinal hernia (through Hesselbach's triangle)

Inguinal canal

Parietal peritoneum

Site of protrusion of indirect hernia

Inferior epigastric vessels

Site of protrusion of direct hernia

Medial umbilical ligaments

Transversalis fascia

Deep inguinal ring

Transversus abdominis

Internal oblique

External oblique

Inguinal ligament

Superficial inguinal ring

Rectus abdominis m.

Pyramidalis m.

Linea alba

Spermatic cord

External spermatic fascia

Cremasteric muscle and fascia

Internal spermatic fascia

(Adapted, with permission, from White JS. *USMLE Road Map: Gross Anatomy,* 1st ed. New York: McGraw-Hill, 2003:69.)

Arterial supply of stomach

Stomach receives main blood supply from branches of the celiac trunk.

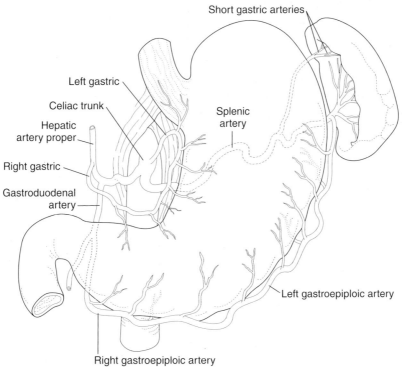

Short gastric arteries

Left gastric

Celiac trunk

Hepatic artery proper

Right gastric

Gastroduodenal artery

Splenic artery

Left gastroepiploic artery

Right gastroepiploic artery

Portal-systemic anastomoses

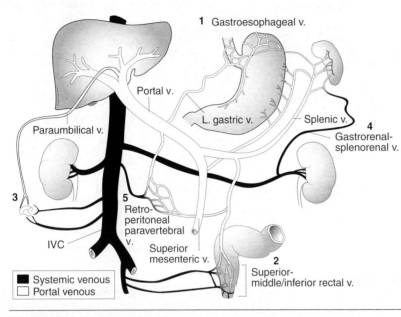

1 Gastroesophageal v.

Portal v.

Paraumbilical v.

L. gastric v.

Splenic v.

4 Gastrorenal-splenorenal v.

3

5 Retroperitoneal paravertebral v.

IVC

Superior mesenteric v.

2 Superior-middle/inferior rectal v.

■ Systemic venous
□ Portal venous

1. Left gastric–azygos → **esophageal varices**
2. Superior–middle/inferior rectal → **hemorrhoids**
3. Paraumbilical–inferior epigastric → **caput medusae** (navel)
4. Retroperitoneal → renal
5. Retroperitoneal → paravertebral

Gut, butt, and **caput,** the anastomoses 3. Commonly seen in alcoholic cirrhosis.

Lymph drainage

Right lymphatic duct | Drains right arm and right half of head.
Thoracic duct | Drains everything else.

Pectinate line

Internal hemorrhoids

External hemorrhoid | Pectinate line

Formed where hindgut meets ectoderm.

Above pectinate line—internal hemorrhoids (not painful), adenocarcinoma. **V**isceral innervation. Arterial supply is from the superior rectal artery (branch of IMA). Venous drainage is to superior rectal vein → inferior mesenteric vein → portal system.

Below pectinate line—external hemorrhoids (painful), squamous cell carcinoma. Somatic innervation. Arterial blood supply is from the inferior rectal artery (branch of internal pudendal artery). Venous drainage is to inferior rectal vein → internal pudendal vein → internal iliac vein → IVC.

Internal hemorrhoids receive visceral innervation.

External hemorrhoids receive somatic innervation and are therefore painful.

Retroperitoneal structures

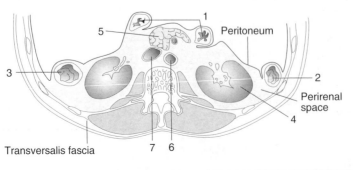

5

1 Peritoneum

3

2

Perirenal space

4

Transversalis fascia

7 6

1. Duodenum (2nd, 3rd, 4th parts)
2. Descending colon
3. Ascending colon
4. Kidney and ureters
5. Pancreas (except tail)
6. Aorta
7. IVC

Adrenal glands and rectum (not shown in diagram)

Digestive tract anatomy

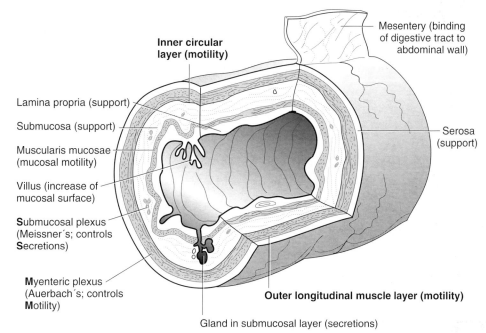

Inner circular layer (motility)

Lamina propria (support)

Submucosa (support)

Muscularis mucosae (mucosal motility)

Villus (increase of mucosal surface)

Submucosal plexus (Meissner´s; controls **S**ecretions)

Myenteric plexus (Auerbach´s; controls **M**otility)

Mesentery (binding of digestive tract to abdominal wall)

Serosa (support)

Outer longitudinal muscle layer (motility)

Gland in submucosal layer (secretions)

(Adapted, with permission, from McPhee S et al. *Pathophysiology of Disease: An Introduction to Clinical Medicine,* 3rd ed. New York: McGraw-Hill, 2000:296.)

| **Gonadal venous drainage** | Left ovary/testis → left gonadal vein → left renal vein → IVC. |
| | Right ovary/testis → right gonadal vein → IVC. |

Enteric plexuses

| **M**yenteric | Coordinates **M**otility along entire gut wall. Also known as Auerbach's plexus. Contains cell bodies of some parasympathetic terminal effector neurons. Located between inner and outer layers (longitudinal and circular) of smooth muscle in GI tract wall. |
| Submucosal | Regulates local **S**ecretions, blood flow, and absorption. Also known as Meissner's plexus. Contains cell bodies of some parasympathetic terminal effector neurons. Located between mucosa and inner layer of smooth muscle in GI tract wall. |

GI blood supply

Artery	**Gut region**	**Structures supplied**
Celiac	Foregut	Stomach to duodenum; liver, gallbladder, pancreas
SMA	Midgut	Duodenum to proximal $^2/_3$ of transverse colon
IMA	Hindgut	Distal $^1/_3$ of transverse colon to upper portion of rectum

Heart

Esophageal regions

Gastric and duodenal regions

Celiac artery

Primordium of liver

Superior mesenteric artery to midgut

Inferior mesenteric artery

Hindgut

Kidney anatomy and glomerular structure

(Adapted, with permission, from McPhee S et al. *Pathophysiology of Disease: An Introduction to Clinical Medicine*, 3rd ed. New York: McGraw-Hill, 2000:384.)

Juxtaglomerular apparatus (JGA)	JGA—JG cells (modified smooth muscle of afferent arteriole) and macula densa (Na^+ sensor, part of the distal convoluted tubule). JG cells secrete renin (leading to ↑ angiotensin II and aldosterone levels) in response to ↓ renal blood pressure, ↓ Na^+ delivery to distal tubule, and ↑ sympathetic tone. JG cells also secrete erythropoietin.	JGA defends glomerular filtration rate via the renin-angiotensin system. *Juxta* = close by.
Ureters: course	Ureters pass **under** uterine artery and **under** ductus deferens (retroperitoneal).	Water (ureters) **under** the bridge (artery, ductus deferens).

Anatomy

Ligaments of the uterus

Suspensory ligament of ovaries	Contains the ovarian vessels.
Transverse cervical (cardinal) ligament	Contains the uterine vessels.
Round ligament of uterus	Contains no important structures.
Broad ligament	Contains the round ligaments of the uterus and ovaries and the uterine tubules and vessels.

Round ligament of uterus — Suspensory ligament of ovary — Uterine tube — Fimbria — Ovary — Broad ligament — Posterior surface of uterus

Autonomic innervation of the male sexual response

Erection is mediated by the **P**arasympathetic nervous system.

Emission is mediated by the **S**ympathetic nervous system.

Ejaculation is mediated by visceral and somatic nerves.

Point and **S**hoot.

Clinically important landmarks

Pudendal nerve block—ischial spine.

Appendix—^{2}/$_3$ of the way from the umbilicus to the anterior superior iliac spine (McBurney's point).

Lumbar puncture—iliac crest.

ANATOMY—HISTOLOGY

Peripheral nerve layers

Nerve trunk — Epineurium — Perineurium — Endoneurium — Nerve fibers

Endoneurium invests single nerve fiber.

Perineurium (permeability barrier) surrounds a fascicle of nerve fibers.

Epineurium (dense connective tissue) surrounds entire nerve (fascicles and blood vessels).

Perineurium—Permeability barrier; must be rejoined in microsurgery for limb reattachment.

Endo = inner.
Peri = around.
Epi = outer.

Corpuscles

Meissner's	Small, encapsulated sensory receptors found in dermis of palm, soles, and digits of skin. Involved in light discriminatory touch of glabrous (hairless) skin.

Pacinian	Large, encapsulated sensory receptors found in deeper layers of skin at ligaments, joint capsules, serous membranes, mesenteries. Involved in pressure, coarse touch, vibration, and tension.

Inner ear

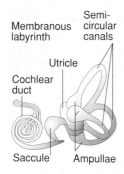

Membranous labyrinth
Semi-circular canals
Utricle
Cochlear duct
Saccule
Ampullae

The bony labyrinth is filled with perilymph (Na$^+$ rich: similar to ECF) and includes the cochlea (hearing), the vestibule (linear acceleration), and the semicircular canals (angular acceleration).

The membranous labyrinth is filled with endolymph (K$^+$ rich: similar to ICF) and contains the cochlear duct, utricle, saccule, and semicircular canals. Hair cells are the sensory elements in both the cochlear and vestibular apparatus.

The base of the cochlea picks up high-frequency sound; the apex, low frequency.

Peri—think outside of cell (Na$^+$).
Endo—think inside of cell (K$^+$).
Endolymph is made by the stria vascularis.
Utricle and saccule contain maculae—for linear acceleration.
Semicircular canals contain ampullae—for angular acceleration.
Hearing loss in the elderly—high frequency → low frequency.

Collagen types

Collagen is the most abundant protein in the human body. Functions to organize and strengthen extracellular matrix.

Type I (90%)—bone, tendon, skin, dentin, fascia, cornea, late wound repair.

Type II—cartilage (including hyaline), vitreous body, nucleus pulposus.

Type III (reticulin)—skin, blood vessels, uterus, fetal tissue, granulation tissue.

Type IV—basement membrane or basal lamina.

Type X—epiphyseal plate.

Type **I**: BONE.

Type **II**: car**TWO**lage.

Type **IV**: Under the **floor** (basement membrane).

Epidermis layers

From surface to base: stratum Corneum, stratum Lucidum, stratum Granulosum, stratum Spinosum, stratum Basalis.

Californians **L**ike **G**irls in **S**tring **B**ikinis.

Epidermis
Dermis

Stratum corneum
Stratum lucidum
Stratum granulosum
Stratum spinosum
Stratum basalis

Epithelial cell junctions

Zona occludens (tight junction)—prevents diffusion across intracellular space

E-cadherin

Actin filaments

Zona adherens (intermediate junction)—surrounds perimeter just below zona occludens

Keratin

Macula adherens (desmosome)—small, discrete sites of attachment

Desmoplakin

Connection with central channel

Gap junction—allows adjacent cells to communicate for electric and metabolic functions

Integrin

Hemidesmosome—connects cells to underlying extracellular matrix

Glomerular basement membrane	Formed from fused endothelial and podocyte basement membranes and coated with negatively charged heparan sulfate. Responsible for actual filtration of plasma according to net charge and size.	In **N**ephrotic syndrome, **N**egative charge is lost (and plasma protein is lost in urine as a consequence).
Cilia structure	9 + 2 arrangement of microtubules. Dynein is an ATPase that links peripheral 9 doublets and causes bending of cilium by differential sliding of doublets.	Kartagener's syndrome is due to a dynein arm defect, resulting in immotile cilia.

Microtubule doublets

Dynein ATPase

Nissl bodies	Nissl bodies (in neurons)—rough ER; not found in axon or axon hillock. Synthesize enzymes (e.g., ChAT) and peptide neurotransmitters.

Functions of Golgi apparatus

1. Distribution center of proteins and lipids from ER to the plasma membrane, lysosomes, and secretory vesicles
2. Modifies N-oligosaccharides on asparagine
3. Adds O-oligosaccharides to serine and threonine residues
4. Proteoglycan assembly from proteoglycan core proteins
5. Sulfation of sugars in proteoglycans and of selected tyrosine on proteins
6. Addition of mannose-6-phosphate to specific lysosomal proteins, which targets the protein to the lysosome

I-cell disease is caused by the failure of addition of mannose-6-phosphate to lysosome proteins, causing these enzymes to be secreted outside the cell instead of being targeted to the lysosome.

(Adapted, with permission, from Junqueira L., Carneiro J. *Basic Histology*, 10th ed., New York: McGraw-Hill, 2003.)

Rough endoplasmic reticulum (RER)	RER is the site of synthesis of secretory (exported) proteins and of N-linked oligosaccharide addition to many proteins.	Mucus-secreting goblet cells of the small intestine and antibody-secreting plasma cells are rich in RER.
Smooth endoplasmic reticulum (SER)	SER is the site of steroid synthesis and detoxification of drugs and poisons.	Liver hepatocytes and steroid hormone–producing cells of the adrenal cortex are rich in SER.
Sinusoids of liver	Irregular "capillaries" with round pores 100–200 nm in diameter. No basement membrane. Allows macromolecules of plasma full access to surface of liver cells through space of Disse.	

Sinusoids of spleen

Long, vascular channels in red pulp with fenestrated "barrel hoop" basement membrane. Macrophages found nearby.

T cells are found in the periarterial lymphatic sheath (PALS) and in the red pulp of the spleen. B cells are found in follicles within the white pulp of the spleen.

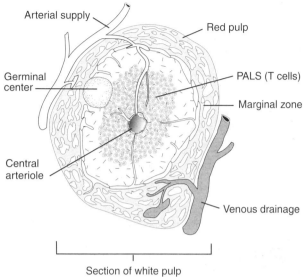

(Adapted, with permission, from Janeway CA, Travers P, Walport M, Capra JD. *Immunobiology: The Immune System in Health and Disease,* 4th ed. New York: Garland, 1999.)

Pancreas endocrine cell types

Islets of Langerhans are collections of endocrine cells (most numerous in tail of pancreas). α = glucagon; β = insulin; δ = somatostatin. Islets arise from pancreatic buds.

Adrenal cortex and medulla

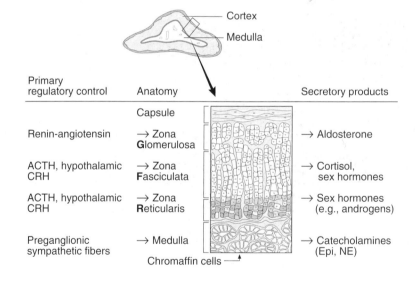

Primary regulatory control	Anatomy	Secretory products
	Capsule	
Renin-angiotensin	→ Zona **G**lomerulosa	→ Aldosterone
ACTH, hypothalamic CRH	→ Zona **F**asciculata	→ Cortisol, sex hormones
ACTH, hypothalamic CRH	→ Zona **R**eticularis	→ Sex hormones (e.g., androgens)
Preganglionic sympathetic fibers	→ Medulla	→ Catecholamines (Epi, NE)

Chromaffin cells →

GFR corresponds with **s**alt (Na⁺), **s**ugar (glucocorticoids), and **s**ex (androgens).

"The deeper you go, the sweeter it gets."

Pheochromocytoma—most common tumor of the adrenal medulla in adults.

Neuroblastoma—most common in children.

Pheochromocytoma causes episodic hypertension; neuroblastoma does not.

Brunner's glands

Secrete alkaline mucus. Located in submucosa of duodenum (the only GI submucosal glands). Duodenal ulcers cause hypertrophy of Brunner's glands.

Lymph node
A 2° lymphoid organ that has many afferents, 1 or more efferents. Encapsulated, with trabeculae. Functions are nonspecific filtration by macrophages, storage/proliferation of B and T cells, antibody production.

Follicle
Site of B-cell localization and proliferation. In outer cortex. 1° follicles are dense and dormant. 2° follicles have pale central germinal centers and are active.

Labels: Subcapsular sinus; Capsule; Capillary supply; Postcapillary (high endothelial) venules; Afferent lymphatic; Medullary sinus (macrophages); Medullary cords (plasma cells); Trabecula; Efferent lymphatic; Artery; Vein; Follicle of cortex (B cells); Paracortex (T cells)

Medulla
Consists of medullary cords (closely packed lymphocytes and plasma cells) and medullary sinuses. Medullary sinuses communicate with efferent lymphatics and contain reticular cells and macrophages.

Paracortex
Houses T cells. Region of cortex between follicles and medulla. Contains high endothelial venules through which T and B cells enter from blood. In an extreme cellular immune response, paracortex becomes greatly enlarged. Not well developed in patients with DiGeorge syndrome.

Paracortex enlarges in an extreme cellular immune response (i.e., viral).

Peyer's patch
Unencapsulated lymphoid tissue found in lamina propria and submucosa of small intestine. Covered by single layer of cuboidal enterocytes (no goblet cells) with specialized M cells interspersed. M cells take up antigen. Stimulated B cells leave Peyer's patch and travel through lymph and blood to lamina propria of intestine, where they differentiate to IgA-secreting plasma cells. IgA receives protective secretory component and is then transported across epithelium to gut to deal with intraluminal antigen.

Think of **IgA,** the **I**ntra-gut **A**ntibody. And always say "secretory IgA."

Lumbar puncture

Cauda equina
Spinous process
L3
L4
L4/5 disk
L5
Needle in subarachnoid space

CSF obtained from lumbar subarachnoid space between L4 and L5 (at the level of iliac crests). Structures pierced as follows:

1. Skin/superficial fascia
2. Ligaments (supraspinous, interspinous, ligamentum flavum)
3. Epidural space
4. Dura mater
5. Subdural space
6. Arachnoid
7. Subarachnoid space—CSF

Pia is not **pier**ced.

Lower extremity nerve injury

Nerve	Deficit in motion	
Common peroneal (L4–S2)	Loss of dorsiflexion (→ foot drop)	**PED** = **P**eroneal **E**verts and **D**orsiflexes.
Tibial (L4–S3)	Loss of plantar flexion	**TIP** = **T**ibial **I**nverts and **P**lantarflexes; if injured, can't stand on **TIP**toes.
Femoral (L2–L4)	Loss of knee jerk	
Obturator (L2–L4)	Loss of hip adduction	

Spinal cord lower extent

In adults, spinal cord extends to lower border of L1–L2; subarachnoid space extends to lower border of S2. Lumbar puncture is usually performed in L3–L4 or L4–L5 interspaces, at level of cauda equina.

To keep the cord alive, keep the spinal needle between L3 and L5.

Spinal nerves

There are 31 spinal nerves altogether: 8 cervical, 12 thoracic, 5 lumbar, 5 sacral, 1 coccygeal.

31, just like 31 flavors! Vertebral disk herniation usually occurs between L5 and S1.

HIGH-YIELD FACTS

Anatomy

CNS/PNS supportive cells

Astrocytes—physical support, repair, K⁺ metabolism.
Microglia—phagocytosis.
Oligodendroglia—central myelin production.
Schwann cells—peripheral myelin production.
Ependymal cells—inner lining of ventricles.

Astrocyte

Oligodendrocyte

Blood-brain barrier

Formed by 3 structures:
1. Choroid plexus epithelium
2. Intracerebral capillary endothelium
3. Arachnoid

Glucose and amino acids cross by carrier-mediated transport mechanism.

Nonpolar/lipid-soluble substances cross more readily than do polar/water-soluble ones.

L-dopa, rather than dopamine, is used to treat parkinsonism because dopamine does not cross the blood-brain barrier.

Blood-brain barrier guarded by **CIA.**

Other barriers include:
1. Blood-gas barrier
2. Blood-testis barrier

Hypothalamus: functions

Thirst and water balance (supraoptic nucleus).
Adenohypophysis control via releasing factors.
Neurohypophysis releases hormones synthesized in hypothalamic nuclei.
Hunger (lateral nucleus) and satiety (ventromedial nucleus).
Autonomic regulation (anterior hypothalamus regulates parasympathetic activity), circadian rhythms (suprachiasmatic nucleus).
Temperature regulation (posterior hypothalamus regulates heat conservation and production when cold; Anterior hypothalamus coordinates Cooling when hot).
Sexual urges and emotions (Septate nucleus).

The hypothalamus wears **TAN HATS.**

If you zap your **ventromedial** nucleus, you grow **vent**rally and **medial**ly (hyperphagia and obesity).

If you zap your **P**osterior hypothalamus, you become a **P**oikilotherm (cold-blooded snake).

A/C = anterior cooling.

Posterior pituitary (neurohypophysis)	Receives hypothalamic axonal projections from supraoptic (ADH) and paraventricular (oxytocin) nuclei.	Oxytocin: *oxys* = quick; *tocos* = birth.

Functions of thalamic nuclei	Lateral geniculate nucleus (LGN)—visual.
	Medial geniculate nucleus (MGN)—auditory.
	Ventral posterior nucleus, lateral part (VPL)
	  —body senses (proprioception, pressure, pain, touch vibration).
	Ventral posterior nucleus, medial part (VPM)
	  —facial sensation, including pain.
	Ventral anterior/lateral (VA/VL) nuclei
	  —motor.
		Lateral to **L**ook.
		Medial for **M**usic.

Limbic system: functions

Responsible for **F**eeding, **F**ighting, **F**eeling, **F**light, and sex.

The famous **5 F's.**

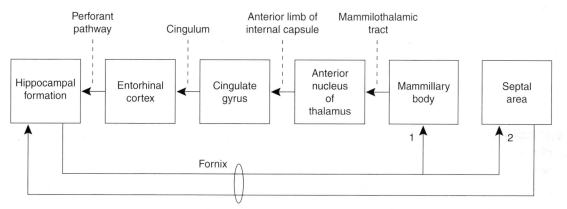

The hippocampus projects to:
1. Subiculum (projecting to mammillary nuclei)
2. Septal area

HIGH-YIELD FACTS

Anatomy

Basal ganglia

Important in voluntary movements and making postural adjustments.

(Adapted, with permission, from Kandel ER, Schwartz JH, Jessell TM. *Principles of Neural Science,* 4th ed. Stamford, CT: Appleton & Lange, 2000:860.)

Chorea	Sudden, jerky, purposeless movements. Characteristic of basal ganglia lesion (e.g., Huntington's disease).	*Chorea* = dancing (Greek). Think choral dancing or choreography.
Athetosis	Slow, writhing movements, especially of fingers. Characteristic of basal ganglia lesion.	*Athetos* = not fixed (Greek). Think snakelike.
Hemiballismus	Sudden, wild flailing of 1 arm. Characteristic of contralateral subthalamic nucleus lesion.	Half ballistic (as in throwing a baseball).

Cerebral cortex functions

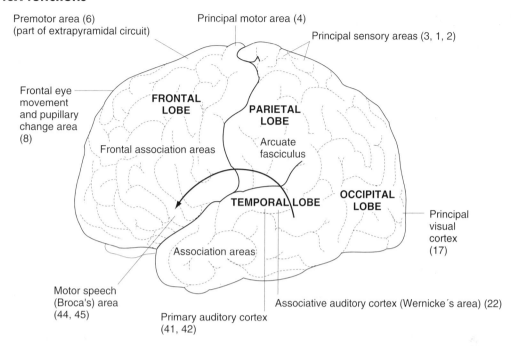

Premotor area (6)
(part of extrapyramidal circuit)

Principal motor area (4)

Principal sensory areas (3, 1, 2)

Frontal eye movement and pupillary change area (8)

FRONTAL LOBE

PARIETAL LOBE

Arcuate fasciculus

Frontal association areas

TEMPORAL LOBE

OCCIPITAL LOBE

Association areas

Principal visual cortex (17)

Motor speech (Broca's) area (44, 45)

Primary auditory cortex (41, 42)

Associative auditory cortex (Wernicke's area) (22)

Brain lesions

Area of lesion	Consequence	
Broca's area	Motor (expressive) aphasia with good comprehension	**BRO**ca's is **BRO**ken speech. Wernicke's is **W**ordy but makes no sense.
Wernicke's area	Sensory (fluent/receptive) aphasia with poor comprehension	
Arcuate fasciculus	Conduction aphasia; poor repetition with good comprehension, fluent speech.	Connects Wernicke's to Broca's area.
Amygdala (bilateral)	Klüver-Bucy syndrome (hyperorality, hypersexuality, disinhibited behavior)	
Frontal lobe	Frontal release signs (e.g., personality changes and deficits in concentration, orientation, judgment)	
Right parietal lobe	Spatial neglect syndrome (agnosia of the contralateral side of the world)	
Reticular activating system	Coma	
Mammillary bodies (bilateral)	Wernicke-Korsakoff's encephalopathy (confabulations, anterograde amnesia)	
Basal ganglia	Tremor at rest	
Cerebellar hemisphere	Intention tremor, limb ataxia	
Cerebellar vermis	Truncal ataxia and dysarthria	

Cavernous sinus

CN III, IV, V_1, V_2, and VI and postganglionic sympathetic fibers en route to the orbit all pass through the cavernous sinus. Only CN VI is "free-floating." Cavernous portion of internal carotid artery is also here.

The nerves that control extraocular muscles (plus V_1 and V_2) pass through the cavernous sinus.

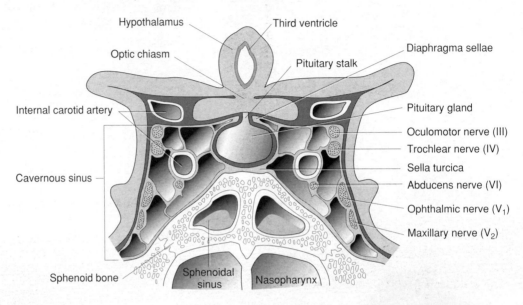

(Adapted, with permission, from Stobo J et al. *The Principles and Practice of Medicine*, 23rd ed. Stamford, CT: Appleton & Lange, 1996:277.)

Foramina: middle cranial fossa (CN II–VI)

1. Optic canal (CN II, ophthalmic artery, central retinal vein)
2. Superior orbital fissure (CN III, IV, V_1, VI, ophthalmic vein)
3. Foramen **R**otundum (CN V_2)
4. Foramen **O**vale (CN V_3)
5. Foramen spinosum (middle meningeal artery)

All structures pass through sphenoid bone. Divisions of CN V exit owing to **S**tanding **R**oom **O**nly (**S**uperior orbital fissure, foramen **R**otundum, foramen **O**vale).

Foramina: posterior cranial fossa (CN VII–XII)

1. Internal auditory meatus (CN VII, VIII)
2. Jugular foramen (CN IX, X, XI, jugular vein)
3. Hypoglossal canal (CN XII)
4. Foramen magnum (spinal roots of CN XI, brain stem, vertebral arteries)

All structures pass through temporal or occipital bones.

Extraocular muscles and nerves

(Note: inferior oblique not in plane of diagram)

Lateral **R**ectus is CN VI, Superior **O**blique is CN IV, the **R**est are CN III.
The "chemical formula" $LR_6SO_4R_3$.
The superior oblique abducts, introverts, depresses.

**Pupillary
light reflex**

Light in either retina sends a signal to pretectal nuclei (dashed lines) in midbrain that activate bilateral Edinger-Westphal nuclei; pupils contract bilaterally (consensual reflex). Note that the illumination of 1 eye results in bilateral pupillary constriction.

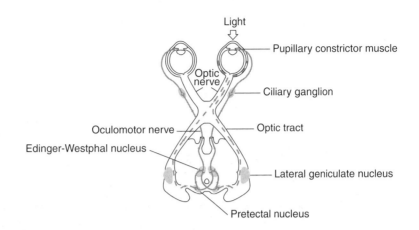

(Adapted, with permission, from Simon RP et al. *Clinical Neurology*, 3rd ed. Stamford, CT: Appleton & Lange, 1996.)

**Internuclear
ophthalmoplegia**

Lesion in the medial longitudinal fasciculus (MLF). Results in medial rectus palsy on attempted lateral gaze. Nystagmus in abducting eye. Convergence is normal. MLF syndrome is seen in many patients with multiple sclerosis.

MLF = MS.

When looking left, the nucleus of CN VI fires, which contracts the left lateral rectus and stimulates the contralateral nucleus of CN III via the MLF to contract the medial rectus.

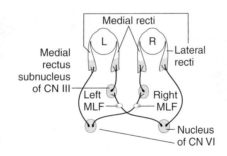

Visual field defects

1. Right anopsia
2. Bitemporal hemianopsia
3. Left homonymous hemianopsia
4. Left upper quadrantic anopsia (right temporal lesion)
5. Left lower quadrantic anopsia (right parietal lesion)
6. Left hemianopsia with macular sparing

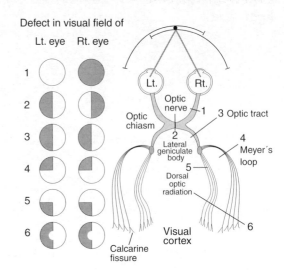

Defect in visual field of

Lt. eye   Rt. eye

Optic nerve — 1
Optic chiasm
2
Lateral geniculate body
Dorsal optic radiation
5
3 Optic tract
4 Meyer's loop
6
Visual cortex
Calcarine fissure

Cranial nerves

Nerve	CN	Function	Type	Mnemonic
Olfactory	I	Smell	Sensory	Some
Optic	II	Sight	Sensory	Say
Oculomotor	III	Eye movement, pupil constriction, accommodation, eyelid opening	Motor	Marry
Trochlear	IV	Eye movement	Motor	Money
Trigeminal	V	Mastication, facial sensation	Both	But
Abducens	VI	Eye movement	Motor	My
Facial	VII	Facial movement, anterior $2/3$ taste, lacrimation, salivation (submaxillary and submandibular salivary glands)	Both	Brother
Vestibulocochlear	VIII	Hearing, balance	Sensory	Says
Glossopharyngeal	IX	Posterior $1/3$ taste, swallowing, salivation (parotid gland), monitoring carotid body and sinus	Both	Big
Vagus	X	Taste, swallowing, palate elevation, talking, thoracoabdominal viscera	Both	Brains
Accessory	XI	Head turning, shoulder shrugging	Motor	Matter
Hypoglossal	XII	Tongue movements	Motor	Most

Cranial nerves and passageways

Cribriform plate	I
Optic canal	II
Superior orbital fissure	III, IV, V_1, VI
Foramen rotundum	V_2
Foramen ovale	V_3
Internal auditory meatus	VII, VIII
Jugular foramen	IX, X, XI
Hypoglossal canal	XII

Brain stem anatomy

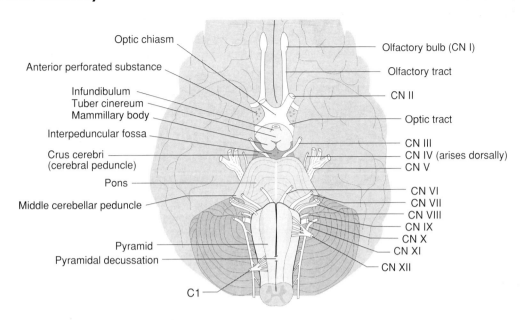

Optic chiasm

Anterior perforated substance

Infundibulum
Tuber cinereum
Mammillary body

Interpeduncular fossa

Crus cerebri
(cerebral peduncle)

Pons

Middle cerebellar peduncle

Pyramid
Pyramidal decussation

C1

Olfactory bulb (CN I)

Olfactory tract

CN II

Optic tract

CN III
CN IV (arises dorsally)
CN V

CN VI
CN VII
CN VIII
CN IX
CN X
CN XI
CN XII

CNs that lie medially at brain stem: III, VI, XII. 3(×2) = 6(×2) = 12.

Dural venous sinuses

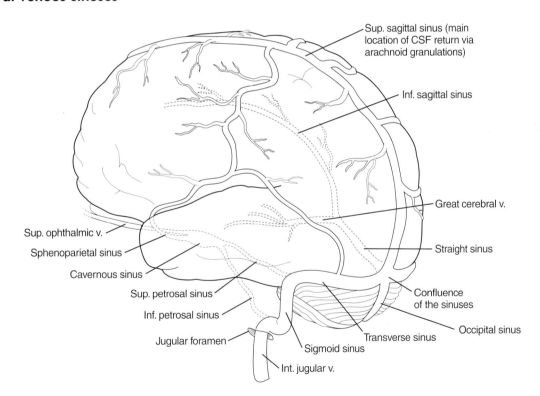

Sup. sagittal sinus (main
location of CSF return via
arachnoid granulations)

Inf. sagittal sinus

Great cerebral v.

Straight sinus

Confluence
of the sinuses

Occipital sinus

Sup. ophthalmic v.

Sphenoparietal sinus

Cavernous sinus

Sup. petrosal sinus

Inf. petrosal sinus

Jugular foramen

Transverse sinus

Sigmoid sinus

Int. jugular v.

(Adapted, with permission, from White JS. *USMLE Road Map: Gross Anatomy*, 1st ed. New York: McGraw-Hill, 2003.)

Homunculus

Topographical representation of sensory and motor areas in the cerebral cortex. Use to localize lesion (e.g., in blood supply) leading to specific defects.

For example, lower extremity deficit in sensation or movement indicates involvement of the anterior cerebral artery (see following entry).

Lateral fissure

Circle of Willis

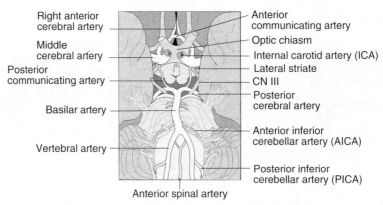

Right anterior cerebral artery
Middle cerebral artery
Posterior communicating artery
Basilar artery
Vertebral artery
Anterior spinal artery

Anterior communicating artery
Optic chiasm
Internal carotid artery (ICA)
Lateral striate
CN III
Posterior cerebral artery
Anterior inferior cerebellar artery (AICA)
Posterior inferior cerebellar artery (PICA)

Anterior cerebral artery—supplies medial surface of the brain, leg-foot area of motor and sensory cortices.

Middle cerebral artery—supplies lateral aspect of brain, Broca's and Wernicke's speech areas.

Anterior communicating artery—most common circle of Willis aneurysm; may cause visual-field defects.

Posterior communicating artery—common area of aneurysm; causes CN III palsy.

Lateral striate—"arteries of stroke"; supply internal capsule, caudate, putamen, globus pallidus.

In general, stroke of anterior circle → general sensory and motor dysfunction, aphasia; stroke of posterior circle → cranial nerve deficits (vertigo, visual deficits), coma, cerebellar deficits (ataxia).

KLM sounds: kuh, la, mi

Kuh-kuh-kuh tests palate elevation (CN X—vagus). Say it aloud.
La-la-la tests tongue (CN XII—hypoglossal).
Mi-mi-mi tests lips (CN VII—facial).

Vagal nuclei

Nucleus Solitarius	Visceral Sensory information (e.g., taste, gut distention, etc.).	VII, IX, **X.**
Nucleus aMbiguus	**M**otor innervation of pharynx, larynx, and upper esophagus.	IX, **X**, XI.
Dorsal motor nucleus	Sends autonomic (parasympathetic) fibers to heart, lungs, and upper GI.	

Lesions and deviations

CN XII lesion (LMN)—tongue deviates **toward** side of lesion (lick your wounds).

CN V motor lesion—jaw deviates **toward** side of lesion.

Unilateral lesion of cerebellum—patient tends to fall **toward** side of lesion.

CN X lesion—uvula deviates **away** from side of lesion.

CN XI lesion—weakness turning head to contralateral side of lesion. Shoulder droop on side of lesion.

Herniation syndromes

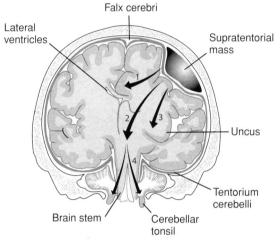

1. Cingulate herniation under falx cerebri
2. Downward transtentorial (central) herniation
3. Uncal herniation
4. Cerebellar tonsillar herniation into the foramen magnum

} Coma and death result when these herniations compress the brain stem

(Adapted, with permission, from Simon RP et al. *Clinical Neurology*, 4th ed. Stamford, CT: Appleton & Lange, 1999:314.)

Uncal herniation

Clinical signs	Cause
Ipsilateral dilated pupil/ptosis	Stretching of CN III
Contralateral homonymous hemianopsia	Compression of ipsilateral posterior cerebral artery
Ipsilateral paresis	Compression of contralateral crus cerebri (Kernohan's notch)
Duret hemorrhages— paramedian artery rupture	Caudal displacement of brain stem

Spinal cord and associated tracts

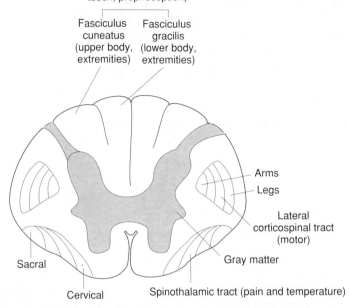

Dorsal columns
(pressure, vibration,
touch, proprioception)

Fasciculus
cuneatus
(upper body,
extremities)

Fasciculus
gracilis
(lower body,
extremities)

Arms

Legs

Lateral
corticospinal tract
(motor)

Gray matter

Sacral

Cervical

Spinothalamic tract (pain and temperature)

Spinal cord lesions

Poliomyelitis/Werdnig-Hoffmann disease: lower motor neuron lesions only, flaccid paralysis

Multiple sclerosis: mostly white matter of cervical region; random and asymmetric lesions

ALS: combined upper and lower motor neuron deficits with no sensory deficit

Complete occlusion of ventral artery; spares dorsal columns

Tabes dorsalis: impaired proprioception and locomotor ataxia resulting from tertiary syphilis

Syringomyelia: ventral white commissure and ventral horns

Vitamin B$_{12}$ neuropathy/Friedreich's ataxia: dorsal columns, lateral corticospinal tracts and spinocerebellar tracts

Dorsal column organization

In dorsal columns, lower limbs are inside to avoid crossing the upper limbs on the outside.

Fasciculus gracilis = legs.

Fasciculus cuneatus = arms.

Dorsal column is organized as you are, with hands at sides—arms outside and legs inside.

Brown-Séquard syndrome	Hemisection of spinal cord. Findings below the lesion:	
 Lesion	1. Ipsilateral motor paralysis and spasticity (pyramidal tract)—not shown 2. Ipsilateral loss of tactile, vibration, proprioception sense (dorsal column) 3. Contralateral pain and temperature loss (spinothalamic tract) 4. Ipsilateral loss of all sensation at level of lesion If lesion occurs above T1, presents with Horner's syndrome.	

Lower motor neuron (LMN) signs	LMN injury signs—atrophy, flaccid paralysis, absent DTRs. Fasciculations may be present.	**Lower** MN ≈ everything lowered (less muscle mass, ↓ muscle tone, ↓ reflexes, downgoing toes).

Upper motor neuron (UMN) signs	UMN injury signs—minor atrophy, spastic paralysis (clonus), hyperactive DTRs, possible positive Babinski.	**Upper** MN ≈ everything **up** (tone, DTRs, toes).

Facial lesions

Central facial	Paralysis of the contralateral lower quadrant.	**AL**exander **Bell** with **STD:**
Bell's palsy	Peripheral ipsilateral facial paralysis with inability to close eye on involved side. Can occur idiopathically. Seen as a complication in **A**IDS, **L**yme disease, **S**arcoidosis, **T**umors, **D**iabetes. Complete destruction of the facial nucleus itself or its branchial efferent fibers (facial nerve proper) paralyzes all ipsilateral facial muscles.	**A**IDS, **L**yme, **S**arcoid, **T**umors, **D**iabetes.
UMN lesion	Lesion to internal capsule causes contralateral weakness of lower face only.	
LMN lesion	Upper and lower lesion paralysis with weakness of upper and lower face.	

Spindle muscle control

Reflex arc

Muscle stretch → intrafusal stretch → stimulates Ia afferent→ stimulates α motor neuron → reflex extrafusal contraction.

Gamma loop

CNS stimulates γ motor neuron → contracts intrafusal fiber → increased sensitivity of reflex arc.

Brachial plexus

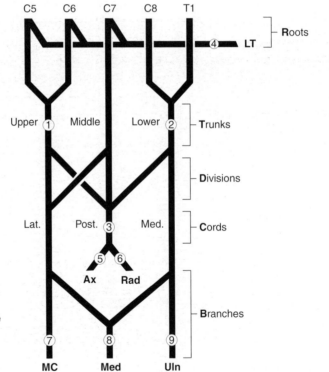

Randy
Travis
Drinks
Cold
Beer.

1. Waiter's tip
2. Claw hand
3. Wrist drop
4. Winged scapula
5. Deltoid paralysis
6. Saturday night palsy
7. Difficulty flexing elbow, variable sensory loss
8. Decreased thumb function, Pope's blessing
9. Intrinsic muscles of hand, claw hand

Rad = radial nerve
Ax = axillary nerve
LT = long thoracic nerve
MC = musculocutaneous nerve
Med = median nerve
Uln = ulnar nerve

HIGH-YIELD FACTS

Anatomy

Upper limb nerve injury

Nerve	Injury/deficit in motion	Deficit in sensation
Radial	Shaft of humerus—loss of triceps brachii (triceps reflex), brachioradialis (brachioradialis reflex), and extensor carpi radialis longus ($\rightarrow$ wrist drop); often 2° to humerus fracture.	Posterior brachial cutaneous. Posterior antebrachial cutaneous. Passes through supinator.
Median	Supracondyle of humerus—no loss of power in any of the arm muscles; loss of forearm pronation, wrist flexion, finger flexion, and several thumb movements; eventually, thenar atrophy.	Loss of sensation over the lateral palm and thumb and the radial $2^1/_2$ fingers. Passes through pronator teres.
Ulnar	Medial epicondyle—impaired wrist flexion and adduction, and impaired adduction of thumb and the ulnar 2 fingers.	Loss of sensation over the medial palm and ulnar $1^1/_2$ fingers. Passes through flexor carpi ulnaris.
Axillary	Surgical neck of humerus or anterior shoulder dislocation—loss of deltoid action.	
Musculocutaneous	Loss of function of coracobrachialis, biceps, and brachialis muscles (biceps reflex).	Passes through coracobrachialis.

Erb-Duchenne palsy

Traction or tear of the superior trunk of the brachial plexus (C5 and C6 roots); follows blow to shoulder or trauma during delivery.

Findings: limb hangs by side (paralysis of abductors), medially rotated (paralysis of lateral rotators), forearm is pronated (loss of biceps).

"Waiter's tip" owing to appearance of arm.

Radial nerve

Known as the "great extensor nerve." Provides innervation of the **B**rachioradialis, **E**xtensors of the wrist and fingers, **S**upinator, and **T**riceps.

Radial nerve innervates the **BEST!**

To **SUP**inate is to move as if carrying a bowl of **SOUP**.

Thoracic outlet syndrome (Klumpke's palsy)

An embryologic defect; can compress subclavian artery and inferior trunk of brachial plexus (C8, T1), resulting in thoracic outlet syndrome:
1. Atrophy of the thenar and hypothenar eminences
2. Atrophy of the interosseous muscles
3. Sensory deficits on the medial side of the forearm and hand
4. Disappearance of the radial pulse upon moving the head toward the opposite side

Clinical reflexes

Biceps = C5 nerve root.

Triceps = C7 nerve root.

Patella = L4 nerve root.

Achilles = S1 nerve root.

Babinski—dorsiflexion of the big toe and fanning of other toes; sign of UMN lesion, but normal reflex in 1st year of life (UMN loss).

Behavioral Science

"It's psychosomatic. You need a lobotomy. I'll get a saw."
—Calvin, "Calvin & Hobbes"

A heterogeneous mix of epidemiology/biostatistics, psychiatry, psychology, sociology, psychopharmacology, and more falls under this heading. Many medical students do not study this discipline diligently because the material is felt to be "easy" or "common sense." In our opinion, this is a missed opportunity. Each question gained in behavioral science is equal to a question in any other section in determining the overall score.

Many students feel that some behavioral science questions are less concrete and require an awareness of the social aspects of medicine. For example: If a patient does or says something, what should you do or say in response? These so-called quote questions now constitute much of the behavioral science section. We have included several examples in the high-yield clinical vignettes. Medical ethics and medical law are also appearing with increasing frequency. In addition, the key aspects of the doctor-patient relationship (e.g., communication skills, open-ended questions, facilitation, silence) are high yield. Basic biostatistics and epidemiology are very learnable and high yield. Be able to apply biostatistical concepts such as specificity and predictive values in a problem-solving format. Also review the clinical presentation of personality disorders.

These abstracted case vignettes are designed to demonstrate the thought processes necessary to answer multistep clinical reasoning questions.

Vignette	Question	Answer
■ Woman with anxiety about a gynecologic exam is told to relax and to imagine going through the steps of the exam.	What process does this exemplify?	Systematic desensitization.
■ 65-year-old man is diagnosed with incurable metastatic pancreatic adenocarcinoma. His family asks you, the doctor, not to tell the patient.	What do you do?	Assess whether telling patient will negatively affect his health. If not, tell him.
■ Man admitted for chest pain is medicated for ventricular tachycardia. The next day he jumps out of bed and does 50 pushups to show the nurses he has not had a heart attack.	What defense mechanism is he using?	Denial.
■ You find yourself attracted to your 26-year-old patient.	What do you say?	Nothing! The tone of the interview must be very professional; it is not acceptable to have any sort of romantic relationship with patients. If you feel your actions may be misinterpreted, invite a chaperone into the room.
■ Large group of people is followed over 10 years. Every 2 years, it is determined who develops heart disease and who does not.	What type of study is this?	Cohort study.
■ Girl can groom herself, can hop on 1 foot, and has an imaginary friend.	How old is she?	Four years old.
■ Man has flashbacks about his girlfriend's death 2 months ago following a hit-and-run accident. He often cries and wishes for the death of the culprit.	What is the diagnosis?	Normal bereavement.
■ 36-year-old woman with a strong family history of breast cancer refuses a mammogram because she heard it hurts.	What do you do?	Discuss the risks and benefits of not having a mammogram. Each patient must give their own informed consent to each procedure; if the patient refuses, you must abide by their wishes.

Vignette	Question	Answer
During a particular stage of sleep, man has variable blood pressure, penile tumescence, and variable EEG.	What stage of sleep is he in?	REM sleep.
15-year-old girl of normal height and weight for her age has enlarged parotid glands but no other complaints. The mother confides that she found laxatives in the daughter's closet.	What is the diagnosis?	Bulimia.
11-year-old girl exhibits Tanner stage 4 sexual development (almost full breasts and pubic hair).	What is the diagnosis?	Advanced stage, early development.
4-year-old girl complains of a burning feeling in her genitalia; otherwise she behaves and sleeps normally. Smear of discharge shows *N. gonorrhoeae*.	How was she infected?	Sexual abuse.
72-year-old man insists on stopping treatment for his heart condition because it makes him feel "funny."	What do you do?	Although you want to encourage the patient to take his medication, the patient has the final say in his own treatment regimen. You should investigate the "funny" feeling and determine if there are drugs available that don't elicit this particular side effect.
Person demands only the best and most famous doctor in town.	What is the personality disorder?	Narcissism.
Nurse has episodes of hypoglycemia; blood analysis reveals no elevation in C protein.	What is the diagnosis?	Factitious disorder; self-scripted insulin.
55-year-old businessman complains of lack of successful sexual contacts with women and lack of ability to reach a full erection. Two years ago he had a heart attack.	What might be the cause of his problem?	Fear of sudden death during intercourse.

Prevalence vs. incidence

Prevalence is the total number of cases in a population at a given time.

Incidence is the number of new cases in a population per unit time.

Prevalence ≅ incidence × disease duration.

Prevalence > incidence for chronic diseases (e.g., diabetes).

Prevalence = incidence for acute disease (e.g., common cold).

Incidence is new **incidents.**

Sensitivity

Number of true positives divided by number of all people with the disease.

False negative ratio is equal to 1 − sensitivity.

High sensitivity is desirable for a screening test.

PID = **P**ositive **I**n **D**isease (note that PID is a **sensitive** topic).

SNOUT = **S**e**N**sitivity rules **OUT.**

Specificity

Number of true negatives divided by number of all people without the disease.

False positive ratio is equal to 1 − specificity.

High specificity is desirable for a confirmatory test.

NIH = **N**egative **I**n **H**ealth.
SPIN = **SP**ecificity rules **IN.**

Predictive value

Positive predictive value (PPV)

Number of true positives divided by number of people who tested positive for the disease.

The probability of having a condition, given a positive test.

Negative predictive value (NPV)

Number of true negatives divided by number of people who tested negative for the disease.

The probability of not having the condition, given a negative test.

Unlike sensitivity and specificity, predictive values are dependent on the prevalence of the disease.

The higher the prevalence of a disease, the higher the positive predictive value of the test.

Disease

		⊕	⊖
Test	⊕	a	b
	⊖	c	d

$$\text{Sensitivity} = \frac{a}{a+c}$$

$$\text{Specificity} = \frac{d}{b+d}$$

$$\text{PPV} = \frac{a}{a+b}$$

$$\text{NPV} = \frac{d}{c+d}$$

Odds ratio and relative risk

Odds ratio (OR)

Approximates the relative risk if the prevalence of the disease is not too high. Used for case-control (retrospective) studies.

OR = ad/bc

Relative risk (RR)

Disease risk in exposed group/disease risk in unexposed group. Used for cohort studies.

Disease

		⊕	⊖
Exposure	⊕	a	b
	⊖	c	d

$$RR = \frac{\left[\frac{a}{a+b}\right]}{\left[\frac{c}{c+d}\right]} \qquad \text{Attributable risk} = \left[\frac{a}{a+b}\right] - \left[\frac{c}{c+d}\right]$$

If the 95% confidence interval for OR or RR includes 1, the study is inconclusive.

| **Standard deviation vs. error** | n = sample size
σ = standard deviation
SEM = standard error of the mean
SEM = σ/√n
Therefore, SEM < σ and SEM decreases as n increases. | Normal (Gaussian) distribution:
 |

Statistical distribution

Terms that describe statistical distributions:

Normal ≈ Gaussian ≈ bell-shaped (mean = median = mode).

Bimodal is simply 2 humps.

Positive skew is asymmetry with tail on the right (mean > median > mode).

Negative skew has tail on the left (mean < median < mode).

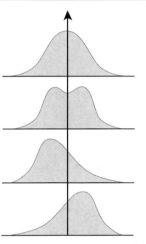

Precision vs. accuracy

Precision is:
1. The consistency and reproducibility of a test (reliability)
2. The absence of random variation in a test

Accuracy is the trueness of test measurements.

Random error—reduced precision in a test.
Systematic error—reduced accuracy in a test.

| Accuracy | Precision | Accuracy and precision | No accuracy, no precision |

Reliability and validity

Reliability—Reproducibility (dependability) of a test.
Validity—whether the test truly measures what it purports to measure. Appropriateness of a test.

Test is reliable if repeat measurements are the same.
Test is valid if it measures what it is supposed to measure.

Correlation coefficient (r)

r is always between −1 and 1. Absolute value indicates strength of correlation between 2 variables.
Coefficient of determination = r^2.

t-test vs. ANOVA vs. χ^2	t-test checks difference between the means of 2 groups. ANOVA checks difference between the means of 3 or more groups. χ^2 checks difference between 2 or more percentages or proportions of categorical outcomes (not mean values).	Mr. **T** is **mean**. ANOVA = **AN**alysis **O**f **VA**riance of 3 or more variables. χ^2 = compare percentages (%) or proportions.
Meta-analysis	Pooling data from several studies (often via a literature search) to achieve greater statistical power.	Cannot overcome limitations of individual studies or bias in study selection.
Case-control study	Observational study. Sample chosen based on presence (cases) or absence (controls) of disease. Information collected about risk factors.	Often retrospective.
Cohort study	Observational study. Sample chosen based on presence or absence of risk factors. Subjects followed over time for development of disease.	The Framingham heart study was a large prospective cohort study.
Clinical trial	Experimental study. Compares therapeutic benefit of 2 or more treatments.	Highest-quality study when randomized and double-blind.
Bias	When one outcome is more likely to occur than another. 1. **Selection bias**—subjects choose group 2. **Recall bias**—knowledge of presence of disorder alters recall by subjects 3. **Sampling bias**—subjects are not representative; therefore the results are not generalizable 4. **Late-look bias**—information gathered at an inappropriate time	Ways to reduce bias: 1. Blind studies (single vs. double) 2. Placebo responses 3. Crossover studies (each subject acts as own control) 4. Randomization

Statistical hypotheses

Null (H_0)	Hypothesis of no difference (e.g., there is no association between the disease and the risk factor in the population).	
Alternative (H_1)	Hypothesis that there is some difference (e.g., there is some association between the disease and the risk factor in the population).	

	Reality	
	H_1	H_0
Study results H_1	Power $(1 - \beta)$	α
Study results H_0	β	

Type I error (α)	Stating that there **is** an effect or difference when none exists (to mistakenly accept the experimental hypothesis and reject the null hypothesis). α is a preset level of significance, usually $p < .05$. p = probability of making a type I error.	If $p < .05$, then there is less than a 5% chance that the data will show something that is not really there. α = you "saw" a difference that did not exist—for example, convicting an innocent man.
Type II error (β)	Stating that there **is not** an effect or difference when one exists (to fail to reject the null hypothesis when in fact H_0 is false). β is the probability of making a type II error.	β = you did not "see" a difference that does exist—for example, setting a guilty man free.
Power	Probability of rejecting null hypothesis when it is in fact false. It depends on: 1. Total number of end points experienced by population 2. Difference in compliance between treatment groups (differences in the mean values between groups)	If you increase sample size, you increase power. There is power in numbers. Power = $1 - \beta$.
Reportable diseases	Only some infectious diseases are reportable in all states, including AIDS, chickenpox, gonorrhea, hepatitis A and B, measles, mumps, rubella, salmonella, shigella, syphilis, and TB. Other diseases (including HIV) vary by state.	**B. A. SSSMMART** **Chicken** or you're **G**one: Hep **B** Hep **A** **S**almonella **S**higella **S**yphilis **M**easles **M**umps **A**IDS **R**ubella **T**uberculosis **C**hickenpox **G**onorrhea

Leading causes of death in the United States by age

Infants	Congenital anomalies, short gestation/low birth weight, sudden infant death syndrome, maternal complications of pregnancy, respiratory distress syndrome.
Age 1–14	Injuries, cancer, congenital anomalies, homicide, heart disease.
Age 15–24	Injuries, homicide, suicide, cancer, heart disease.
Age 25–64	Cancer, heart disease, injuries, suicide, stroke.
Age 65+	Heart disease, cancer, stroke, COPD, pneumonia, influenza.

HIGH-YIELD FACTS

Behavioral Science

Disease prevention
1°—Prevent disease occurrence (e.g., vaccination).
2°—Early detection of disease (e.g., Pap smear).
3°—Reduce disability from disease (e.g., exogenous insulin for diabetes).

Additional Services for Specific Groups

Risk factor	Preventive service(s) needed
Diabetes	Eye, foot exams; urine test
Drug abuse	HIV, TB tests; hepatitis immunization
Alcoholism	Influenza, pneumococcal immunizations; TB test
Overweight	Blood sugar test (test for diabetes mellitus)
Homeless, recent refugee or immigrant	TB test
High-risk sexual behavior	HIV, hep B, syphilis, gonorrhea, chlamydia tests

Risk factors for suicide completion
White, male, alone, prior attempts, presence and lethality of plan, medical illness, alcohol or drug use, 3 or more prescription medications.
Women try more often; men succeed more often.

SAD PERSONS: **S**ex (male), **A**ge, **D**epression, **P**revious attempt, **E**thanol, **R**ational thought, **S**ickness, **O**rganized plan, **N**o spouse, **S**ocial support lacking.

Medicare, Medicaid
Medicare and Medicaid are federal programs that originated from amendments to the Social Security Act.
Medicare Part A = hospital; Part B = doctor bills.
Medicaid is federal and state assistance for very poor people.

Medicar**E** is for **E**lderly.
Medicai**D** is for **D**estitute.

BEHAVIORAL SCIENCE — ETHICS

Autonomy
Obligation to respect patients as individuals and to honor their preferences in medical care.

Informed consent
Legally requires:
1. Discussion of pertinent information
2. Patient's agreement to the plan of care
3. Freedom from coercion

Patients must understand the risks, benefits, and alternatives, which include no intervention.

Exceptions to informed consent
1. Patient lacks decision-making capacity (not legally competent)
2. Implied consent in an emergency
3. Therapeutic privilege—withholding information when disclosure would severely harm the patient or undermine informed decision-making capacity
4. Waiver—patient waives the right of informed consent

Decision-making capacity	1. Patient makes and communicates a choice 2. Patient is informed 3. Decision remains stable over time 4. Decision consistent with patient's values and goals 5. Decision not a result of delusions or hallucinations	The patient's family cannot require that a doctor withhold information from the patient.
Oral advance directive	Incapacitated patient's prior oral statements commonly used as guide. Problems arise from variance in interpretation. However, if patient was informed, directive is specific, patient makes a choice, and decision is repeated over time, the oral directive is more valid.	
Written advance directive	Living wills—patient directs physician to withhold or withdraw life-sustaining treatment if the patient develops a terminal disease or enters a persistent vegetative state. Durable power of attorney—patient designates a surrogate to make medical decisions in the event that the patient loses decision-making capacity. Patient may also specify decisions in clinical situations. Surrogate retains power unless revoked by patient. More flexible than a living will.	
Nonmaleficence	"Do no harm." However, if benefits of an intervention outweigh the risks, a patient may make an informed decision to proceed.	
Beneficence	Physicians have a special ethical responsibility to act in the patient's best interest ("physician is a fiduciary"). Patient autonomy may conflict with beneficence. If the patient makes an informed decision, ultimately the patient has the right to decide.	
Confidentiality	Confidentiality respects patient privacy and autonomy. Disclosing information to family and friends should be guided by what the patient would want. The patient may also waive the right to confidentiality (e.g., insurance companies).	

Exceptions to confidentiality	1. Potential harm to others is serious
	2. Likelihood of harm to self is great
	3. No alternative means exist to warn or to protect those at risk
	4. Physicians can take steps to prevent harm
	   Examples include:
	     1. Infectious diseases—physicians may have a duty to warn public officials and identifiable people at risk
	     2. The Tarasoff decision—law requiring physician to directly inform and protect potential victim from harm; may involve breach of confidentiality
	     3. Child and/or elder abuse
	     4. Impaired automobile drivers
	     5. Suicidal/homicidal patient—physician may hold patient involuntarily for a period of time	

Ethical situations

Situation	Appropriate response
Patient is noncompliant.	Work to improve the physician-patient relationship.
Patient has difficulty taking medications.	Provide written instructions; attempt to simplify treatment regimens.
Family members ask for information about patient's prognosis.	Avoid discussing issues with relatives without the permission of the patient.
A 17-year-old girl is pregnant and asks for an abortion.	Inform the patient that most states require parental consent for minors for an abortion. Parental consent is **not** required for emergency situations, treatment of STDs, medical care during pregnancy, prescriptions for contraceptives, and management of drug addiction.
A terminally ill patient requests physician assistance in ending his life.	Refuse involvement in any form of euthanasia (physician-assisted suicide). Physician may, however, prescribe medically appropriate analgesics that coincidentally shorten the patient's life.
Patient states that he finds you attractive.	Ask direct, closed-ended questions and use a chaperone if necessary. Romantic relationships with patients are **never** appropriate.
Patient refuses a necessary procedure or desires an unnecessary one.	Attempt to understand why the patient wants/does not want the procedure. Address the underlying concerns. Avoid performing unnecessary procedures.
Patient is angry about the amount of time he spent in the waiting room.	Apologize to the patient for any inconvenience. Stay away from efforts to explain the delay.
Patient is upset with the way he was treated by another doctor.	Suggest that the patient speak directly to that physician regarding his concerns. If the problem is with a member of the office staff, tell the patient you will speak to that individual.
A child wishes to know more about his illness.	Ask what the parents have told the child about his illness. Parents of a child decide what information can be relayed about the illness.
Patient continues to smoke, believing that cigarettes are good for him.	Ask how the patient feels about his smoking. Offer advice on cessation if the patient seems willing to make an effort to quit.

Malpractice

Civil suit under negligence requires:
1. Physician breach of duty to patient (**D**ereliction)
2. Patient suffers harm (**D**amage)
3. Breach of duty causes harm (**D**irect)

The most common factor leading to litigation is poor communication between physician and patient.

The **3 D's.**

Unlike a criminal suit, in which the burden of proof is "beyond a reasonable doubt," the burden of proof in a malpractice suit is "more likely than not."

Apgar score (at birth)	Score 0–2 at 1 and 5 minutes in each of 5 categories: 1. Color (blue/pale, trunk pink, all pink) 2. Heart rate (0, < 100, 100+) 3. Reflex irritability (0, grimace, grimace + cough) 4. Muscle tone (limp, some, active) 5. Respiratory effort (0, irregular, regular) 10 is perfect score.	After Virginia **Apgar,** a famous anesthesiologist. **APGAR:** **A**ppearance (color) **P**ulse **G**rimace **A**ctivity **R**espiration
Low birth weight	Defined as < 2500 g. Associated with greater incidence of physical and emotional problems. Caused by prematurity or intrauterine growth retardation. Complications include infections, respiratory distress syndrome, necrotizing enterocolitis, intraventricular hemorrhage, and persistent fetal circulation.	
Infant deprivation effects	Long-term deprivation of affection results in: 1. Decreased muscle tone 2. Poor language skills 3. Poor socialization skills 4. Lack of basic trust 5. Anaclitic depression 6. Weight loss 7. Physical illness Severe deprivation can result in infant death.	The **4 W's:** Weak, Wordless, Wanting (socially), Wary. Deprivation for > 6 months can lead to irreversible changes.
Anaclitic depression	Depression in an infant owing to continued separation from caregiver—can result in failure to thrive. Infant becomes withdrawn and unresponsive.	
Regression in children	Children regress to younger behavior under stress: physical illness, punishment, birth of a new sibling, tiredness. An example is bed-wetting in a previously toilet-trained child when hospitalized.	

Child abuse

	Physical abuse	Sexual abuse
Evidence	Healed fractures on x-ray, cigarette burns, subdural hematomas, multiple bruises, retinal hemorrhage or detachment	Genital/anal trauma, STDs, UTIs
Abuser	Usually female and the 1° caregiver	Known to victim, usually male
Epidemiology	~3000 deaths/year in the United States	Peak incidence 9–12 years of age

HIGH-YIELD FACTS

Behavioral Science

Developmental milestones

Approximate age	Motor milestone	Cognitive/social milestone
Infant		
3 mo	Holds head up, Moro reflex disappears	Social smile
4–5 mo	Rolls front to back, sits when propped	Recognizes people
7–9 mo	Sits alone	Stranger anxiety, orients to voice
12–14 mo	Upgoing Babinski disappears	
15 mo	Walks	Few words, separation anxiety
Toddler		
12–24 mo	Climbs stairs, stacks 3 blocks	Object permanence
18–24 mo	Stacks 6 blocks	Rapprochement
24–48 mo		Parallel play
24–36 mo		Core gender identity
Preschool		
30–36 mo		Toilet training
3 yrs	Rides tricycle, copies line or circle drawing	Group play
4 yrs	Simple drawings (stick figure), hops on 1 foot	Cooperative play
School age		
6–11 yrs		Development of conscience (superego), same-sex friends, identification with same-sex parent
Adolescence (puberty)		
11 yrs (girls)		Abstract reasoning (formal operations), formation of personality
13 yrs (boys)		

Reflexes present at birth	1. Moro reflex—extension of limbs when startled 2. Rooting reflex—nipple seeking 3. Palmar reflex—grasps objects in palm 4. Babinski reflex—large toe dorsiflexes with plantar stimulation	Normally disappear within 1st year.
Changes in the elderly	1. Sexual changes—sexual interest does not decrease Men: slower erection/ejaculation, longer refractory period Women: vaginal shortening, thinning, and dryness 2. Sleep patterns— ↓ REM sleep, ↓ slow-wave sleep, ↑ sleep latency, ↑ awakenings during the night 3. Common medical conditions—arthritis, hypertension, heart disease 4. Psychiatric problems (e.g., depression) become more prevalent 5. Suicide rate increases	
Kübler-Ross dying stages	Denial, Anger, Bargaining, Grieving, Acceptance. Stages do not necessarily occur in this order, and > 1 stage can be present at once.	**D**eath **A**rrives **B**ringing **G**rave **A**djustments.

Grief	Normal bereavement characterized by shock, denial, guilt, and somatic symptoms. Typically lasts 6 months to 1 year.
	Pathologic grief includes excessively intense or prolonged grief or grief that is delayed, inhibited, or denied.

Neurotransmitter changes with disease

Anxiety—↑ NE, ↓ GABA, ↓ serotonin.
Depression—↓ NE and serotonin (5-HT).
Alzheimer's dementia—↓ **A**Ch.
Huntington's disease—↓ GABA, ↓ ACh.
Schizophrenia—↑ dopamine.
Parkinson's disease—↓ dopamine.

Frontal lobe functions

Concentration, orientation, language, abstraction, judgment, motor regulation, mood.
Lack of social judgment is most notable in frontal lobe lesion.

Sleep stages

Stage (% of total sleep time in young adults)	Description	Waveform
	Awake (eyes open), alert, active mental concentration	**B**eta (highest frequency, lowest amplitude)
	Awake (eyes closed)	**A**lpha
1 (5%)	Light sleep	**T**heta
2 (45%)	Deeper sleep	**S**leep spindles and K complexes
3–4 (25%)	Deepest, non-REM sleep; sleepwalking; night terrors, bed-wetting (slow-wave sleep)	**D**elta (lowest frequency, highest amplitude)
REM (25%)	Dreaming, loss of motor tone, possibly a memory processing function, erections, ↑ brain O_2 use	**B**eta
		At night, **BATS** Drink **B**lood.

1. Serotonergic predominance of raphe nucleus key to initiating sleep
2. NE reduces REM sleep
3. Extraocular movements during REM due to activity of PPRF (paramedian pontine reticular formation/conjugate gaze center)
4. REM sleep having the same EEG pattern as while awake and alert has spawned the terms "paradoxical sleep" and "desynchronized sleep"
5. Benzodiazepines shorten stage 4 sleep; thus useful for night terrors and sleepwalking
6. Imipramine is used to treat enuresis because it decreases stage 4 sleep

REM sleep

↑ and variable pulse, REM, ↑ and variable blood pressure, penile/clitoral tumescence. 25% of total sleep. Occurs every 90 minutes; duration ↑ through the night. REM sleep ↓ with age. ACh is the principal neurotransmitter involved in REM sleep.

REM sleep is like sex: ↑ pulse, penile/clitoral tumescence, ↓ with age.

Sleep apnea

Central sleep apnea—no respiratory effort.
Obstructive sleep apnea—respiratory effort against airway obstruction.
Person stops breathing for at least 10 seconds repeatedly during sleep.
Associated with obesity, loud snoring, systemic/ pulmonary hypertension, arrhythmias, and possibly sudden death.
Individuals may become chronically tired.

Treatment: weight loss, CPAP, surgery.

Narcolepsy

Person falls asleep suddenly. May include hypnagogic (just before sleep) or hypnopompic (just before awakening) hallucinations. The person's nocturnal and narcoleptic sleep episodes start off with REM sleep. **Cataplexy** (sudden collapse while awake) in some patients. Strong genetic component. Treat with stimulants (e.g., amphetamines).

Sleep patterns of depressed patients

Patients with depression typically have the following changes in their sleep stages:
1. ↓ slow-wave sleep
2. ↓ REM latency
3. Early-morning awakening (important screening question)

Stress effects

Stress induces production of free fatty acids, 17-OH corticosteroids, lipids, cholesterol, catecholamines; affects water absorption, muscular tonicity, gastrocolic reflex, and mucosal circulation.

Sexual dysfunction

Differential diagnosis includes:
1. Drugs (e.g., antihypertensives, neuroleptics, SSRIs, ethanol)
2. Diseases (e.g., depression, diabetes)
3. Psychological (e.g., performance anxiety)

Body-mass index (BMI)

BMI is a measure of weight adjusted for height.

$$BMI = \frac{\text{weight in kg}}{(\text{height in meters})^2}$$

< 18.5 underweight;
18.5–24.9 normal;
25.0–29.9 overweight;
> 30.0 obese.

Orientation	Is the patient aware of him- or herself as a person? Does the patient know his or her own name? Anosognosia—unaware that one is ill. Autotopagnosia—unable to locate one's own body parts. Depersonalization—body seems unreal or dissociated.	Order of loss: 1st—time; 2nd—place; last—person.
Amnesia types	*Antero*grade amnesia is the inability to remember things that occurred after a CNS insult (no new memory). Korsakoff's amnesia is a classic anterograde amnesia that is caused by thiamine deficiency (bilateral destruction of the mammillary bodies), is seen in alcoholics, and is associated with confabulations. *Retro*grade amnesia is inability to remember things that occurred before a CNS insult. Complication of ECT.	*Antero* = after. *Retro* = before.
Substance dependence	Maladaptive pattern of substance use defined as 3 or more of the following signs in 1 year: 1. Tolerance 2. Withdrawal 3. Substance taken in larger amounts than intended 4. Persistent desire or attempts to cut down 5. Lots of energy spent trying to obtain substance 6. Important social, occupational, or recreational activities given up or reduced because of substance use 7. Use continued in spite of knowing the problems that it causes	
Substance abuse	Maladaptive pattern leading to clinically significant impairment or distress. Symptoms have not met criteria for substance dependence. 1 or more of the following in 1 year: 1. Recurrent use resulting in failure to fulfill major obligations at work, school, or home 2. Recurrent use in physically hazardous situations 3. Recurrent substance-related legal problems 4. Continued use in spite of persistent problems caused by use	

Signs and symptoms of substance abuse

Drug	Intoxication	Withdrawal
Alcohol	Disinhibition, emotional lability, slurred speech, ataxia, coma, blackouts.	Tremor, tachycardia, hypertension, malaise, nausea, seizures, delirium tremens (DTs), tremulousness, agitation, hallucinations
Opioids	CNS depression, nausea and vomiting, constipation, pupillary constriction (pinpoint pupils), seizures (overdose is life-threatening).	Anxiety, insomnia, anorexia, sweating, dilated pupils, piloerection ("cold turkey"), fever, rhinorrhea, nausea, stomach cramps, diarrhea ("flu-like" symptoms), yawning
Amphetamines	Psychomotor agitation, impaired judgment, pupillary dilation, hypertension, tachycardia, euphoria, prolonged wakefulness and attention, cardiac arrhythmias, delusions, hallucinations, fever.	Post-use "crash," including depression, lethargy, headache, stomach cramps, hunger, hypersomnolence
Cocaine	Euphoria, psychomotor agitation, impaired judgment, tachycardia, pupillary dilation, hypertension, hallucinations (including tactile), paranoid ideations, angina, sudden cardiac death.	Post-use "crash," including severe depression and suicidality, hypersomnolence, fatigue, malaise, severe psychological craving
PCP	Belligerence, impulsiveness, fever, psychomotor agitation, vertical and horizontal nystagmus, tachycardia, ataxia, homicidality, psychosis, delirium.	Recurrence of intoxication symptoms due to reabsorption in GI tract; sudden onset of severe, random, homicidal violence
LSD	Marked anxiety or depression, delusions, visual hallucinations, flashbacks, pupil dilation.	
Marijuana	Euphoria, anxiety, paranoid delusions, perception of slowed time, impaired judgment, social withdrawal, increased appetite, dry mouth, hallucinations.	
Barbiturates	Low safety margin, respiratory depression.	Anxiety, seizures, delirium, life-threatening cardiovascular collapse
Benzodiazepines	Amnesia, ataxia, somnolence, minor respiratory depression. Additive effects with alcohol. Greater safety margin.	Rebound anxiety, seizures, tremor, insomnia
Caffeine	Restlessness, insomnia, increased diuresis, muscle twitching, cardiac arrhythmias.	Headache, lethargy, depression, weight gain
Nicotine	Restlessness, insomnia, anxiety, arrhythmias.	Irritability, headache, anxiety, weight gain, craving, tachycardia

Delirium tremens	Life-threatening alcohol withdrawal syndrome that peaks 2–5 days after last drink. In order of appearance—autonomic system hyperactivity (tachycardia, tremors, anxiety), psychotic symptoms (hallucinations, delusions), confusion. Treat with benzodiazepines.

HIGH-YIELD FACTS

Behavioral Science

Heroin addiction	Approximately 500,000 U.S. addicts. Heroin is Schedule I (not prescribable). Also look for track marks (needle sticks in veins). Related diagnoses are hepatitis, abscesses, overdose, hemorrhoids, AIDS, and right-sided endocarditis.	Naloxone (Narcan) and naltrexone competitively inhibit opioids. Methadone (long-acting oral opiate) for heroin detoxification or long-term maintenance.
Delirium	↓ attention span and level of arousal, disorganized thinking, hallucinations, illusions, misperceptions, disturbance in sleep-wake cycle, cognitive dysfunction. Key to diagnosis: waxing and waning level of consciousness; develops rapidly. Often due to substance use/abuse or medical illness.	DeliRIUM = changes in sensoRIUM. Most common psychiatric illness on medical and surgical floors. Often reversible. Check for drugs with anticholinergic effects.
Dementia	Development of multiple cognitive deficits—memory, aphasia, apraxia, agnosia, loss of abstract thought, behavioral/personality changes, impaired judgment. Key to diagnosis: rule out delirium—patient is alert, no change in level of consciousness. More often gradual onset. In elderly patients, depression may present like dementia.	DeMEMtia characterized by MEMory loss. Commonly irreversible.
Major depressive episode	Characterized by 5 of the following for 2 weeks, including (1) depressed mood or (2) anhedonia: 1. **S**leep disturbances 2. Loss of **I**nterest 3. **G**uilt 4. Loss of **E**nergy 5. Loss of **C**oncentration 6. Change in **A**ppetite 7. **P**sychomotor retardation 8. **S**uicidal ideations 9. Depressed mood Major depressive disorder, recurrent—requires 2 or more episodes with a symptom-free interval of 2 months. Lifetime prevalence—5–12% male, 10–25% female. **Dysthymia** is a milder form of depression lasting at least 2 years.	**SIG E CAPS.**
Electroconvulsive therapy	Treatment option for major depressive disorder refractory to other treatment. ECT is painless and produces a seizure. Complications can result from anesthesia. The major adverse effects of ECT are disorientation and anterograde and retrograde amnesia.	

Manic episode

Distinct period of abnormally and persistently elevated, expansive, or irritable mood lasting at least 1 week.
During mood disturbance, 3 or more of the following are present:

1. **D**istractibility   DIG FAST.
2. **I**nsomnia— ↓ need for sleep
3. **G**randiosity—inflated self-esteem
4. **F**light of ideas
5. Increase in goal-directed **A**ctivity/ psychomotor **A**gitation
6. Pressured **S**peech
7. **T**houghtlessness—seeks pleasure without regard to consequences

Hypomanic episode

Like manic episode except mood disturbance not severe enough to cause marked impairment in social and/or occupational functioning or to necessitate hospitalization; there are no psychotic features.

Bipolar disorder

6 separate criteria sets exist for bipolar disorders with combinations of manic (bipolar I), hypomanic (bipolar II), and depressed episodes. 1 manic or hypomanic episode defines bipolar disorder. Lithium is drug of choice.
Cyclothymic disorder is a milder form lasting at least 2 years.

Malingering

Patient consciously fakes or claims to have a disorder in order to attain a specific gain (e.g., financial).

Factitious disorder

Consciously creates symptoms in order to assume "sick role" and to get medical attention.
Munchausen's syndrome is manifested by a chronic history of multiple hospital admissions and willingness to receive invasive procedures. **Munchausen's syndrome by proxy** is seen when illness in a child is caused by the parent. Motivation is unconscious.

Somatoform disorders

Both illness production and motivation are unconscious drives. More common in women. Several types:

1. Conversion—symptoms suggest motor or sensory neurologic or physical disorder, but tests and physical exam are negative
2. Somatoform pain disorder—prolonged pain that is not explained completely by illness
3. Hypochondriasis—misinterpretation of normal physical findings, leading to preoccupation with and fear of having a serious illness in spite of medical reassurance
4. Somatization disorder—variety of complaints in multiple organ systems
5. Body dysmorphic disorder—patient convinced that part of own anatomy is malformed
6. Pseudocyesis—false belief of being pregnant associated with objective physical signs of pregnancy

Gain: 1°, 2°, 3°	1° gain—what the symptom does for the patient's internal psychic economy. 2° gain—what the symptom gets the patient (sympathy, attention). 3° gain—what the caretaker gets (like an MD on an interesting case).

Panic disorder	Discrete periods of intense fear and discomfort peaking
	    in 10 minutes with 4 of the following:
	      1. **P**alpitations **PANIC.**
	      2. **A**bdominal distress
	      3. **N**ausea
	      4. **I**ncreased perspiration
	      5. **C**hest pain, **C**hills, and **C**hoking
	Panic disorder must be diagnosed in context of
	    occurrence (e.g., panic disorder with agoraphobia).
	    High prevalence during Step 1 exam.

Specific phobia	Fear that is excessive or unreasonable, cued by presence or anticipation of a specific
	    object or entity. Exposure provokes anxiety response. Person recognizes fear is
	    excessive (insight). Fear interferes with normal routine. Treatment options
	    include systematic desensitization. Examples include:
	      1. Gamophobia (*gam* = gamete)—fear of marriage
	      2. Algophobia (*alg* = pain)—fear of pain
	      3. Acrophobia (*acro* = height)—fear of heights
	      4. Agoraphobia (*agora* = open market)—fear of open places

Post-traumatic stress disorder	Person experienced or witnessed event that involved actual or threatened death or serious
	    injury. Response involves intense fear, helplessness, or horror. Traumatic event is
	    persistently reexperienced; person persistently avoids stimuli associated with the trauma
	    and experiences persistent symptoms of increased arousal. Disturbance lasts > 1 month
	    and causes distress or social/occupational impairment. PTSD often follows acute stress
	    disorder, which lasts 2–4 weeks.

Other anxiety disorders	Adjustment disorder—emotional symptoms (anxiety, depression) causing impairment
	    following an identifiable psychosocial stressor (e.g., divorce, moving) and lasting
	    < 6 months.
	Generalized anxiety disorder—uncontrollable anxiety unrelated to a specific person,
	    situation, or event. GI symptoms, fatigue, and difficulty concentrating are common.

Personality	Personality trait—an enduring pattern of perceiving, relating to, and thinking about the
	    environment and oneself that is exhibited in a wide range of important social and
	    personal contexts.
	Personality disorder—when these patterns become inflexible and maladaptive, causing
	    impairment in social or occupational functioning or subjective distress; person is usually
	    not aware of problem.

HIGH-YIELD FACTS

Behavioral Science

Cluster A personality disorders

Odd or eccentric; cannot develop meaningful social relationships. No psychosis; genetic association with schizophrenia.

Types:

1. Paranoid—distrust and suspiciousness; projection is main defense mechanism
2. Schizoid—voluntary social withdrawal, limited emotional expression
3. Schizotypal—interpersonal awkwardness, odd thought patterns and appearance

"Weird."

Cluster B personality disorders

Dramatic, emotional, or erratic; genetic association with mood disorders.

Types:

1. Antisocial—disregard for and violation of rights of others, criminality; males > females; conduct disorder if < 18 years
2. Borderline—unstable mood and behavior, impulsiveness, sense of emptiness; females > males
3. Histrionic—excessive emotionality, somatization, attention seeking, sexually provocative
4. Narcissistic—grandiosity, sense of entitlement; may demand "top" physician/best health care

"Wild."

Cluster C personality disorders

Anxious or fearful; genetic association with anxiety disorders.

Types:

1. Avoidant—sensitive to rejection, socially inhibited, timid, feelings of inadequacy
2. Obsessive-compulsive—preoccupation with order, perfectionism, and control
3. Dependent—submissive and clinging, excessive need to be taken care of, low self-confidence

"Worried."

Childhood disorders	Autistic disorder—patients have severe communication problems and difficulty forming relationships. Characterized by repetitive behavior, unusual abilities (savants), and below-normal intelligence. Treatment: ↑ communication and social skills. Asperger syndrome—a milder form of autism involving problems with social relationships and repetitive behavior. Children are of normal intelligence and lack social or cognitive deficits. Rett disorder—X-linked disorder seen only in girls (affected males die in utero). Characterized by loss of development and mental retardation appearing at approximately age 4. Attention-deficit hyperactivity disorder (ADHD)—limited attention span and hyperactivity. Children are emotionally labile, impulsive, and prone to accidents. Normal intelligence. Treatment: methylphenidate (Ritalin). Conduct disorder—continued behavior violating social norms. Oppositional defiant disorder is seen when child is noncompliant in the absence of criminality. Tourette's syndrome—motor/vocal tics and involuntary profanity. Onset < 18 years. Treatment: haloperidol. Separation anxiety disorder—fear of loss of attachment figure leading to factitious physical complaints to avoid going to school. Common in children age 7–8.
Eating disorders	Anorexia nervosa—abnormal eating habits (excessive dieting), body image distortion, and ↑ exercise. Severe weight loss, amenorrhea, anemia, and electrolyte disturbances can follow. Seen primarily in adolescent girls. Bulimia nervosa—binge eating followed by self-induced vomiting or use of laxatives. Body weight is normal. Parotitis, enamel erosion, ↑ amylase, and esophageal varices from vomiting.
Hallucination vs. illusion vs. delusion	Hallucinations are perceptions in the absence of external stimuli. Illusions are misinterpretations of actual external stimuli. Delusions are false beliefs not shared with other members of culture/subculture that are firmly maintained in spite of obvious proof to the contrary.
Delusion vs. loose association	A delusion is a disorder in the content of thought (the actual idea). A loose association is a disorder in the form of thought (the way ideas are tied together).
Hallucination types	Visual and auditory hallucinations are common in schizophrenia. Olfactory hallucination often occurs as an aura of a psychomotor epilepsy. Gustatory hallucination is rare. Tactile hallucination (e.g., formication) is common in DTs. Also seen in cocaine abusers ("cocaine bugs"). Hypnagogic hallucination occurs while going to sleep. Hypnopompic hallucination occurs while waking from sleep.

Schizophrenia

Periods of psychosis and disturbed behavior lasting > 6 months.

Positive symptoms—hallucinations, delusions, strange behavior, loose associations.

Negative symptoms—flat affect, social withdrawal, thought blocking, lack of motivation.

The **4 A's** described by Bleuler:

1. **A**mbivalence (uncertainty)
2. **A**utism (self-preoccupation and lack of communication)
3. **A**ffect (blunted)
4. **A**ssociations (loose)

5th A should be **A**uditory hallucinations.

Genetic factors outweigh environmental factors in the etiology of schizophrenia.

Lifetime prevalence—1.5% (males > females, blacks > whites). Presents earlier in men.

5 subtypes:

1. Disorganized
2. Catatonic
3. Paranoid
4. Undifferentiated
5. Residual

Schizoaffective disorder—a combination of schizophrenia and a mood disorder.

BEHAVIORAL SCIENCE—PSYCHOLOGY

Structural theory of the mind

Freud's 3 structures of the mind.

Id — Primal urges, sex, and aggression. (I want it.)

Superego — Moral values, conscience. (You know you can't have it.)

Ego — Bridge and mediator between the unconscious mind and the external world. (Deals with the conflict.)

Topographic theory of the mind

Conscious—what you are aware of.

Preconscious—what you are able to make conscious with effort (like your phone number).

Unconscious—what you are not aware of; the central goal of Freudian psychoanalysis is to make the patient aware of what is hidden in his/her unconscious.

Oedipus complex

Repressed sexual feelings of a child for the opposite-sex parent, accompanied by rivalry with same-sex parent. First described by Freud.

Ego defenses

All ego defenses are automatic and unconscious reactions to psychological stress.

Mature

Altruism	Guilty feelings alleviated by unsolicited generosity toward others.	Mafia boss makes large donation to charity.
Humor	Appreciating the amusing nature of an anxiety-provoking or adverse situation.	Nervous medical student jokes about the boards.
Sublimation	Process whereby one replaces an unacceptable wish with a course of action that is similar to the wish but does not conflict with one's value system.	Aggressive impulses used to succeed in business ventures.
Suppression	Voluntary (unlike other defenses) withholding of an idea or feeling from conscious awareness.	Choosing not to think about the USMLE until the week of the exam.

Mature women wear a **SASH: S**ublimation, **A**ltruism, **S**uppression, **H**umor.

Immature

Acting out	Unacceptable feelings and thoughts are expressed through actions.	Tantrums.
Dissociation	Temporary, drastic change in personality, memory, consciousness, or motor behavior to avoid emotional stress.	Extreme forms can result in multiple personalities (dissociative identity disorder).
Denial	Avoidance of awareness of some painful reality.	A common reaction in newly diagnosed AIDS and cancer patients.
Displacement	Process whereby avoided ideas and feelings are transferred to some neutral person or object.	Mother yells at child because she is angry at her husband.
Fixation	Partially remaining at a more childish level of development.	Men fixating on sports games.
Identification	Modeling behavior after another person.	Abused child becomes an abuser.
Isolation	Separation of feelings from ideas and events.	Describing murder in graphic detail with no emotional response.
Projection	An unacceptable internal impulse is attributed to an external source.	A man who wants another woman thinks his wife is cheating on him.
Rationalization	Proclaiming logical reasons for actions actually performed for other reasons, usually to avoid self-blame.	Saying the job was not important anyway, after getting fired.
Reaction formation	Process whereby a warded-off idea or feeling is replaced by an (unconsciously derived) emphasis on its opposite.	A patient with libidinous thoughts enters a monastery.
Regression	Turning back the maturational clock and going back to earlier modes of dealing with the world.	Seen in children under stress (e.g., bed-wetting) and in patients on dialysis (e.g., crying).
Repression	Involuntary withholding of an idea or feeling from conscious awareness. The basic mechanism underlying all others.	
Splitting	Belief that people are either good or bad.	A patient says that all the nurses are cold and insensitive but that the doctors are warm and friendly.

Transference and countertransference

Transference	Patient projects feelings stemming from personal life onto physician.
Countertransference	Doctor projects feelings stemming from personal life onto patient.

Classical conditioning

Learning in which a natural response (salivation) is elicited by a conditioned (learned) stimulus (bell) that previously was presented in conjunction with an unconditioned stimulus (food).

Programmed by association, not necessarily reward. As in Pavlov's classical experiments with dogs (ringing the bell provoked salivation).

Operant conditioning

Learning in which a particular action is elicited because it produces a reward.

Positive reinforcement—desired reward produces action (mouse presses button to get food).

Negative reinforcement—removal of aversive stimulus increases behavior (mouse presses button to avoid shock). Do not confuse with punishment.

Reinforcement schedules

Pattern of reinforcement determines how quickly a behavior is learned and extinguished.

Continuous	Behavior shows the most rapid extinction when not rewarded.	This explains why people continue to play slot machines at casinos (variable ratio) and yet get upset when vending machines (continuous) don't work.
Variable ratio	Behavior shows the slowest extinction when not rewarded.	

Intelligence testing

Stanford-Binet and Wechsler are the most famous tests.

Stanford-Binet calculates IQ as mental age/chronological age × 100.

Wechsler Adult Intelligence Scale uses 11 subtests (6 verbal, 5 performance).

Mean is defined at 100, with standard deviation of 15.

IQ < 70 (or 2 standard deviations below the mean) is one of the criteria for diagnosis of mental retardation (MR). IQ < 40—severe MR. IQ < 20—profound MR.

IQ scores are correlated with genetic factors but are more highly correlated with school achievement.

Intelligence tests are objective (not projective) tests.

Biochemistry

"Biochemistry is the study of carbon compounds that crawl."
—Mike Adams

This high-yield material includes molecular biology, genetics, cell biology, and principles of metabolism (especially vitamins, cofactors, minerals, and single-enzyme-deficiency diseases). When studying metabolic pathways, emphasize important regulatory steps and enzyme deficiencies that result in disease. For example, understanding the defect in Lesch-Nyhan syndrome and its clinical consequences is higher yield than memorizing every intermediate in the purine salvage pathway. Do not spend time on hard-core organic chemistry, mechanisms, and physical chemistry. Detailed chemical structures are infrequently tested. Familiarity with the latest biochemical techniques that have medical relevance—such as enzyme-linked immunosorbent assay (ELISA), immunoelectrophoresis, Southern blotting, and PCR—is useful. Beware if you placed out of your medical school's biochemistry class, for the emphasis of the test differs from the emphasis of many undergraduate courses. Review the related biochemistry when studying pharmacology or genetic diseases as a way to reinforce and integrate the material.

High-Yield Clinical Vignettes

DNA/RNA

Lab Tests/Techniques

Genetics

Cellular

Metabolism

Nutrition

These abstracted case vignettes are designed to demonstrate the thought processes necessary to answer multistep clinical reasoning questions.

Vignette	Question	Answer
■ Full-term neonate of uneventful delivery becomes mentally retarded and hyperactive and has a musty odor.	What is the diagnosis?	PKU.
■ Stressed executive comes home from work, consumes 7 or 8 martinis in rapid succession before dinner, and becomes hypoglycemic.	What is the mechanism?	NADH increase prevents gluconeogenesis by shunting pyruvate and oxaloacetate to lactate and malate.
■ 2-year-old girl has an ↑ in abdominal girth, failure to thrive, and skin and hair depigmentation.	What is the diagnosis?	Kwashiorkor.
■ Alcoholic develops a rash, diarrhea, and altered mental status.	What is the vitamin deficiency?	Vitamin B_3 (pellagra).
■ 20-year-old male presents with idiopathic hyperbilirubinemia.	What is the most common cause?	Gilbert's disease.
■ 51-year-old man has black spots in his sclera and has noted that his urine turns black when he is standing.	What is the diagnosis?	Alkaptonuria.
■ 25-year-old male complains of severe chest pain and has xanthomas of his Achilles tendons.	What is the disease, and where is the defect?	Familial hypercholesterolemia; LDL receptor.

Chromatin structure	Condensed by (−) charged DNA looped twice around (+) charged H2A, H2B, H3, and H4 histones (nucleosome bead). H1 ties nucleosomes together in a string (30-nm fiber). In mitosis, DNA condenses to form mitotic chromosomes.	Think of beads on a string.
Heterochromatin	Condensed, transcriptionally inactive.	
Euchromatin	Less condensed, transcriptionally active.	*Eu* = true, "truly transcribed."

Nucleotides	Purines (**A, G**) have 2 rings. Pyrimidines (**C, T, U**) have 1 ring. Guanine has a ketone. Thymine has a methyl. Deamination of cytosine makes uracil. Uracil found in RNA; thymine in DNA. G-C bond (3 H-bonds) stronger than A-T bond (2 H-bonds). ↑ G-C content → ↑ melting temperature.	**PUR**e **A**s **G**old: **PUR**ines. **CUT** the **PY** (pie): **PY**rimidines. **THY**mine has a me**THY**l.

Nucleotides are linked by 3′-5′ phosphodiesterase bond.

Transition vs. transversion	Transition—substituting purine for purine or pyrimidine for pyrimidine. Transversion—substituting purine for pyrimidine or vice versa.	Transversion— **Trans**conversion (1 type to another).

Genetic code features	Unambiguous—each codon specifies only 1 amino acid. Degenerate—more than 1 codon may code for same amino acid. Commaless, nonoverlapping (except some viruses). Universal (exceptions include mitochondria, archaeobacteria, *Mycoplasma*, and some yeasts).

HIGH-YIELD FACTS

Biochemistry

HIGH-YIELD FACTS

Biochemistry

Mutations in DNA

Silent—same aa, often base change in 3rd position of codon.

Missense—changed aa (conservative—new aa is similar in chemical structure).

Nonsense—change resulting in early stop codon.

Frame shift—change resulting in misreading of all nucleotides downstream, usually resulting in a truncated protein.

Severity of damage: nonsense > missense > silent.

Prokaryotic DNA replication and DNA polymerases

Origin of replication—continuous DNA synthesis on leading strand and discontinuous (Okazaki fragments) on lagging strand. **Primase** makes an RNA **primer** on which DNA polymerase III can initiate replication. **DNA polymerase III** reaches primer of preceding fragment; $5' \rightarrow 3'$ exonuclease activity of DNA polymerase I degrades RNA primer; **DNA ligase** seals; $3' \rightarrow 5'$ exonuclease activity of DNA polymerase III "proofreads" each added nucleotide.

DNA topoisomerases create a nick in the helix to relieve supercoils.

Eukaryotic genome has multiple origins of replication. Bacteria, viruses, and plasmids have only 1 origin of replication.

DNA polymerase III has $5' \rightarrow 3'$ synthesis and $3' \rightarrow 5'$ exonuclease proofreading ability.

DNA polymerase I excises RNA primer.

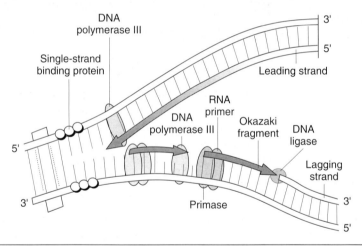

Eukaryotic DNA polymerases

α replicates lagging strand; synthesizes RNA primer.
β repairs DNA.
γ replicates mitochondrial DNA.
δ replicates leading-strand DNA.
ε repairs DNA.

DNA repair: single strand

Single-strand, excision repair–specific glycosylase recognizes and removes damaged base. Endonuclease makes a break several bases to the 5' side. Exonuclease removes short stretch of nucleotides. DNA polymerase fills gap. DNA ligase seals.

If both strands are damaged, repair may proceed via recombination with undamaged homologous chromosome.

DNA repair defects	Xeroderma pigmentosum (skin sensitivity to UV light), ataxia-telangiectasia (x-rays), Bloom's syndrome (radiation), and Fanconi's anemia (cross-linking agents).	
Xeroderma pigmentosum	Defective excision repair such as uvr ABC endonuclease. Results in inability to repair thymidine dimers, which form in DNA when exposed to UV light. Associated with dry skin and with melanoma and other cancers.	Autosomal recessive.
DNA/RNA/protein synthesis direction	DNA and RNA are both synthesized 5′ → 3′. Remember that the 5′ of the incoming nucleotide bears the triphosphate (energy source for bond). The 3′ hydroxyl of the nascent chain is the target. Protein synthesis also proceeds in the 5′ to 3′ direction.	Imagine the incoming nucleotide bringing a gift (triphosphate) to the 3′ host. "**BYOP** (phosphate) from **5** to **3**." Amino acids are linked N to C.
Types of RNA	mRNA is the **largest** type of RNA. rRNA is the most **abundant** type of RNA. tRNA is the **smallest** type of RNA.	**M**assive, **R**ampant, **T**iny.

RNA polymerases

Eukaryotes	RNA polymerase I makes **r**RNA. RNA polymerase II makes **m**RNA. RNA polymerase III makes **t**RNA. No proofreading function, but can initiate chains. RNA polymerase II opens DNA at promoter site (A-T-rich upstream sequence—TATA and CAAT). α-amanitin inhibits RNA polymerase II.	I, II, and III are numbered as their products are used in protein synthesis. OR **1, 2, 3 = RMT** (rhyme).
Prokaryotes	RNA polymerase makes all 3 kinds of RNA.	

Start and stop codons	AUG (or rarely GUG) is the mRNA initiation codon. AUG codes for methionine, which may be removed before translation is completed. In prokaryotes the initial AUG codes for a formyl-methionine (f-met). Stop codons: UGA, UAA, UAG.	**AUG** in**AUG**urates protein synthesis. **UGA** = **U** **G**o **A**way. **UAA** = **U** **A**re **A**way. **UAG** = **U** **A**re **G**one.

Regulation of gene expression

Promoter	Site where RNA polymerase and multiple other transcription factors bind to DNA upstream from gene locus.	Promoter mutation commonly results in dramatic ↓ in amount of gene transcribed.
Enhancer	Stretch of DNA that alters gene expression by binding transcription factors. May be located close to, far from, or even within (in an intron) the gene whose expression it regulates.	

Introns vs. exons	Exons contain the actual genetic information coding for protein. Introns are intervening noncoding segments of DNA.	**IN**trons stay **IN** the nucleus, whereas **EX**ons **EX**it and are **EX**pressed.

Splicing of mRNA	Introns are precisely spliced out of 1° mRNA transcripts. A lariat-shaped intermediate is formed. Small nuclear ribonucleoprotein particles (snRNP) facilitate splicing by binding to 1° mRNA transcripts and forming spliceosomes.	
RNA processing (eukaryotes)	Occurs in nucleus. After transcription: 1. Capping on 5′ end (7-methyl-G) 2. Polyadenylation on 3′ end (≈ 200 A's) 3. Splicing out of introns Initial transcript is called heterogeneous nuclear RNA (hnRNA). Capped and tailed transcript is called mRNA.	Only processed RNA is transported out of the nucleus.
tRNA structure	75–90 nucleotides, cloverleaf form, anticodon end is opposite 3′ aminoacyl end. All tRNAs, both eukaryotic and prokaryotic, have CCA at 3′ end along with a high percentage of chemically modified bases. The amino acid is covalently bound to the 3′ end of the tRNA.	
tRNA charging	Aminoacyl-tRNA synthetase (1 per aa, uses ATP) scrutinizes aa before and after it binds to tRNA. If incorrect, bond is hydrolyzed by synthetase. The aa-tRNA bond has energy for formation of peptide bond. A mischarged tRNA reads usual codon but inserts wrong amino acid.	Aminoacyl-tRNA synthetase and binding of charged tRNA to the codon are responsible for accuracy of amino acid selection.
tRNA wobble	Accurate base pairing is required only in the first 2 nucleotide positions of an mRNA codon, so codons differing in the 3rd "wobble" position may code for the same tRNA/amino acid.	
Protein synthesis: ATP vs. GTP	P site—peptidyl; A site—aminoacyl. ATP is used in tRNA charging, whereas GTP is used in binding of tRNA to ribosome and for translocation.	**ATP**—tRNA **A**ctivation. **GTP**—tRNA **G**ripping and **G**oing places.

Polymerase chain reaction (PCR)	Molecular biology laboratory procedure that is used to synthesize many copies of a desired fragment of DNA. Steps: 1. DNA is denatured by heating to generate 2 separate strands 2. During cooling, excess premade DNA primers anneal to a specific sequence on each strand to be amplified 3. Heat-stable DNA polymerase replicates the DNA sequence following each primer These steps are repeated multiple times for DNA sequence amplification.	

Molecular biology techniques

Southern blot	A **DNA** sample is electrophoresed on a gel and then transferred to a filter. The filter is then soaked in a denaturant and subsequently exposed to a labeled DNA probe that recognizes and anneals to its complementary strand. The resulting double-stranded labeled piece of DNA is visualized when the filter is exposed to film.	DNA-DNA hybridization. **S**outhern = **S**ame.
Northern blot	Similar technique, except that Northern blotting involves radioactive DNA probe binding to sample **RNA.**	DNA-RNA hybridization.
Western blot	Sample protein is separated via gel electrophoresis and transferred to a filter. Labeled antibody is used to bind to relevant **protein.**	Antibody-protein hybridization.
Southwestern blot	Protein sample is run on a gel, transferred to a filter, and exposed to labeled DNA. Used to detect DNA-protein interactions as with transcription factors (e.g., *p53, jun*).	DNA-protein interaction.

Enzyme-linked immunosorbent assay (ELISA)	A rapid immunologic technique in which an antibody or an antigen is coupled to an enzyme as a means of detecting an antigenic match—it is a test of **antigen-antibody** reactivity. The test challenges patients' blood samples either with an antigen to see if their immune system recognizes it or with an antibody to see whether a particular antigen is present in their system. If the target substance is present in the sample, the test solution will have an intense color reaction indicating a positive test result.	ELISA is used in many laboratories to determine whether a particular antibody (e.g., anti-HIV) is present in a patient's blood sample. Both the sensitivity and the specificity of ELISA approach 100%, but both false-positive and false-negative results do occur.

HIGH-YIELD FACTS

Biochemistry

Modes of inheritance

Autosomal dominant

Often due to defects in structural genes. Many generations, both male and female, affected.

Often pleiotropic and, in many cases, present clinically after puberty. Family history crucial to diagnosis.

Autosomal recessive

25% of offspring from 2 carrier parents are affected. Often due to enzyme deficiencies. Usually seen in only 1 generation.

Commonly more severe than dominant disorders; patients often present in childhood.

X-linked recessive

Sons of heterozygous mothers have a 50% chance of being affected. No male-to-male transmission.

Commonly more severe in males. Heterozygous females may be affected.

Mitochondrial inheritance

Transmitted only through mother. All offspring of affected females may show signs of disease.

Leber's hereditary optic neuropathy; mitochondrial myopathies.

Genetic terms

Variable expression	Nature and severity of the phenotype varies from 1 individual to another.
Incomplete penetrance	Not all individuals with a mutant genotype show the mutant phenotype.
Pleiotropy	1 gene has > 1 effect on an individual's phenotype.
Imprinting	Differences in phenotype depend on whether the mutation is of maternal or paternal origin (e.g., Angelman's syndrome [maternal], Prader-Willi syndrome [paternal]).
Anticipation	Severity of disease worsens or age of onset of disease is earlier in succeeding generations (e.g., Huntington's disease).
Loss of heterozygosity	If a patient inherits or develops a mutation in a tumor suppressor gene, the complementary allele must be deleted/mutated before cancer develops. This is not true of oncogenes.
Dominant negative mutation	Exerts a **dominant** effect because the body cannot produce enough of the normal gene product with only 1 allele functioning normally (e.g., *COL1A1* gene mutation associated with osteogenesis imperfecta).
Linkage disequilibrium	Tendency for certain alleles at 2 linked loci to occur together more often than expected by chance. Measured in a population, not in a family, and often varies in different populations.
Mosaicism	Occurs when cells in the body have different genetic makeup.

Hardy-Weinberg population genetics

If a population is in Hardy-Weinberg equilibrium, then:

$$p^2 + 2pq + q^2 = 1$$
$$p + q = 1$$

p and q are separate alleles; 2pq = heterozygote prevalence.

Hardy-Weinberg law assumes:

1. There is no mutation occurring at the locus
2. There is no selection for any of the genotypes at the locus
3. Mating is completely random
4. There is no migration into or out of the population being considered

Genetic errors

Disorder	Phenotype	Genetic mechanism	Prevalence
Down syndrome	Mental and growth retardation, dysmorphic features, internal organ anomalies	Chromosomal imbalance caused by trisomy 21	≈ 1:800; ↑ risk with advanced maternal age
Fragile X–associated mental retardation	Mental retardation, characteristic facial features, large testes	X-linked; progressive expansion of unstable DNA causes failure to express gene-encoding RNA-binding protein	≈ 1:1500 males; can be manifest in females; multistep mechanism
Sickle cell anemia	Recurrent painful crises, ↑ susceptibility to infections	Autosomal recessive; caused by a single missense mutation in β globin	≈ 1:400 African-Americans
Cystic fibrosis	Recurrent pulmonary infections, exocrine pancreatic insufficiency, infertility	Autosomal recessive; caused by multiple loss-of-function mutations in a chloride channel	≈ 1:2000 whites; very rare in Asians
Neurofibromatosis	Multiple café-au-lait spots, neurofibromas, ↑ tumor susceptibility	Autosomal dominant; caused by multiple loss-of-function mutations in a signaling molecule	≈ 1:3000; about 50% are new mutations
Duchenne's muscular dystrophy	Muscular weakness and degeneration	X-linked recessive; caused by multiple loss-of-function mutations in a muscle protein	≈ 1:3000; about 33% are new mutations
Osteogenesis imperfecta	↑ susceptibility to fractures, connective tissue fragility	Phenotypically and genetically heterogeneous	≈ 1:10,000
Phenylketonuria	Mental and growth retardation	Autosomal recessive; caused by multiple loss-of-function mutations in phenylalanine hydroxylase	≈ 1:10,000

(Adapted, with permission, from McPhee S et al. *Pathophysiology of Disease: An Introduction to Clinical Medicine,* 3rd ed. New York: McGraw-Hill, 2000:7.)

Trinucleotide repeat expansion diseases

Friedreich's ataxia, Huntington's chorea, myotonic dystrophy, fragile X syndrome.

Lysosomal storage diseases

Each is caused by a deficiency in one of the many lysosomal enzymes.

Sphingolipidoses

Fabry's disease	Caused by deficiency of α-galactosidase A, resulting in accumulation of ceramide trihexoside. Finding: renal failure.	X-linked recessive.
Krabbe's disease	Absence of galactosylceramide β-galactosidase leads to the accumulation of galactocerebroside in the brain. Optic atrophy, spasticity, early death.	Autosomal recessive.
Gaucher's disease	Caused by deficiency of β-glucocerebrosidase, leading to glucocerebroside accumulation in brain, liver, spleen, and bone marrow (Gaucher's cells with characteristic "crinkled paper" enlarged cytoplasm). Type I, the more common form, is compatible with a normal life span.	Autosomal recessive.
Niemann-Pick disease	Deficiency of sphingomyelinase causes buildup of **sphingo**myelin and cholesterol in reticuloendothelial and parenchymal cells and tissues. Patients die by age 3.	Autosomal recessive. No **man** PICKs (Niemann-PICK) his nose with his **sphing**er.
Tay-Sachs disease	Absence of hexosaminidase A results in GM_2 ganglioside accumulation. Death occurs by age 3. Cherry-red spot visible on macula. Carrier rate is 1:30 in Jews of European descent (1:300 for others).	Autosomal recessive. **Tay-saX** lacks he**X**osaminidase.
Metachromatic leukodystrophy	Deficiency of arylsulfatase A results in the accumulation of sulfatide in the brain, kidney, liver, and peripheral nerves.	Autosomal recessive.

Mucopolysaccharidoses

Hurler's syndrome	Deficiency of α-L-iduronidase results in corneal clouding and mental retardation.	Autosomal recessive.
Hunter's syndrome	Deficiency of iduronate sulfatase. Mild form of Hurler's with no corneal clouding and mild mental retardation.	**X**-linked recessive. Hunters aim for the **X.**

GM_1
$\downarrow$
GM_2
Tay-Sachs ―┼―   Globoside
$\downarrow$ $\downarrow$
GM_3 Ceramide trihexoside
            ―┼― Fabry's
Sulfatides   Lactosyl cerebroside
Metachromatic ―┼― $\downarrow$
leukodystrophy
Galactocerebroside   Glucocerebroside
                    ―┼― Gaucher's
Krabbe's ―╳― $\downarrow$ ―┼― Sphingomyelin
            Cerebroside ◄―   Niemann-Pick

Enzyme kinetics

$$K_m = [S] \text{ at } \tfrac{1}{2} V_{max}$$

$$\text{slope} = \frac{K_m}{V_{max}}$$

The lower the K_m, the higher the affinity.

Competitive inhibitors— resemble substrates; bind reversibly to active sites of enzymes. High substrate concentration overcomes effect of inhibitor. V_{max} remains unchanged; K_m ↑ compared to uninhibited.

Noncompetitive inhibitors— do not resemble substrate; bind to enzyme but not necessarily at active site. Inhibition cannot be overcome by high substrate concentration. V_{max} ↓; K_m remains unchanged compared to uninhibited.

HINT: Competitive inhibitors cross each other competitively, while noncompetitive inhibitors do not.

Enzyme regulation methods

Enzyme concentration alteration (synthesis and/or destruction), covalent modification (e.g., phosphorylation), proteolytic modification (zymogen), allosteric regulation (e.g., feedback inhibition), and transcriptional regulation (e.g., steroid hormones).

Cell cycle phases

M (mitosis: prophase–metaphase– anaphase–telophase)
G_1 (growth)
S (synthesis of DNA)
G_2 (growth)
G_0 (quiescent G_1 phase)
G_1 and G_0 are of variable duration. Mitosis is usually shortest phase. Most cells are in G_0.
Rapidly dividing cells have a shorter G_1.

G stands for Gap or Growth; S for Synthesis.

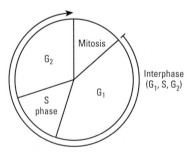

Plasma membrane composition

Plasma membranes contain cholesterol (≈ 50%, promotes membrane stability), phospholipids (≈ 50%), sphingolipids, glycolipids, and proteins. Only noncytoplasmic side of membrane contains glycosylated lipids or proteins (i.e., the plasma membrane is an asymmetric, fluid bilayer).

Phosphatidylcholine function

Phosphatidylcholine (lecithin) is a major component of RBC membranes, of myelin, of bile, and of surfactant (DPPC—dipalmitoyl phosphatidylcholine). Also used in esterification of cholesterol.

Sodium pump

Na^+-K^+ATPase is located in the plasma membrane with ATP site on cytoplasmic side. For each ATP consumed, 3 Na^+ go out and 2 K^+ come in. During cycle, pump is phosphorylated. Ouabain inhibits by binding to K^+ site. Cardiac glycosides (digoxin, digitoxin) also inhibit the Na^+-K^+ATPase, causing ↑ cardiac contractility.

G-protein-linked 2nd messengers

Receptor	G-protein class	Major functions
α_1	q	↑ vascular smooth muscle contraction
α_2	i	↓ sympathetic outflow, ↓ insulin release
β_1	s	↑ heart rate, ↑ contractility, ↑ renin release, ↑ lipolysis, ↑ aqueous humor formation
β_2	s	Vasodilation, bronchodilation, ↑ glucagon release
M_1	q	CNS
M_2	i	↓ heart rate
M_3	q	↑ exocrine gland secretions
D_1	s	Relaxes renal vascular smooth muscle
D_2	i	Modulates transmitter release, especially in brain
H_1	q	↑ nasal and bronchial mucus production, contraction of bronchioles, pruritus, and pain
H_2	s	↑ gastric acid secretion
V_1	q	↑ vascular smooth muscle contraction
V_2	s	↑ H_2O permeability and reabsorption in the collecting tubules of the kidney

α_1, M_1, M_3, H_1, V_1 Receptor $\xrightarrow{G_q}$ Phospholipase C ⟶ Lipids ↓ PIP_2 ⟶ IP_3 ⟶ ↑ $[Ca^{2+}]_{in}$; PIP_2 ⟶ DAG ⟶ Protein kinase C

β_1, β_2, D_1, H_2, V_2 Receptor $\xrightarrow{G_s}$ Adenylcyclase ⟶ ATP ↓ cAMP ⟶ Protein kinase A

α_2, M_2, D_2 Receptor $\xrightarrow{G_i}$ Adenylcyclase ⟶ cAMP ↓ ⟶ Protein kinase A ↓

HIGH-YIELD FACTS

Biochemistry

Arachidonic acid products

Phospholipase A_2 liberates arachidonic acid from cell membrane.

Lipoxygenase pathway yields Leukotrienes.

LT B_4 is a neutrophil chemotactic agent.

LT C_4, D_4, and E_4 (SRS-A) function in bronchoconstriction, vasoconstriction, contraction of smooth muscle, and ↑ vascular permeability.

Cyclooxygenase pathway yields thromboxanes, prostaglandins, and prostacyclin.

Tx A_2 stimulates platelet aggregation and vasoconstriction.

PGI$_2$ inhibits platelet aggregation and promotes vasodilation.

L for **L**ipoxygenase and **L**eukotriene.

Platelet-**G**athering **I**nhibitor.

Microtubule

24 nm

Cylindrical structure 24 nm in diameter and of variable length. A helical array of polymerized dimers of α- and β-tubulin (13 per circumference). Each dimer has 2 GTP bound. Incorporated into flagella, cilia, mitotic spindles. Grows slowly, collapses quickly. Microtubules are also involved in slow axoplasmic transport in neurons.

Drugs that act on microtubules:
1. Mebendazole/thiabendazole (antihelminthic)
2. Taxol (anti–breast cancer)
3. Griseofulvin (antifungal)
4. Vincristine/vinblastine (anti-cancer)
5. Colchicine (anti-gout)

Collagen synthesis and structure

Hydroxylation of specific prolyl and lysyl residues in the endoplasmic reticulum requires vitamin C.

Procollagen molecules are exocytosed into extracellular space. Procollagen peptidases cleave terminal regions of procollagen, transforming procollagen into insoluble tropocollagen, which aggregates to form collagen fibrils.

Fibrillar structure is reinforced by the formation of covalent lysine-hydroxylysine cross-links between tropocollagen molecules.

Collagen fibril—many staggered collagen molecules (linked by lysyl oxidase). Collagen molecule—3 collagen α chains (usually Gly-X-Y, X and Y—proline, hydroxyproline, or hydroxylysine).

Ehlers-Danlos syndrome

Faulty collagen synthesis causing:
1. Hyperextensible skin
2. Tendency to bleed
3. Hypermobile joints

10 types. Inheritance varies from autosomal dominant (type IV) to autosomal recessive (type VI) to X-linked recessive (type IX). Associated with berry aneurysms.

| Osteogenesis imperfecta | Clinically characterized by **multiple fractures** occurring with minimal trauma (brittle bone disease), which may occur during the birth process, as well as by **blue sclerae** due to the translucency of the connective tissue over the choroid. Caused by a variety of gene defects resulting in abnormal collagen synthesis.

The most common form is autosomal dominant with abnormal collagen type I synthesis. | May be confused with child abuse. |

BIOCHEMISTRY—METABOLISM

| ATP | Base (adenine), ribose, 3 phosphoryls. 2 phosphoanhydride bonds, 7 kcal/mol each.
Aerobic metabolism of glucose produces 38 ATP via malate shuttle, 36 ATP via G3P shuttle.
Anaerobic glycolysis produces only 2 ATP per glucose molecule.
ATP hydrolysis can be coupled to energetically unfavorable reactions. | |

| Activated carriers | Phosphoryl (ATP)
Electrons (NADH, NADPH, $FADH_2$)
Acyl (coenzyme A, lipoamide)
CO_2 (biotin)
1-carbon units (tetrahydrofolates)
CH_3 groups (SAM)
Aldehydes (TPP)
Glucose (UDP-glucose)
Choline (CDP-choline) | |

| *S*-adenosyl-methionine | ATP + methionine → **SAM.** SAM transfers methyl units to a wide variety of acceptors (e.g., in synthesis of phosphocreatine, a high-energy phosphate active in muscle ATP production). Regeneration of methionine (and thus SAM) is dependent on vitamin B_{12}. | **SAM** the methyl donor man. |

Signal molecule precursors

ATP → cAMP via adenylate cyclase.

GTP → cGMP via guanylate cyclase.

Glutamate → GABA via glutamate decarboxylase (requires vitamin B_6).

Choline → ACh via choline acetyltransferase (ChAT).

Arachidonate → prostaglandins, thromboxanes, leukotrienes via cyclooxygenase/lipoxygenase.

Fructose-6-P → fructose-1,6-bis-P via phosphofructokinase (PFK), the rate-limiting enzyme of glycolysis.

1,3-BPG → 2,3-BPG via bisphosphoglycerate mutase.

NAD^+/NADPH

NAD^+ is generally used in **catabolic** processes to carry reducing equivalents away as NADH. **NADPH** is used in **anabolic** processes as a supply of reducing equivalents.

NADPH is a product of the HMP shunt and the malate dehydrogenase reaction.

NADPH is used in:
1. Anabolic processes
2. Respiratory burst
3. P-450

Oxygen-dependent respiratory burst

SOD = superoxide dismutase
MPO = myeloperoxidase
G6P = glucose-6-phosphate dehydrogenase

GSH/GSSG = glutathione (reduced/oxidized)
HOCl• = bleach

Hexokinase vs. glucokinase

Hexokinase is found throughout body.

Glucokinase (lower affinity [↑ K_m] but higher capacity [↑ V_{max}]) is predominantly found in the liver.

Only hexokinase is feedback inhibited by G6P.

Glycolysis regulation, irreversible enzymes	D-glucose $\xrightarrow[\text{Hexokinase/glucokinase}^*]{}$ Glucose-6-phosphate	Glucose-6-P $\ominus$
	Fructose-6-P $\xrightarrow[\substack{\text{Phosphofructokinase}\\\text{(rate-limiting step)}}]{}$ Fructose-1,6-BP	ATP $\ominus$, AMP $\oplus$, citrate $\ominus$, fructose-2,6-BP $\oplus$
	Phosphoenolpyruvate $\xrightarrow[\text{Pyruvate kinase}]{}$ Pyruvate	ATP $\ominus$, alanine $\ominus$, fructose-1,6-BP $\oplus$
	Pyruvate $\xrightarrow[\substack{\text{Pyruvate}\\\text{dehydrogenase}}]{}$ Acetyl-CoA	ATP $\ominus$, NADH $\ominus$, acetyl-CoA $\ominus$

* Glucokinase in liver; hexokinase in all other tissues.

Glycolytic enzyme deficiency	Hexokinase, glucose phosphate isomerase, aldolase, triosephosphate isomerase, phosphate glycerate kinase, enolase, and pyruvate kinase deficiencies are associated with hemolytic anemia.	RBCs metabolize glucose anaerobically (no mitochondria) and thus depend solely on glycolysis.
Pyruvate dehydrogenase complex	The complex contains 3 enzymes that require 5 cofactors: pyrophosphate (from thiamine), lipoic acid, CoA (from pantothenate), FAD (riboflavin), NAD (niacin). Reaction: pyruvate + NAD$^+$ + CoA $\rightarrow$ acetyl-CoA + CO$_2$ + NADH.	The complex is similar to the α-ketoglutarate dehydrogenase complex (same cofactors, similar substrate and action). Cofactors are the first 4 B vitamins plus lipoic acid: B$_1$ (thiamine; TPP) B$_2$ (FAD) B$_3$ (NAD) B$_5$ (pantothenate $\rightarrow$ CoA) Lipoic acid
Pyruvate dehydrogenase deficiency	Causes backup of substrate (pyruvate and alanine), resulting in lactic acidosis. Can be seen in alcoholics due to B$_1$ deficiency. Findings: neurologic defects. Treatment: $\uparrow$ intake of ketogenic nutrients (e.g., high fat content).	**L**ysine and **L**eucine—the only purely ketogenic amino acids.

Pyruvate metabolism

6 ATP equivalents are needed to generate glucose from pyruvate.

Alanine serves as carrier of amino groups from muscle to liver.

Oxaloacetate can be used to replenish TCA cycle or in gluconeogenesis.

Cori cycle

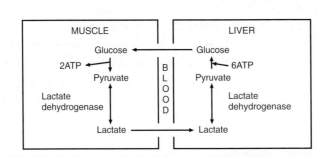

Transfers excess reducing equivalents from RBCs and muscle to liver, allowing muscle to function anaerobically (net 2 ATP).

TCA cycle

Produces 3 NADH, 1 FADH$_2$, 2 CO$_2$, 1 GTP per acetyl-CoA = 12 ATP/acetyl-CoA (2× everything per glucose)

α-ketoglutarate dehydrogenase complex requires same cofactors as the pyruvate dehydrogenase complex.

Cindy **I**s **K**inky **S**o **S**he **F**ornicates **M**ore **O**ften.

Biochemistry

HIGH-YIELD FACTS

Electron transport chain and oxidative phosphorylation

| Electron transport chain | $1 \text{ NADH} \rightarrow 3 \text{ ATP}; 1 \text{ FADH}_2 \rightarrow 2 \text{ ATP}$ |

Oxidative phosphorylation poisons

1. Electron transport inhibitors (rotenone, antimycin A, CN^-, CO) directly inhibit electron transport, causing a $\downarrow$ of proton gradient and block of ATP synthesis.
2. ATPase inhibitor (oligomycin) directly inhibits mitochondrial ATPase, causing an $\uparrow$ of proton gradient, but no ATP is produced because electron transport stops.
3. Uncoupling agents (2,4-DNP) increase permeability of membrane, causing a $\downarrow$ of proton gradient and $\uparrow$ O_2 consumption. ATP synthesis stops. Electron transport continues.

Gluconeogenesis, irreversible enzymes

Pyruvate carboxylase	In mitochondria. Pyruvate $\rightarrow$ oxaloacetate.	Requires biotin, ATP. Activated by acetyl-CoA.
PEP carboxykinase	In cytosol. Oxaloacetate $\rightarrow$ phosphoenolpyruvate.	Requires GTP.
Fructose-1,6-bisphosphatase	In cytosol. Fructose-1,6-bisphosphate $\rightarrow$ fructose-6-P.	
Glucose-6-phosphatase	In cytosol. Glucose-6-P $\rightarrow$ glucose.	Pathway Produces Fresh Glucose.

Above enzymes found only in liver, kidney, intestinal epithelium. Muscle cannot participate in gluconeogenesis.

Hypoglycemia is caused by a deficiency of the key gluconeogenic enzymes listed above (e.g., von Gierke's disease, which is caused by a lack of glucose-6-phosphatase in the liver).

Pentose phosphate pathway (HMP shunt)

Produces ribose-5-P from G6P for nucleotide synthesis.

Produces NADPH from $NADP^+$ for fatty acid and steroid biosynthesis and for maintaining reduced glutathione inside RBCs.

All reactions of this pathway occur in the cytoplasm.

Sites: lactating mammary glands, liver, adrenal cortex—all sites of fatty acid or steroid synthesis.

Glucose-6-phosphate dehydrogenase deficiency

G6PD is a rate-limiting enzyme in HMP shunt (which yields NADPH). NADPH is necessary to keep glutathione reduced, which in turn detoxifies free radicals and peroxides. ↓ NADPH in RBCs leads to **hemolytic anemia** due to poor RBC defense against oxidizing agents (fava beans, sulfonamides, primaquine) and antituberculosis drugs. X-linked recessive disorder.

G6PD deficiency is more prevalent among blacks.

Heinz bodies—altered **H**emoglobin precipitates within RBCs.

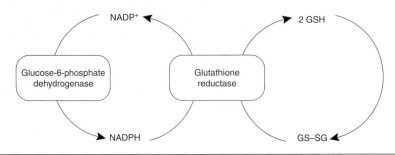

Disorders of fructose metabolism

Fructose intolerance
Hereditary deficiency of aldolase B (recessive). Fructose-1-phosphate accumulates, causing a ↓ in available phosphate, which results in inhibition of glycogenolysis and gluconeogenesis.

Symptoms: hypoglycemia, jaundice, cirrhosis.

Treatment: must ↓ intake of both fructose and sucrose (glucose + fructose).

Essential fructosuria
Involves a defect in fructokinase and is a benign, asymptomatic condition.

Symptoms: fructose appears in blood and urine.

FRUCTOSE METABOLISM (LIVER)

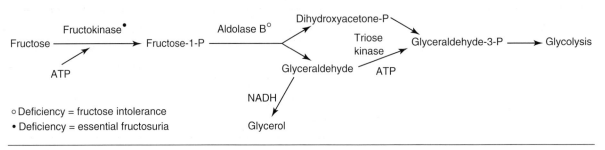

○ Deficiency = fructose intolerance
• Deficiency = essential fructosuria

Disorders of galactose metabolism

Galactosemia

Absence of galactose-1-phosphate uridyltransferase. Autosomal recessive. Damage is caused by accumulation of toxic substances (including galactitol) rather than absence of an essential compound.

Symptoms: cataracts, hepatosplenomegaly, mental retardation.

Treatment: exclude galactose and lactose (galactose + glucose) from diet.

Galactokinase deficiency

Causes galactosemia and galactosuria, galactitol accumulation if galactose is present in diet.

GALACTOSE METABOLISM

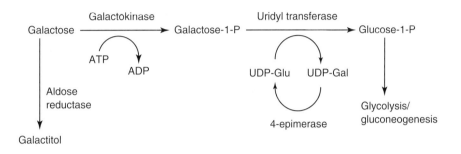

Lactase deficiency

Age-dependent and/or hereditary lactose intolerance (blacks, Asians).

Symptoms: bloating, cramps, osmotic diarrhea.

Treatment: avoid milk or add lactase pills to diet.

Essential amino acids

Ketogenic: **Leu, Lys.**

Glucogenic/ketogenic: **Ile, Phe, Trp.**

Glucogenic: **Met, Thr, Val, Arg, His.**

All essential amino acids: **PriVaTe TIM HALL.** Arg and His are required during periods of growth.

Acidic and basic amino acids

At body pH (7.4), acidic amino acids Asp and Glu are negatively charged; basic amino acids Arg and Lys are positively charged. Basic amino acid His at pH 7.4 has no net charge.

Arginine is the most basic amino acid. Arg and Lys are found in high amounts in histones, which bind to negatively charged DNA.

Asp = aspartic ACID, Glu = glutamic ACID.

Arg and Lys have an extra NH_3 group.

Transport of ammonium by alanine and glutamine

Urea cycle

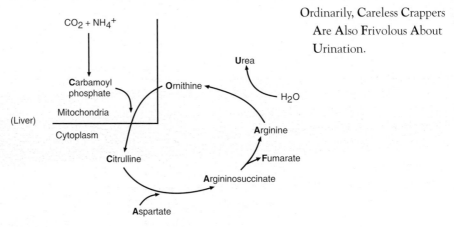

Ordinarily, Careless Crappers Are Also Frivolous About Urination.

Amino acid derivatives

Phenylalanine ⟶ Tyrosine ⟶ Dopa ⟶ Dopamine
- Tyrosine ⟶ Thyroxine
- Dopamine ⟶ NE ⟶ Epi
- Dopamine ⟶ Melanin

Tryptophan
- ⟶ Niacin ⟶ $NAD^+/NADP^+$
- ⟶ Serotonin
- ⟶ Melatonin

Histidine ⟶ Histamine

Glycine ⟶ Porphyrin ⟶ Heme

Arginine
- ⟶ Creatine
- ⟶ Urea
- ⟶ Nitric oxide

158

Phenylketonuria

Normally, phenylalanine is converted into tyrosine (nonessential aa). In PKU, there is ↓ phenylalanine hydroxylase or ↓ tetrahydrobiopterin cofactor. Tyrosine becomes essential and phenylalanine builds up, leading to excess phenylketones.

Findings: mental retardation, fair skin, eczema, musty body odor.

Treatment: ↓ phenylalanine (contained in Nutrasweet) and ↑ tyrosine in diet.

Screened for at birth. Phenylketones—phenylacetate, phenyllactate, and phenylpyruvate in urine.

Alkaptonuria

Congenital deficiency of homogentisic acid oxidase in the degradative pathway of tyrosine. Resulting alkapton bodies cause **dark urine.** Also, the connective tissue is dark. Benign disease. May have arthralgias.

Albinism

Congenital deficiency of tyrosinase. Results in an inability to synthesize melanin from tyrosine. Can result from a lack of migration of neural crest cells.

Lack of melanin results in an ↑ risk of skin cancer.

Homocystinuria

Defect in cystathionine synthase and/or methionine synthase. 2 forms:
1. Deficiency (treatment: ↓ Met and ↑ Cys in diet)
2. ↓ affinity of synthase for pyridoxal phosphate (treatment: ↑↑ vitamin B_6 in diet)

Results in excess homocysteine in the urine. Cysteine becomes essential.

Can cause mental retardation, osteoporosis, and lens dislocation.

Cystinuria

Common (1:7000) inherited defect of tubular amino acid transporter for **C**ystine, **O**rnithine, **L**ysine, and **A**rginine in kidneys. Excess cystine in urine can lead to the precipitation of cystine kidney stones.

COLA.
Treat with acetazolamide to alkalinize the urine.

Maple syrup urine disease

Blocked degradation of **branched** amino acids (Ile, Val, Leu) due to ↓ α-ketoacid dehydrogenase.

Causes severe CNS defects, mental retardation, and death.

Urine smells like maple syrup.
I Love **V**ermont maple syrup.

Purine salvage deficiencies

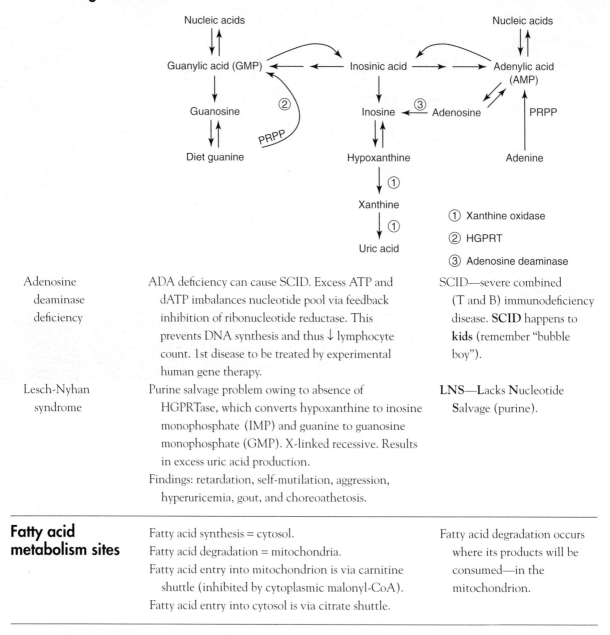

① Xanthine oxidase

② HGPRT

③ Adenosine deaminase

Adenosine deaminase deficiency	ADA deficiency can cause SCID. Excess ATP and dATP imbalances nucleotide pool via feedback inhibition of ribonucleotide reductase. This prevents DNA synthesis and thus ↓ lymphocyte count. 1st disease to be treated by experimental human gene therapy.	SCID—severe combined (T and B) immunodeficiency disease. **SCID** happens to **kids** (remember "bubble boy").
Lesch-Nyhan syndrome	Purine salvage problem owing to absence of HGPRTase, which converts hypoxanthine to inosine monophosphate (IMP) and guanine to guanosine monophosphate (GMP). X-linked recessive. Results in excess uric acid production. Findings: retardation, self-mutilation, aggression, hyperuricemia, gout, and choreoathetosis.	**LNS**—**L**acks **N**ucleotide **S**alvage (purine).

| **Fatty acid metabolism sites** | Fatty acid synthesis = cytosol.
Fatty acid degradation = mitochondria.
Fatty acid entry into mitochondrion is via carnitine shuttle (inhibited by cytoplasmic malonyl-CoA).
Fatty acid entry into cytosol is via citrate shuttle. | Fatty acid degradation occurs where its products will be consumed—in the mitochondrion. |

Liver: fed state vs. fasting state

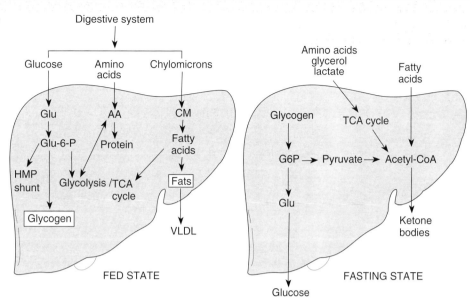

Glycogen storage diseases

12 types, all resulting in abnormal glycogen metabolism and an accumulation of glycogen within cells.

Type I

Von Gierke's disease—glucose-6-phosphatase deficiency.
Findings: severe fasting hypoglycemia, ↑↑ glycogen in liver.

The liver becomes a muscle. (Think about it.)

Type II

Pompe's disease—lysosomal α-1,4-glucosidase deficiency.
Findings: cardiomegaly and systemic findings, leading to early death.

Pompe's trashes the Pump (heart, liver, and muscle).

Type III

Cori's—deficiency of debranching enzyme α-1,6-glucosidase.

Type V

McArdle's disease—skeletal muscle glycogen phosphorylase deficiency.
Findings: ↑ glycogen in muscle but cannot break it down, leading to painful cramps, myoglobinuria with strenuous exercise.

McArdle's: Muscle.

Very Poor Carbohydrate Metabolism.

Ketone bodies

In liver: fatty acid and amino acids → acetoacetate + β-hydroxybutyrate (to be used in muscle and brain). Ketone bodies found in prolonged starvation and diabetic ketoacidosis. Excreted in urine. Made from HMG-CoA. Ketone bodies are metabolized by the brain to 2 molecules of acetyl-CoA.

Breath smells like acetone (fruity odor). Urine test for ketones does not detect β-hydroxybutyrate (favored by high redox state).

Insulin

Made in β cells of pancreas. No effect on glucose uptake by brain, RBCs, and hepatocytes. Required for adipose and skeletal muscle uptake of glucose. GLUT2 receptors are found in β cells and GLUT4 in muscle and fat. Inhibits glucagon release by α cells of pancreas. Serum C-peptide is not present with exogenous insulin intake.

Brain, liver, and RBCs take up glucose independent of insulin. Insulin moves glucose Into cells.

Insulin vs. glucagon	Glucagon phosphorylates stuff → turns glycogen synthase OFF and phosphorylase ON. Insulin dephosphorylates stuff → turns glycogen synthase ON and phosphorylase OFF.

Cholesterol synthesis	Rate-limiting step is catalyzed by HMG-CoA reductase, which converts HMG-CoA to mevalonate. ⅔ of plasma cholesterol is esterified by lecithin-cholesterol acyltransferase (LCAT).	Lovastatin inhibits HMG-CoA reductase.

Lipoproteins

TG = triglyceride, CE = cholesterol, FFA = free fatty acid

Lipoprotein lipase—fatty acid uptake into cells from chylomicrons and VLDLs.
Hormone-sensitive lipase—degradation of stored triacylglycerols.

Major apolipoproteins	A-I—Activates LCAT. B-100—Binds to LDL receptor. C-II—Cofactor for lipoprotein lipase. E—Mediates Extra (remnant) uptake.

Lipoprotein functions

	Function and route	Apolipoproteins
Chylomicron	Delivers dietary triglycerides to peripheral tissues and dietary cholesterol to liver. Secreted by intestinal epithelial cells. Excess causes pancreatitis, lipemia retinalis, and eruptive xanthomas.	B-48 mediates secretion. A's are used for formation of new HDL. C-II activates lipoprotein lipase. E mediates remnant uptake by liver.
VLDL	Delivers hepatic triglycerides to peripheral tissues. Secreted by liver. Excess causes pancreatitis.	B-100 mediates secretion. C-II activates lipoprotein lipase. E mediates remnant uptake by liver.
LDL	Delivers hepatic cholesterol to peripheral tissues. Formed by lipoprotein lipase modification of VLDL in the peripheral tissue. Taken up by target cells via receptor-mediated endocytosis. Excess causes atherosclerosis, xanthomas, and arcus corneae.	B-100 mediates binding to cell surface receptor for endocytosis.
HDL	Mediates centripetal transport of cholesterol (reverse cholesterol transport, from periphery to liver). Acts as a repository for apoC and apoE (which are needed for chylomicron and VLDL metabolism). Secreted from both liver and intestine.	A's help form HDL structure. A-I in particular activates LCAT (which catalyzes esterification of cholesterol). CETP mediates transfer of cholesteryl esters to other lipoprotein particles.
	LDL and HDL carry most cholesterol. LDL transports cholesterol from liver to tissue; HDL transports it from periphery to liver.	**HDL** is **H**ealthy. **LDL** is **L**ousy.

Familial dyslipidemias

Type	Increased	Elevated blood levels	Pathophysiology
I—hyperchylomicronemia	Chylomicrons	TG	Lipoprotein lipase deficiency or altered apolipoprotein C-II
IIa—hypercholesterolemia	LDL	Cholesterol	↓ LDL receptors
IIb—combined hyperlipidemia	LDL, VLDL	TG, cholesterol	Hepatic ↑ synthesis of VLDL
III—dysbetalipoproteinemia	IDL, VLDL	TG, cholesterol	Altered apolipoprotein E
IV—hypertriglyceridemia	VLDL	TG	Hepatic overproduction of VLDL
V—mixed hypertriglyceridemia	VLDL, chylomicrons	TG, cholesterol	↑ production/↓ clearance of VLDL and chylomicrons

Metabolism sites

Mitochondria	Fatty acid oxidation (β-oxidation), acetyl-CoA production, Krebs cycle.
Cytoplasm	Glycolysis, fatty acid synthesis, HMP shunt, protein synthesis (RER), steroid synthesis (SER).
Both	Gluconeogenesis, urea cycle, heme synthesis.

Regulation of metabolic pathways

Pathway	Major Regulatory Enzyme(s)	Activator	Inhibitor	Effector Hormone	Remarks
Citric acid cycle	Citrate synthase		ATP, long-chain acyl-CoA		Regulated mainly by the need for ATP and therefore by the supply of NAD+
Glycolysis and pyruvate oxidation	Phospho-fructokinase-1	AMP, fructose-2,6-bisphosphate in liver, fructose-1,6-bisphosphate in muscle	Citrate (fatty acids, ketone bodies), ATP, cAMP	Glucagon ↓	Induced by insulin
	Pyruvate dehydrogenase	CoA, NAD, ADP, pyruvate	Acetyl-CoA, NADH, ATP (fatty acids, ketone bodies)	Insulin ↑ (in adipose tissue)	Also important in regulating the citric acid cycle
Gluconeogenesis	Pyruvate carboxylase Phosphoenolpyruvate carboxykinase	Acetyl-CoA	ADP		Induced by glu-cocorticoids, glucagon, cAMP
	Fructose-1,6-bisphosphatase	cAMP	AMP, fructose-2,6-bisphosphate	Glucagon	Suppressed by insulin
Glycogenesis	Glycogen synthase		Phosphorylase (in liver) cAMP, Ca²⁺ (muscle)	Insulin ↑ Glucagon ↓ (liver) Epinephrine ↓	Induced by insulin
Glycogenolysis	Phosphorylase	cAMP, Ca²⁺ (muscle)		Insulin ↓ Glucagon ↑ (liver) Epinephrine ↑	
Pentose phosphate pathway	Glucose-6-phosphate dehydrogenase	NADP+	NADPH		Induced by insulin
Lipogenesis	Acetyl-CoA carboxylase	Citrate	Long-chain acyl-CoA, cAMP	Insulin ↑ Glucagon ↓ (liver)	Induced by insulin
Cholesterol synthesis	HMG-CoA reductase		Cholesterol, cAMP	Insulin ↑ Glucagon ↓ (liver)	Inhibited by certain drugs, e.g., lovastatin

Aminolevulinate (ALA) synthase	Rate-limiting step for heme synthesis. The end-product (heme) feedback inhibits this enzyme. Found in the mitochondria, where it converts succinyl-CoA and glycine to ALA.	
Heme synthesis	Occurs in the liver and bone marrow. Committed step is glycine + succinyl-CoA → δ-aminolevulinate. Catalyzed by ALA synthase. Accumulation of intermediates causes porphyrias.	Underproduction of heme causes microcytic hypochromic anemia.

Porphyrias

Acute intermittent porphyria	Deficiency in uroporphyrinogen I synthetase, leading to accumulation of δ-ALA and porphobilinogen in urine. Symptoms include abdominal pain and neuropsychiatric disturbances.	
Lead poisoning	Lead inhibits ferrochelatase and ALA dehydratase, leading to ALA and coproporphyrin III accumulation in urine and anemia (prevents iron incorporation).	
Porphyria cutanea tarda	Deficiency in uroporphyrinogen decarboxylase. Uroporphyrin seen in urine. Most common porphyria.	

Heme catabolism	Heme is scavenged from RBCs and Fe^{2+} is reused. Heme → biliverdin → bilirubin (sparingly water soluble, toxic to CNS, transported by albumin). Bilirubin is removed from blood by liver, conjugated with glucuronate, and excreted in bile. In the intestine it is processed into its excreted form. Some urobilinogen, an intestinal intermediate, is reabsorbed into blood and excreted as urobilin into urine.	
Hemoglobin	Hemoglobin is composed of 4 polypeptide subunits (2 α and 2 β) and exists in 2 forms: 1. T (taut) form has low affinity for O_2. 2. R (relaxed) form has high affinity for O_2 (300×). Hemoglobin exhibits positive cooperativity and negative allostery (accounts for the sigmoid-shaped O_2 dissociation curve for hemoglobin), unlike myoglobin.	Carbon monoxide has 200× greater affinity for hemoglobin than for O_2.
Hb structure regulation	↑ Cl^-, H^+, CO_2, DPG, and temperature favor T form over **R** form (shifts dissociation curve to right, leading to ↑ O_2 unloading). T form has low affinity for O_2.	When you're **R**elaxed, you do your job better (carry O_2).
Methemo-globinemia	Iron in hemoglobin is in a reduced state (ferrous, Fe^{2+}). Methemoglobin is an oxidized form of hemoglobin (ferric, Fe^{3+}) that does not bind O_2 as readily.	
CO_2 transport in blood	CO_2 binds to amino acids in globin chain (at N terminus) but not to heme. CO_2 binding favors T (taut) form of hemoglobin (and thus promotes O_2 unloading).	CO_2 must be transported from tissue to lungs, the reverse of O_2.

Vitamins

Vitamins: fat soluble	A, D, E, K. Absorption dependent on gut (ileum) and pancreas. Toxicity more common than for water-soluble vitamins, because these accumulate in fat.	Malabsorption syndromes (steatorrhea), such as cystic fibrosis and sprue, or mineral oil intake can cause fat-soluble vitamin deficiencies.
Vitamins: water soluble	B_1 (thiamine: TPP) B_2 (riboflavin: FAD, FMN) B_3 (niacin: NAD^+) B_5 (pantothenate: CoA) B_6 (pyridoxine: PP) B_{12} (cobalamin) C (ascorbic acid) Biotin Folate	All wash out easily from body except B_{12} (stored in liver). B-complex deficiencies often result in dermatitis, glossitis, and diarrhea.

Vitamin A (retinol)

Deficiency	Night blindness and dry skin.	**Retinol** is vitamin **A,** so think
Function	Constituent of visual pigments (retinal).	**Retin-A** (used topically for
Excess	Arthralgias, fatigue, headaches, skin changes, sore throat, alopecia.	wrinkles and acne).

Vitamin B_1 (thiamine)

Deficiency	Beriberi and Wernicke-Korsakoff syndrome. Seen in alcoholism and malnutrition.	Beriberi characterized by polyneuritis, cardiac pathology, and edema. Spell
Function	In thiamine pyrophosphate, a cofactor for oxidative decarboxylation of α-keto acids (pyruvate, α-ketoglutarate) and a cofactor for transketolase in the HMP shunt.	beriberi as **Ber1Ber1.** Wet beriberi may lead to high-output cardiac failure (dilated cardiomyopathy).

Vitamin B$_2$ (riboflavin)

Deficiency	Angular stomatitis, **C**heilosis, **C**orneal vascularization.	The 2 **C**'s.
Function	Cofactor in oxidation and reduction (e.g., FADH$_2$).	**FAD** and **FMN** are derived from ribo**F**lavin (B$_2$ = 2 ATP).

Vitamin B$_3$ (niacin)

Deficiency	Pellagra can be caused by Hartnup disease, malignant carcinoid syndrome, and INH.	Pellagra's symptoms are the **3 D's:** **D**iarrhea, **D**ermatitis, **D**ementia (also beefy glossitis).
Function	Constituent of NAD$^+$, NADP$^+$ (used in redox reactions). Derived from tryptophan.	**NAD** derived from **N**iacin (B$_3$ = 3 ATP).

Vitamin B$_5$ (pantothenate)

Deficiency	Dermatitis, enteritis, alopecia, adrenal insufficiency.	
Function	Constituent of CoA, part of fatty acid synthase. Cofactor for acyl transfers.	Pantothen-**A** is in Co-**A**.

Vitamin B$_6$ (pyridoxine)

Deficiency	Convulsions, hyperirritability (deficiency inducible by INH and oral contraceptives).
Function	Converted to pyridoxal phosphate, a cofactor used in transamination (e.g., ALT and AST), decarboxylation, and trans-sulfuration.

Biotin

Deficiency	Dermatitis, enteritis. Caused by antibiotic use, ingestion of raw eggs.	"**AVID**in in egg whites **AVID**ly binds biotin."
Function	Cofactor for carboxylations: 1. Pyruvate → oxaloacetate 2. Acetyl-CoA → malonyl-CoA 3. Proprionyl-CoA → methylmalonyl-CoA	

Folic acid

Deficiency	Most common vitamin deficiency in the United States. Macrocytic, megaloblastic anemia (often no neurologic symptoms, as opposed to vitamin B$_{12}$ deficiency), sprue.	**FOL**ate from **FOL**iage. Eat green leaves (because folic acid is not stored very long). Supplemental folic acid in early pregnancy reduces neural tube defects.
Function	Coenzyme for 1-carbon transfer; involved in methylation reactions. Important for the synthesis of nitrogenous bases in DNA and RNA.	PABA is the folic acid precursor in bacteria. Sulfa drugs and dapsone are PABA analogs.

Vitamin B₁₂ (cobalamin)

Deficiency   Macrocytic, megaloblastic anemia; neurologic symptoms (optic neuropathy, subacute combined degeneration, paresthesia); glossitis.

Function   Cofactor for homocysteine methylation and methylmalonyl-CoA handling.
Stored primarily in the liver.
Synthesized only by microorganisms.

Found only in animal products.
Vitamin B₁₂ deficiency is usually caused by malabsorption (sprue, enteritis, *Diphyllobothrium latum*), lack of intrinsic factor (pernicious anemia), or absence of terminal ileum (Crohn's disease).
Use Schilling test to detect deficiency.

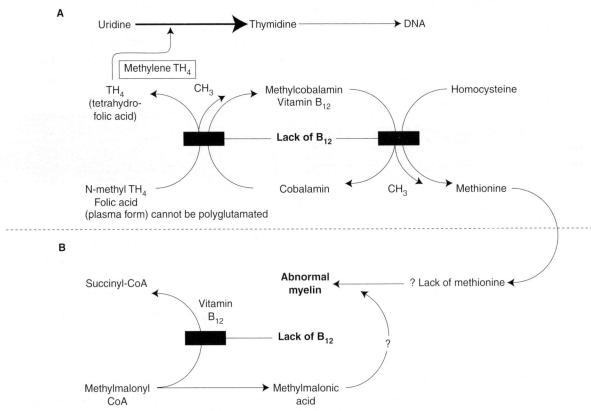

(**A.** Adapted, with permission, from McPhee S et al. *Pathophysiology of Disease: An Introduction to Clinical Medicine*, 3rd ed. New York: McGraw-Hill, 2000:113.
B. Adapted, with permission, from McPhee S et al. *Pathophysiology of Disease: An Introduction to Clinical Medicine*, 3rd ed. New York: McGraw-Hill, 2000:113, as modified from Chandrasoma P et al. *Concise Pathology*, 3rd ed. Stamford, CT: Appleton & Lange, 1998.)

Vitamin C (ascorbic acid)

Deficiency	Scurvy.	Vitamin **C** Cross-links **C**ollagen. British sailors carried limes to prevent scurvy (origin of the word "limey").
Function	Necessary for hydroxylation of proline and lysine in collagen synthesis.	
	Facilitates iron absorption by keeping iron in Fe^{+2} reduced state (more absorbable)	
	Necessary as a cofactor for dopamine $\rightarrow$ NE.	
	Scurvy findings: swollen gums, bruising, anemia, poor wound healing.	

Vitamin D

	D_2 = ergocalciferol, consumed in milk.	Remember that drinking milk (fortified with vitamin D) is good for bones.
	D_3 = cholecalciferol, formed in sun-exposed skin.	
	25-OH D_3 = storage form.	
	1,25 $(OH)_2$ D_3 = active form.	Causes of hypercalcemia:
Deficiency	Rickets in children (bending bones), osteomalacia in adults (soft bones), and hypocalcemic tetany.	1. Vitamin D intoxication 2. Malignancy
Function	↑ intestinal absorption of calcium and phosphate.	3. Hyperparathyroidism
Excess	Hypercalcemia, loss of appetite, stupor. Seen in sarcoidosis, a disease where the epithelioid macrophages convert vitamin D into its active form.	4. Milk-alkali syndrome 5. Sarcoidosis 6. Paget's disease of bone

Vitamin E

Deficiency	Increased fragility of erythrocytes.	Vitamin **E** is for **E**rythrocytes.
Function	Antioxidant (protects erythrocytes from hemolysis).	

Vitamin K

Deficiency	Neonatal hemorrhage with ↑ PT and ↑ aPTT but normal bleeding time.	**K** for **K**oagulation. Note that the vitamin K–dependent clotting factors are II, VII, IX, X, and protein C and S. Warfarin is a vitamin K antagonist.
Function	Catalyzes γ-carboxylation of glutamic acid residues on various proteins concerned with blood clotting. Synthesized by intestinal flora. Therefore, vitamin K deficiency can occur after the prolonged use of broad-spectrum antibiotics.	

Ethanol metabolism

Alcohol dehydrogenase: Ethanol $\rightarrow$ Acetaldehyde ($NAD^+ \rightarrow NADH$)

Acetaldehyde dehydrogenase: Acetaldehyde $\rightarrow$ Acetate ($NAD^+ \rightarrow NADH$)

NAD^+ is the limiting reagent.
Alcohol dehydrogenase operates via zero-order kinetics.

Disulfiram (Antabuse) inhibits acetaldehyde dehydrogenase (acetaldehyde accumulates, contributing to hangover symptoms).

Ethanol hypoglycemia

Ethanol metabolism ↑ NADH/NAD$^+$ ratio in liver, causing diversion of pyruvate to lactate and OAA to malate, thereby inhibiting gluconeogenesis and leading to hypoglycemia. This altered NADH/NAD+ ratio is responsible for the hepatic fatty change (hepatocellular steatosis) seen in chronic alcoholics (shunting away from glycolysis and toward fatty acid synthesis).

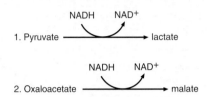

1. Pyruvate → lactate (NADH → NAD$^+$)

2. Oxaloacetate → malate (NADH → NAD$^+$)

Kwashiorkor vs. marasmus

Kwashiorkor—protein malnutrition resulting in skin lesions, edema, liver malfunction (fatty change). Clinical picture is small child with swollen belly.
Marasmus—protein-calorie malnutrition resulting in tissue wasting.

Kwashiorkor results from a protein-deficient **MEAL:**
Malabsorption
Edema
Anemia
Liver (fatty)

Summary of pathways

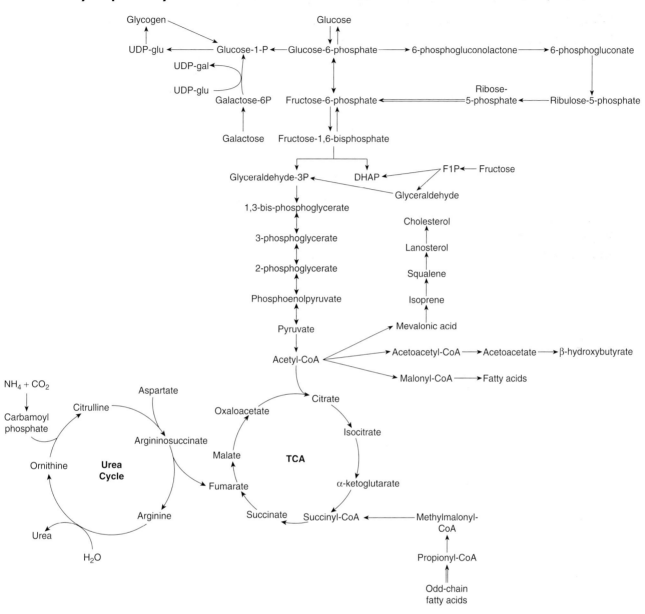

Microbiology

"What lies behind us and what lies ahead of us are tiny matters compared to what lives within us."
—Oliver Wendell Holmes

This high-yield material covers the basic concepts of microbiology and immunology. The emphasis in previous examinations has been approximately 40% bacteriology (20% basic, 20% quasi-clinical), 25% immunology, 25% virology (10% basic, 15% quasi-clinical), 5% parasitology, and 5% mycology. Learning the distinguishing characteristics, target organs, and method of spread of—as well as relevant laboratory tests for—major pathogens can improve your score substantially.

Many students preparing for this part of the boards make the mistake of studying bacteriology thoroughly without devoting sufficient time to the other topics. For this reason, learning immunology and virology thoroughly is high yield. Learn the components and mechanistic details of the immune response, including T cells, B cells, and the structure and function of immunoglobulins. Also learn the major immunodeficiency diseases (e.g., AIDS, agammaglobulinemia, DiGeorge syndrome). Knowledge of viral structures and genomes remains important as well.

High-Yield Clinical Vignettes

Clinical Bacteriology

Bacteriology

Mycology

Parasitology

Virology

Systems

Immunology

These abstracted case vignettes are designed to demonstrate the thought processes necessary to answer multistep clinical reasoning questions.

Vignette	Question	Answer
■ Alcoholic vomits gastric contents and develops foul-smelling sputum.	What organisms are most likely?	Anaerobes.
■ Middle-age male presents with acute-onset monoarticular joint pain and bilateral Bell's palsy.	What is the likely disease and how did he get it?	Lyme disease; bite from *Ixodes* tick.
■ Patient with *Mycoplasma pneumoniae* exhibits cryoagglutinins during recovery phase.	What types of immunoglobulins are reacting?	IgM.
■ UA of patient shows WBC casts.	What is the diagnosis?	Pyelonephritis.
■ Young child presents with tetany and candidiasis. Hypocalcemia and immunosuppression are found.	What cell is deficient?	T cell (DiGeorge).
■ Patient presents with "rose gardener's" scenario (thorn prick with ulcers along lymphatic drainage).	What is the infectious bug?	*Sporothrix schenckii*.
■ 25-year-old medical student has a burning feeling in his gut after meals. Biopsy of gastric mucosa shows gram-negative rods.	What is the likely organism?	*H. pylori*.
■ 32-year-old male has "cauliflower" skin lesions. Tissue biopsy shows broad-based budding yeasts.	What is the likely organism?	*Blastomyces*.
■ Breast-feeding woman suddenly develops redness and swelling of her right breast. On examination, it is found to be a fluctuant mass.	What is the diagnosis?	Mastitis caused by *S. aureus*.
■ Young child has recurrent lung infections and granulomatous lesions.	What is the defect in neutrophils?	NADPH oxidase (chronic granulomatous disease).
■ 20-year-old college student presents with lymphadenopathy, fever, and hepatosplenomegaly. His serum agglutinates sheep RBCs.	What cell is infected?	B cell (EBV; infectious mononucleosis).

Vignette	Question	Answer
■ 1 hour after eating custard at a picnic, a whole family began to vomit. After 10 hours, they were better.	What is the organism?	*S. aureus* (produces preformed enterotoxin).
■ Infant becomes flaccid after eating honey.	What organism is implicated, and what is the mechanism of action?	*Clostridium botulinum;* inhibited release of ACh.
■ Man presents with squamous cell carcinoma of the penis.	He had exposure to what virus?	HPV.
■ Patient develops endocarditis 3 weeks after receiving a prosthetic heart valve.	What organism is suspected?	*S. aureus* or *S. epidermidis*.

Bacterial structures

Structure	Function	Chemical composition
Peptidoglycan	Gives rigid support, protects against osmotic pressure.	Sugar backbone with cross-linked peptide side chains.
Cell wall/cell membrane (gram positives)	Major surface antigen.	Teichoic acid induces TNF and IL-1.
Outer membrane (gram negatives)	Site of endotoxin (lipopolysaccharide); major surface antigen.	Lipid A induces TNF and IL-1; polysaccharide is the antigen.
Plasma membrane	Site of oxidative and transport enzymes.	Lipoprotein bilayer.
Ribosome	Protein synthesis.	RNA and protein in 50S and 30S subunits.
Periplasm	Space between the cytoplasmic membrane and outer membrane in gram-negative bacteria.	Contains many hydrolytic enzymes, including β-lactamases.
Capsule	Protects against phagocytosis.	Polysaccharide (except *Bacillus anthracis*, which contains D-glutamate).
Pilus/fimbria	Mediates adherence of bacteria to cell surface; sex pilus forms attachment between 2 bacteria during conjugation.	Glycoprotein.
Flagellum	Motility.	Protein.
Spore	Provides resistance to dehydration, heat, and chemicals.	Keratin-like coat; dipicolinic acid.
Plasmid	Contains a variety of genes for antibiotic resistance, enzymes, and toxins.	DNA.
Glycocalyx	Mediates adherence to surfaces, especially foreign surfaces (e.g., indwelling catheters).	Polysaccharide.

Cell walls

(Adapted, with permission, from Levinson W, Jawetz E. *Medical Microbiology and Immunology: Examination and Board Review*, 6th ed. New York: McGraw-Hill, 2000:7.)

Bacterial growth curve

Lag—metabolic activity without division.

Log—rapid cell division.

Stationary—nutrient depletion slows growth.

Death—prolonged nutrient depletion and buildup of waste products lead to death.

(Adapted, with permission, from Levinson W, Jawetz E. *Medical Microbiology and Immunology: Examination and Board Review*, 6th ed. New York: McGraw-Hill, 2000:14.)

Main features of exotoxins and endotoxins

Property	Exotoxin	Endotoxin
Source	Certain species of some gram-positive and gram-negative bacteria	Cell wall of most gram-negative bacteria
Secreted from cell	Yes	No
Chemistry	Polypeptide	Lipopolysaccharide
Location of genes	Plasmid or bacteriophage	Bacterial chromosome
Toxicity	High (fatal dose on the order of 1 μg)	Low (fatal dose on the order of hundreds of micrograms)
Clinical effects	Various effects (see text)	Fever, shock
Mode of action	Various modes (see text)	Includes TNF and IL-1
Antigenicity	Induces high-titer antibodies called antitoxins	Poorly antigenic
Vaccines	Toxoids used as vaccines	No toxoids formed and no vaccine available
Heat stability	Destroyed rapidly at 60°C (except staphylococcal enterotoxin)	Stable at 100°C for 1 hour
Typical diseases	Tetanus, botulism, diphtheria	Meningococcemia, sepsis by gram-negative rods

(Adapted, with permission, from Levinson W, Jawetz E. *Medical Microbiology and Immunology: Examination and Board Review*, 6th ed. New York: McGraw-Hill, 2000:34.)

Bugs with exotoxins

Gram-positive bugs	Mode of action
Corynebacterium diphtheriae	Inactivates EF-2 by ADP ribosylation (similar to exotoxin A of *Pseudomonas*); causes pharyngitis and "pseudomembrane" in throat.
Clostridium tetani	Blocks the release of the inhibitory neurotransmitter glycine; causes "lockjaw."
C. botulinum	Blocks the release of ACh; causes anticholinergic symptoms, CNS paralysis; spores found in canned food, honey (causes floppy baby).
C. perfringens	α toxin is a lecithinase; causes gas gangrene; get double zone of hemolysis on blood agar.
Bacillus anthracis	1 toxin in the toxin complex is an adenylate cyclase.
S. aureus	Toxin is a superantigen that binds to MHC II protein and T-cell receptor, inducing IL-1 and IL-2 synthesis in toxic shock syndrome; also causes food poisoning.
Streptococcus pyogenes	Erythrogenic toxin (causes rash of scarlet fever) and streptolysin O (antigen for ASO antibody is found in rheumatic fever). Erythrogenic toxin is a superantigen; streptolysin O is a hemolysin.

Gram-negative bugs	
E. coli	Heat-labile toxin stimulates adenylate cyclase by ADP ribosylation of G protein; causes watery diarrhea. Heat-stable toxin stimulates guanylate cyclase.
Vibrio cholerae	Stimulates adenylate cyclase by ADP ribosylation of G protein; increases pumping of Cl⁻ and H_2O into gut; causes voluminous rice-water diarrhea.
Bordetella pertussis	Stimulates adenylate cyclase by ADP ribosylation; causes whooping cough; inhibits chemokine receptor, causing lymphocytosis.

Endotoxin

A lipopolysaccharide found in cell wall of gram-negative bacteria.

N-dotoxin is an integral part of gram-**N**egative cell wall. Endotoxin is heat stable.

(Adapted, with permission, from Levinson W, Jawetz E. *Medical Microbiology and Immunology: Examination and Board Review*, 6th ed. New York: McGraw-Hill, 2000:39.)

Gram stain limitations

These bugs do not Gram stain well:

Treponema (too thin to be visualized).

These **R**ascals **M**ay **M**icroscopically **L**ack **C**olor.

Treponemes—darkfield microscopy and fluorescent antibody staining.

Rickettsia (intracellular parasite).

Mycobacteria (high-lipid-content cell wall requires acid-fast stain).

Mycobacteria—acid fast.

Mycoplasma (no cell wall).

Legionella pneumophila (primarily intracellular).

Legionella—silver stain.

Chlamydia (intracellular parasite).

Fermentation patterns of *Neisseria*	The pathogenic *Neisseria* species are differentiated on the basis of sugar fermentation.	MeninGococci ferment Maltose and Glucose. Gonococci ferment Glucose.
Pigment-producing bacteria	*S. aureus* produces a yellow pigment. *Pseudomonas aeruginosa* produces a blue-green pigment. *Serratia marcescens* produces a red pigment.	*Aureus* (Latin) = gold. *Serratia marcescens* = maraschino cherries are red.
IgA proteases	IgA proteases allow these organisms to colonize mucosal surfaces: *Streptococcus pneumoniae*, *Neisseria meningitidis*, *N. gonorrhoeae*, *Haemophilus influenzae*.	

Gram-positive lab algorithm

Important pathogens are in **bold type**.
Note: *Enterococcus* is either α- or γ-hemolytic.

HIGH-YIELD FACTS

Microbiology

Gram-negative lab algorithm

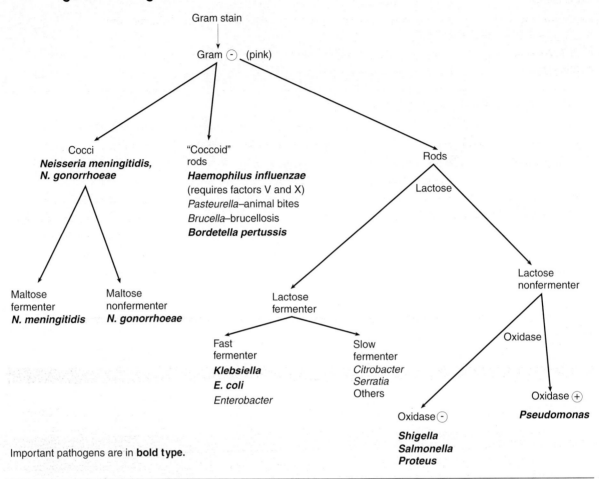

Gram stain

Gram ⊖ (pink)

Cocci
**Neisseria meningitidis,
N. gonorrhoeae**

"Coccoid"
rods
Haemophilus influenzae
(requires factors V and X)
Pasteurella–animal bites
Brucella–brucellosis
Bordetella pertussis

Rods

Lactose

Maltose
fermenter
N. meningitidis

Maltose
nonfermenter
N. gonorrhoeae

Lactose
fermenter

Lactose
nonfermenter

Fast
fermenter
Klebsiella
E. coli
Enterobacter

Slow
fermenter
Citrobacter
Serratia
Others

Oxidase

Oxidase ⊖
**Shigella
Salmonella
Proteus**

Oxidase ⊕
Pseudomonas

Important pathogens are in **bold type.**

Special culture requirements

Bug	Media used for isolation
H. influenzae	Chocolate agar with factors V (NAD) and X (hematin)
N. gonorrhoeae	Thayer-Martin (VCN) media
B. pertussis	Bordet-Gengou (potato) agar
C. diphtheriae	Tellurite plate, Loffler's medium, blood agar
M. tuberculosis	Löwenstein-Jensen agar
Lactose-fermenting enterics (e.g., *Escherichia, Klebsiella,* and *Enterobacter*)	Pink colonies on MacConkey's agar
Legionella pneumophila	Charcoal yeast extract agar buffered with increased iron and cysteine
Fungi	Sabouraud's agar

Stains

Congo red	Amyloid; apple-green birefringence in polarized light.
Giemsa's	*Borrelia, Plasmodium,* trypanosomes, *Chlamydia.*
PAS (periodic acid Schiff)	Stains glycogen, mucopolysaccharides; used to diagnose Whipple's disease.
Ziehl-Neelsen	Acid-fast bacteria.
India ink	*Cryptococcus neoformans.*

Conjugation, transduction, and transformation

Transfer procedure	Transfer process	Types of cells involved	Nature of DNA transferred
Conjugation	DNA transferred from 1 bacterium to another	Prokaryotic	Chromosomal or plasmid
Transduction	DNA transferred by a virus from 1 cell to another	Prokaryotic	Any gene in generalized transduction; only certain genes in specialized transduction
Transformation	Purified DNA taken up by a cell	Prokaryotic or eukaryotic (e.g., human)	Any DNA

(Adapted, with permission, from Levinson W, Jawetz E. *Medical Microbiology and Immunology: Examination and Board Review,* 6th ed. New York: McGraw-Hill, 2000:18.)

MICROBIOLOGY—BACTERIOLOGY

Obligate aerobes	Use an O_2-dependent system to generate ATP. Examples include **N**ocardia, **P**seudomonas aeruginosa, **M**ycobacterium tuberculosis, and **B**acillus. M. tuberculosis has a predilection for the apices of the lung, which have the highest PO_2.	P. **AER**uginosa is an **AER**obe seen in burn wounds, nosocomial pneumonia, and pneumonias in cystic fibrosis patients. **N**agging **P**ests **M**ust **B**reathe.
Obligate anaerobes	Examples include *Clostridium, Bacteroides,* and *Actinomyces.* They lack catalase and/or superoxide dismutase and thus are susceptible to oxidative damage. They are generally foul smelling (short-chain fatty acids), are difficult to culture, and produce gas in tissue (CO_2 and H_2).	Anaerobes are normal flora in GI tract, pathogenic elsewhere. AminO_2glycosides are ineffective against anaerobes because these antibiotics require O_2 to enter into bacterial cell.

Intracellular bugs

Obligate intracellular	*Rickettsia, Chlamydia.* Can't make own ATP.	Stay inside (cells) when it is **R**eally **C**old.
Facultative intracellular	*Mycobacterium, Brucella, Francisella, Listeria, Yersinia, Legionella, Salmonella.*	

HIGH-YIELD FACTS

Microbiology

Encapsulated bacteria

Examples are *Streptococcus pneumoniae* (pneumococcus), *Haemophilus influenzae* (especially B serotype), *Neisseria meningitidis* (meningococcus), and *Klebsiella pneumoniae*.

Polysaccharide capsule is an antiphagocytic virulence factor.

Positive **Quellung** reaction: If encapsulated bug is present, capsule **swells** when specific anticapsular antisera are added.

IgG_2 necessary for immune response. Capsule serves as antigen in vaccines (Pneumovax, *H. influenzae* B, meningococcal vaccines).

Quellung = capsular **"swellung."**

Pneumococcus associated with "rusty" sputum, sepsis in sickle cell anemia, and splenectomy.

Spores: bacterial

Only certain gram-positive rods form spores when nutrients are limited. Spores are highly resistant to destruction by heat and chemicals. Have dipicolinic acid in their core. Have no metabolic activity. Must autoclave to kill spores (as is done to surgical equipment).

Gram-positive soil bugs ≈ spore formers (*Bacillus anthracis*, *Clostridium perfringens*, *C. tetani*).

α-hemolytic bacteria

Include the following organisms:
1. *Streptococcus pneumoniae* (catalase negative and optochin sensitive)
2. Viridans streptococci (catalase negative and optochin resistant)

β-hemolytic bacteria

Include the following organisms:
1. *Staphylococcus aureus* (catalase and coagulase positive)
2. *Streptococcus pyogenes* (catalase negative and bacitracin sensitive)
3. *Streptococcus agalactiae* (catalase negative and bacitracin resistant)
4. *Listeria monocytogenes* (tumbling motility, meningitis in newborns, unpasteurized milk)

Catalase/coagulase (gram-positive cocci)

Catalase degrades H_2O_2, an antimicrobial product of PMNs. H_2O_2 is a substrate for myeloperoxidase. Staphylococci make catalase, whereas streptococci do not.

S. aureus makes coagulase, whereas *S. epidermidis* and *S. saprophyticus* do not.

Staph make catalase because they have more "staff." Bad staph (*aureus*, because *epidermidis* is skin flora) make coagulase and toxins.

Staphylococcus aureus

Protein A (virulence factor) binds Fc-IgG, inhibiting complement fixation and phagocytosis.

Causes:
1. Inflammatory disease—skin infections, organ abscesses, pneumonia
2. Toxin-mediated disease—toxic shock syndrome (TSST-1 toxin), scalded skin syndrome (exfoliative toxin), rapid-onset food poisoning (enterotoxins)

TSST is a superantigen that binds to MHC II and T-cell receptor, resulting in polyclonal T-cell activation.

S. aureus food poisoning is due to ingestion of preformed toxin.

Causes acute bacterial endocarditis.

***Streptococcus pyogenes* (group A β-hemolytic streptococci) sequelae**	Causes:
	  1. Pyogenic—pharyngitis, cellulitis, impetigo
	  2. Toxigenic—scarlet fever, toxic shock syndrome
	  3. Immunologic—rheumatic fever, acute glomerulonephritis
	Bacitracin sensitive. Antibody to **M protein** enhances host defenses against *S. pyogenes*.
		Pharyngitis gives you rheumatic "phever."
		Rheumatic fever = **PECCS:** Polyarthritis, Erythema marginatum, Chorea, Carditis, Subcutaneous nodules.

Enterococci 	Enterococci (*Enterococcus faecalis* and *E. faecium*) are penicillin G resistant and cause UTI and subacute endocarditis. Lancefield group D includes the enterococci and the nonenterococcal group D streptococci. Lancefield grouping is based on differences in the C carbohydrate on the bacterial cell wall. Variable hemolysis.	*Entero* = intestine, *faecalis* = feces, *strepto* = twisted (chains), *coccus* = berry. Enterococci, hardier than nonenterococcal group D, can thus grow in 6.5% NaCl (lab test).
Viridans group streptococci	Viridans streptococci are α-hemolytic. They are normal flora of the oropharynx and cause dental caries (*Streptococcus mutans*) and subacute bacterial endocarditis (*S. sanguis*). Resistant to optochin, differentiating them from *S. pneumoniae*, which is α-hemolytic but is optochin sensitive.	*Sanguis* (Latin) = blood. There is lots of blood in the heart (endocarditis). Viridans group strep live in the mouth because they are not afraid **of-the-chin** (**op-to-chin** resistant).
Clostridia (with exotoxins)	Gram-positive, spore-forming, obligate anaerobic bacilli. *Clostridium tetani* produces an exotoxin causing tetanus. *C. botulinum* produces a preformed, heat-labile toxin that inhibits ACh release, causing botulism. *C. perfringens* produces α toxin, lecithinase that causes myonecrosis, gas gangrene or hemolysis. *C. difficile* produces a cytotoxin, an exotoxin that kills enterocytes, causing pseudomembranous colitis. Often 2° to antibiotic use, especially clindamycin or ampicillin.	**TET**anus is **TET**anic paralysis (blocks glycine release [inhibitory neurotransmitter]) from Renshaw cells in spinal cord. *BOT*ulinum is from bad **BOT**tles of food (causes a flaccid paralysis). *PERF*ringens **PERF**orates a gangrenous leg. *DI*fficile causes **DI**arrhea. Treat with metronidazole.

Diphtheria (and exotoxin)	Caused by *Corynebacterium diphtheriae* via exotoxin encoded by β-prophage. Potent exotoxin inhibits protein synthesis via ADP ribosylation of EF-2. Symptoms include pseudomembranous pharyngitis (grayish-white membrane) with lymphadenopathy. Lab diagnosis based on gram-positive rods with metachromatic granules.	*Coryne* = club shaped.
		Grows on tellurite agar.
		ABCDEFG:
		  ADP ribosylation
		  Beta-prophage
		  *C*orynebacterium
		  *D*iphtheriae
		  Elongation **F**actor 2
		  Granules

HIGH-YIELD FACTS

Microbiology

Anthrax	Caused by *Bacillus anthracis*, a gram-positive, spore-forming rod that produces anthrax toxin. Contact → malignant pustule (painless ulcer); can progress to bacteremia and death. Inhalation of spores can cause life-threatening pneumonia (woolsorters' disease).	Black skin lesions—vesicular papules covered by black eschar.
Actinomyces* vs. *Nocardia	Both are gram-positive rods forming long branching filaments resembling fungi. *Actinomyces israelii*, a gram-positive anaerobe, causes oral/facial abscesses with "sulfur granules" that may drain through sinus tracts in skin. Normal oral flora. *Nocardia asteroides*, a gram-positive and also a weakly acid-fast aerobe in soil, causes pulmonary infection in immunocompromised patients.	*A. israelii* forms yellow "sulfur granules" in sinus tracts. **SNAP:** **S**ulfa for **N**ocardia; **A**ctinomyces use **P**enicillin
Penicillin and gram-negative bugs	Gram-negative bugs are resistant to benzyl penicillin G but may be susceptible to penicillin derivatives such as ampicillin. The gram-negative outer membrane layer inhibits entry of penicillin G and vancomycin.	
Bugs causing food poisoning	*Vibrio parahaemolyticus and V. vulnificus* in contaminated seafood. *Bacillus cereus* in reheated rice. *S. aureus* in meats, mayonnaise, custard. *Clostridium perfringens* in reheated meat dishes. *C. botulinum* in improperly canned foods (bulging cans). *E. coli* 0157:H7 in undercooked meat. *Salmonella* in poultry, meat, and eggs.	*S. aureus* food poisoning starts quickly and ends quickly. "Food poisoning from reheated rice? **Be serious!**" **(B. cereus).**

Diarrhea

Species	Typical findings
E. coli	Ferments lactose
Vibrio cholerae	Comma-shaped organisms
Salmonella	Does not ferment lactose, motile
Shigella	Does not ferment lactose, nonmotile, very low ID_{50}
Campylobacter jejuni	Comma- or S-shaped organisms; growth at 42°C
Vibrio parahaemolyticus	Transmitted by seafood
Yersinia enterocolitica	Usually transmitted from pet feces (e.g., puppies)

Bugs causing watery diarrhea	Include *Vibrio cholerae* (associated with rice-water stools), enterotoxigenic *E. coli*, viruses (e.g., rotaviruses), and protozoans (e.g., *Cryptosporidium* and *Giardia*).
Bugs causing bloody diarrhea	Include *Salmonella, Shigella, Campylobacter jejuni*, enterohemorrhagic/enteroinvasive (0157:H7) *E. coli, Yersinia enterocolitica*, and *Entamoeba histolytica* (a protozoan).

Enterobacteriaceae	Diverse family including *E. coli*, *Salmonella*, *Klebsiella*, *Enterobacter*, *Serratia*, *Proteus*. All species have somatic (O) antigen (which is the polysaccharide of endotoxin). The capsular (K) antigen is related to the virulence of the bug. The flagellar (H) antigen is found in motile species. All ferment glucose and are oxidase negative.	Think **COFFEe**: **C**apsular **O** antigen **F**lagellar antigen **F**erment glucose **E**nterobacteriaceae
Haemophilus influenzae	*Ha**EMOP**hilus* causes **E**piglottitis, **M**eningitis, **O**titis media, and **P**neumonia. Small gram-negative (coccobacillary) rod. Aerosol transmission. Most invasive disease caused by capsular type B. Produces IgA protease. Culture on chocolate agar requires factors **V** (NAD) and **X** (hematin) for growth. Treat meningitis with ceftriaxone. Rifampin prophylaxis in close contacts. Does not cause the flu (influenza virus does).	When a child has "flu," mom goes to five (**V**) and dime (**X**) store to buy some chocolate. Vaccine contains type B capsular polysaccharide conjugated to diphtheria toxoid or other protein. Given between 2 and 18 months of age.
Legionella pneumophila	Legionnaires' disease. Gram-negative rod. Gram stains poorly—use silver stain. Grow on charcoal yeast extract culture with iron and cysteine. Aerosol transmission from environmental water source habitat. No person-to-person transmission. Treat with erythromycin.	Think of a French legionnaire (soldier) with his silver helmet, sitting around a campfire (charcoal) with his iron dagger—he is no sissy (cysteine).
Pseudomonas aeruginosa	*PSEUdomonas* causes wound and burn infections, **P**neumonia (especially in cystic fibrosis), **S**epsis (black lesions on skin), **E**xternal otitis (swimmer's ear), **U**TI, and hot tub folliculitis. Aerobic gram-negative rod. Non–lactose fermenting, oxidase positive. Produces pyocyanin (blue-green) pigment. Water source. Produces endotoxin (fever, shock) and exotoxin A (inactivates EF-2). Treat with aminoglycoside plus extended-spectrum penicillin (e.g., piperacillin, ticarcillin).	**AER**uginosa—**AER**obic. Think water connection and blue-green pigment. Think *Pseudomonas* in burn victims.
Helicobacter pylori	Causes gastritis and up to 90% of duodenal ulcers. Risk factor for peptic ulcer and gastric carcinoma. Gram-negative rod. Urease positive (e.g., urease breath test). Creates alkaline environment. Treat with triple therapy: (1) bismuth (Pepto-Bismol), metronidazole, and either tetracycline or amoxicillin; or (2) (more costly) metronidazole, omeprazole, and clarithromycin.	Pylori—think pylorus of stomach. *Proteus* and *H. pylori* are both urease positive (cleave urea to ammonia).
Lactose-fermenting enteric bacteria	These bacteria grow pink colonies on MacConkey's agar. Examples include *Klebsiella*, *E. coli*, *Enterobacter*, and *Citrobacter*.	Lactose is **KEE**.

Salmonella vs. *Shigella*

Both are non–lactose fermenters; both invade intestinal mucosa and can cause bloody diarrhea. Only *Sal**M**onella* is **M**otile and can invade further and disseminate hematogenously. Symptoms of salmonellosis may be prolonged with antibiotic treatments, and there is typically a monocyte response. *Shigella* is more virulent (10^1 organisms) than *Salmonella* (10^5 organisms).

Salmon swim (motile and disseminate). *Salmonella* has an animal reservoir; *Shigella* does not and is transmitted via "**F**ood, **F**ingers, **F**eces, and **F**lies."

Cholera and pertussis toxins

Vibrio cholerae toxin permanently activates G_s, causing rice-water diarrhea.

Pertussis toxin permanently disables G_i, causing whooping cough.

Both toxins act via ADP ribosylation that permanently activates adenyl cyclase (resulting in increased cAMP).

Cholera turns the "on" on. Pertussis turns the "off" off. Pertussis toxin also promotes lymphocytosis by inhibiting chemokine receptors.

Zoonotic bacteria

Species	Disease	Transmission and source
Borrelia burgdorferi	Lyme disease	Tick bite; *Ixodes* ticks that live on deer and mice
Brucella spp.	Brucellosis/ Undulant fever	Dairy products, contact with animals
Francisella tularensis	Tularemia	Tick bite; rabbits, deer
Yersinia pestis	Plague	Flea bite; rodents, especially prairie dogs
Pasteurella multocida	Cellulitis	Animal bite; cats, dogs

Bugs **F**rom **Y**our **P**et **U**ndulate and **U**npasteurized dairy products give you **U**ndulant fever.

Gardnerella vaginalis

A pleomorphic, gram-variable rod that causes vaginosis—greenish vaginal discharge with fishy smell; nonpainful. *Mobiluncus, an anaerobe, is also involved.* Treat with metronidazole. Clue cells, or vaginal epithelial cells covered with bacteria, are visible under the microscope.

Neisseria

Gram-negative cocci.

Gonococci	Meningococci
No polysaccharide capsule	Polysaccharide capsule
No maltose fermentation	Maltose fermentation
No vaccine	Vaccine
Causes: gonorrhea, septic arthritis, neonatal conjunctivitis, PID	Causes: meningococcemia and meningitis, Waterhouse-Friderichsen syndrome

1° and 2° tuberculosis

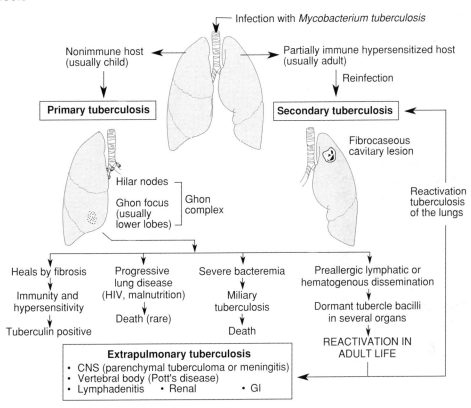

Infection with *Mycobacterium tuberculosis*

Nonimmune host (usually child) ← → Partially immune hypersensitized host (usually adult)

| Reinfection

Primary tuberculosis   **Secondary tuberculosis** ←

Fibrocaseous cavitary lesion

Hilar nodes
Ghon focus (usually lower lobes) } Ghon complex

Reactivation tuberculosis of the lungs

Heals by fibrosis → Immunity and hypersensitivity → Tuberculin positive

Progressive lung disease (HIV, malnutrition) → Death (rare)

Severe bacteremia → Miliary tuberculosis → Death

Preallergic lymphatic or hematogenous dissemination → Dormant tubercle bacilli in several organs → REACTIVATION IN ADULT LIFE

Extrapulmonary tuberculosis
- CNS (parenchymal tuberculoma or meningitis)
- Vertebral body (Pott's disease)
- Lymphadenitis   • Renal   • GI

(Adapted, with permission, from Chandrasoma P, Taylor CR. *Concise Pathology*, 3rd ed. Stamford, CT: Appleton & Lange, 1998:523.)

Mycobacteria	*Mycobacterium tuberculosis* (TB, often resistant to multiple drugs). M. *kansasii* (pulmonary TB-like symptoms). M. *scrofulaceum* (cervical lymphadenitis in kids). M. *avium–intracellulare* (often resistant to multiple drugs; causes disseminated disease in AIDS). All mycobacteria are acid-fast organisms.	TB symptoms include fever, night sweats, weight loss, and hemoptysis.
Leprosy (Hansen's disease)	Caused by *Mycobacterium leprae*, an acid-fast bacillus that likes cool temperatures (infects skin and superficial nerves) and cannot be grown in vitro. Reservoir in United States: armadillos. Treatment: long-term oral dapsone; toxicity is hemolysis and methemoglobinemia. Alternate treatments include rifampin and combination of clofazimine and dapsone.	Hansen's disease has two forms: lepromatous and tuberculoid; lepromatous is worse (failed cell-mediated immunity), tuberculoid is self-limited. **LE**promatous = **LE**thal.

HIGH-YIELD FACTS

Microbiology

Rickettsiae

Rickettsiae are obligate intracellular parasites and need CoA and NAD. All except *Coxiella* are transmitted by an arthropod vector and cause headache, fever, and rash; *Coxiella* is an atypical rickettsia because it is transmitted by aerosol and causes pneumonia.

Tetracycline is the treatment of choice for most rickettsial infections.

Classic triad—headache, fever, rash (vasculitis).

Rickettsial diseases and vectors

Rocky Mountain spotted fever (tick)—*Rickettsia rickettsii*.
Endemic typhus (fleas)—*R. typhi*.
Epidemic typhus (human body louse)—*R. prowazekii*.
Q fever (inhaled aerosols)—*Coxiella burnetii*.
Treatment for all: tetracycline.

Ty**PH**us has centri**PH**ugal (outward) spread of rash; s**P**otted fever is centri**P**etal (inward). **Q** fever is **Q**ueer because it has no rash, has no vector, and has negative Weil-Felix, and its causative organism can survive outside for a long time and does not have *Rickettsia* as its genus name.

Rocky Mountain spotted fever

Caused by *Rickettsia rickettsii*.
Symptoms: rash on palms and soles (migrating to wrists, ankles, then trunk), headache, fever.
Endemic to East Coast (in spite of name).

Palm and sole rash is seen in Rocky Mountain spotted fever, syphilis, and coxsackievirus A infection (hand, foot, and mouth disease).

Weil-Felix reaction

Weil-Felix reaction assays for antirickettsial antibodies, which cross-react with *Proteus* antigen. Weil-Felix is usually positive for typhus and Rocky Mountain spotted fever but negative for Q fever.

Mycoplasma pneumoniae

Classic cause of atypical "walking" pneumonia (insidious onset, headache, nonproductive cough, diffuse interstitial infiltrate). X-ray looks worse than patient. High titer of cold agglutinins (IgM). Grown on Eaton's agar.
Treatment: tetracycline or erythromycin (bugs are penicillin resistant because they have no cell wall).

No cell wall.
Only bacterial membrane containing cholesterol.
Mycoplasma pneumonia is more common in patients < 30 years of age.
Frequent outbreaks in military recruits and prisons.

Chlamydiae

Chlamydiae are obligate intracellular parasites that cause mucosal infections. 2 forms:

1. **E**lementary body (small, dense), which **E**nters cell via endocytosis
2. Initial or **R**eticulate body, which **R**eplicates in cell by fission

Chlamydiae cause arthritis, conjunctivitis, pneumonia, and nongonococcal urethritis. The peptidoglycan wall is unusual in that it lacks muramic acid.

Treatment: erythromycin or tetracycline.

Chlamys = cloak (intracellular).
Chlamydia psittaci—notable for an avian reservoir.
C. trachomatis and *C. pneumoniae*—infect only humans.
C. trachomatis causes arthritis. *C. pneumoniae* causes atypical pneumonia; transmitted by aerosol.
Lab diagnosis: cytoplasmic inclusions seen on Giemsa or fluorescent antibody–stained smear.

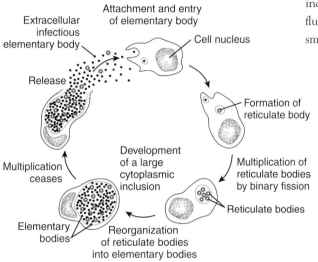

Chlamydia trachomatis serotypes

Types A, B, and C—chronic infection, causes blindness in Africa.

Types D–K—urethritis/PID, ectopic pregnancy, neonatal pneumonia, or neonatal conjunctivitis.

Types L1, L2, and L3—lymphogranuloma venereum (acute lymphadenitis—positive Frei test).

ABC = **A**frica/**B**lindness/**C**hronic infection.
L1–3 = **L**ymphogranuloma venereum.
D–K = everything else.

Neonatal disease acquired by passage through infected birth canal. Treat with erythromycin eye drops.

Spirochetes

The spirochetes are spiral-shaped bacteria with axial filaments and include **B**orrelia (big size), **L**eptospira, and **T**reponema. Only *Borrelia* can be visualized using aniline dyes (Wright's or Giemsa stain) in light microscopy. *Treponema* is visualized by dark-field microscopy.

BLT. B is **B**ig.

HIGH-YIELD FACTS

Microbiology

Lyme disease

Classic symptom is erythema chronicum migrans, an expanding "bull's eye" red rash with central clearing. Also affects joints, CNS, and heart.

Caused by *Borrelia burgdorferi*, which is transmitted by the tick *Ixodes*.

Mice are important reservoirs. Deer required for tick life cycle.

Treat with tetracycline.

Named after Lyme, Connecticut; disease is common in northeastern United States.

Transmission is most common in summer months.

3 stages of Lyme disease:
Stage 1—erythema chronicum migrans, flu-like symptoms.
Stage 2—neurologic and cardiac manifestations.
Stage 3—autoimmune migratory polyarthritis.

Treponemal disease

Treponemes are spirochetes.

Treponema pallidum causes syphilis.

T. pertenue causes yaws (a tropical infection that is not an STD, although VDRL test is positive).

Syphilis

Caused by spirochete *Treponema pallidum*.

Treat with penicillin G.

1° syphilis — Presents with painless chancre (localized disease).

2° syphilis — Disseminated disease with constitutional symptoms, maculopapular rash, condylomata lata.

Secondary syphilis = **S**ystemic.

3° syphilis — Gummas, aortitis, neurosyphilis (tabes dorsalis), Argyll Robertson pupil.

VDRL vs. FTA-ABS

FTA-ABS is specific for treponemes, turns positive earliest in disease, and remains positive longest during disease. VDRL is less specific.

FTA-ABS = **F**ind **T**he **A**ntibody-**ABS**olutely:
1. Most specific
2. Earliest positive
3. Remains positive the longest

VDRL false positives

VDRL detects nonspecific antibody that reacts with beef cardiolipin. Used for diagnosis of syphilis, but many biologic false positives, including viral infection (mononucleosis, hepatitis), some drugs, rheumatic fever, rheumatoid arthritis, SLE, and leprosy.

VDRL:
Viruses (mono, hepatitis)
Drugs
Rheumatic fever and rheumatic arthritis
Lupus and leprosy

Spores: fungal

Most fungal spores are asexual. Both coccidioidomycosis and histoplasmosis are transmitted by inhalation of asexual spores.

Conidia—asexual fungal spores (e.g., blastoconidia, arthroconidia).

Candida albicans

Systemic or superficial fungal infection (budding yeast with pseudohyphae in culture at 20°C; germ tube formation at 37°C).

Thrush in throat with immunocompromised patients (neonates, steroids, diabetes, AIDS), endocarditis in IV drug users, vaginitis (post-antibiotic), diaper rash.

Treatment: nystatin for superficial infection; amphotericin B for serious systemic infection.

Alba = white.

Systemic mycoses

Disease	Endemic location	Notes
Coccidioidomycosis	Southwestern United States, California.	San Joaquin Valley or desert (desert bumps) "valley fever"
Histoplasmosis	Mississippi and Ohio river valleys.	Bird or bat droppings; intracellular (frequently seen inside macrophages)
Paracoccidioidomy-cosis	Rural Latin America.	"Captain's wheel" appearance
Blastomycosis Broad-based budding	States east of Mississippi River and Central America.	**B**ig, **B**road-**B**ased **B**udding

All of the above are caused by **dimorphic** fungi, which are mold in soil (at lower temperature) and yeast in tissue (at higher/body temperature: 37°C) except coccidioidomycosis, which is a spherule in tissue. Treat with fluconazole or ketoconazole for local infection; amphotericin B for systemic infection. Systemic mycoses can mimic TB (granuloma formation).

Cold = Mold
Heat = Yeast
Culture on Sabouraud's agar

Cutaneous mycoses

Tinea versicolor	Caused by *Malassezia furfur*. Causes hypopigmented skin lesions. Occurs in hot, humid weather. Treat with topical miconazole, selenium sulfide (Selsun).
Tinea nigra	Caused by *Cladosporium werneckii*. Infection of keratinized layer of skin. Appears as brownish spot. Treat with topical salicylic acid.
Tinea pedis, tinea cruris, tinea corporis, tinea capitis	Pruritic lesions with central clearing resembling a ring, caused by dermatophytes (*Microsporum*, *Trichophyton*, and *Epidermophyton*). See mold hyphae in KOH prep, not dimorphic. Pets are a reservoir for *Microsporum* and can be treated with topical azoles.

HIGH-YIELD FACTS

Microbiology

Opportunistic fungal infections

Candida albicans	Thrush in immunocompromised (neonates, steroids, diabetes, AIDS), vulvovaginitis (high pH, diabetes, use of antibiotics), disseminated candidiasis (to any organ), chronic mucocutaneous candidiasis.
Aspergillus fumigatus	Allergic bronchopulmonary aspergillosis, lung cavity aspergilloma ("fungus ball"), invasive aspergillosis. **Mold** with septate hyphae that branch at a V-shaped (45°) angle. Not dimorphic.
Cryptococcus neoformans	Cryptococcal meningitis, cryptococcosis. Heavily encapsulated **yeast.** Not dimorphic. Found in soil, pigeon droppings. Culture on Sabouraud's agar. Stains with India ink. Latex agglutination test detects polysaccharide capsular antigen.
Mucor and *Rhizopus* spp.	Mucormycosis. **Mold** with irregular nonseptate hyphae branching at wide angles (≥ 90°). Disease mostly in ketoacidotic diabetic and leukemic patients. Fungi also proliferate in the walls of blood vessels and cause infarction of distal tissue.

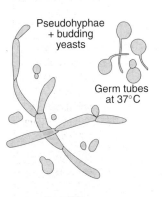

Pseudohyphae + budding yeasts

Germ tubes at 37°C

Candida

45° angle branching septate hyphae

Aspergillus

Rare fruiting bodies

5–10-μm yeasts with wide capsular halo

Narrow-based unequal budding

Cryptoccus

Irregular broad (empty-looking) nonseptate hyphae, wide-angle branching

Mucor

Pneumocystis carinii

Causes diffuse interstitial pneumonia (PCP). Yeast (originally classified as protozoan). Inhaled. Most infections asymptomatic. Immunosuppression (e.g., AIDS) predisposes to disease. Diagnosed by lung biopsy or lavage. Identified by methenamine silver stain of lung tissue. Treat with TMP-SMX, pentamidine, dapsone. Start prophylaxis when CD4 drops < 200 cells/mL in HIV patients.

Sporothrix schenckii

Yeast forms, unequal budding

Sporotrichosis. Dimorphic fungus that lives on vegetation. When traumatically introduced into the skin, typically by a thorn ("rose gardener's" disease), causes local pustule or ulcer with nodules along draining lymphatics (ascending lymphangitis). Little systemic illness. Cigar-shaped budding yeast visible in pus. Treat with itraconazole or potassium iodide.

Medically important protozoa

Organism	Disease	Transmission	Diagnosis	Treatment
Entamoeba histolytica	Amebiasis: bloody diarrhea, (dysentery), liver abscess, RUQ pain	Cysts in water	Serology and/or trophozoites or cysts in stool	Metronidazole and iodoquinol
Giardia lamblia	Giardiasis: bloating, flatulence, foul-smelling diarrhea	Cysts in water	Trophozoites or cysts in stool	Metronidazole
Cryptosporidium	Severe diarrhea in AIDS Mild disease (watery diarrhea) in non-HIV	Cysts in water	Cysts on acid-fast stain	None
Toxoplasma	Brain abscess in HIV, birth defects	Cysts in meat or cat feces	Serology, biopsy	Sulfadiazine + pyrimethamine
Plasmodium *P. vivax* *P. ovale* *P. malariae* *P. falciparum*	Malaria: cyclic fever, headache, anemia, splenomegaly Malaria—severe (cerebral)	Mosquito (*Anopheles*)	Blood smear	Chloroquine (primaquine for *P. vivax*, *P. ovale*), sulfadoxine + pyrimethamine, mefloquine, quinine
Trichomonas vaginalis	Vaginitis: foul-smelling, greenish discharge; itching and burning	Sexual	Trophozoites on wet mount	Metronidazole
Trypanosoma cruzi	Chagas' disease (heart disease)	Reduviid bug	Blood smear	Nifurtimox
Trypanosoma *T. gambiense* *T. rhodesiense*	African sleeping sickness	Tsetse fly	Blood smear	Suramin for blood-borne disease or melarsoprol for CNS penetration
Leishmania donovani	Visceral leishmaniasis (kala-azar)	Sandfly	Macrophages containing amastigotes	Sodium stibogluconate
Babesia	Babesiosis	*Ixodes* tick	Blood smear, no RBC pigment, appears as "maltese cross"	Quinine, clindamycin
Naegleria	Rapidly fatal meningoencephalitis	Swimming in freshwater lakes	Amebas in spinal fluid	None

HIGH-YIELD FACTS

Microbiology

Medically important helminths

Organism	Transmission/disease	Treatment
Cestodes (tapeworms)		
Taenia solium	Undercooked pork tapeworm; causes mass lesions in the brain, cysticercosis.	Praziquantel/niclosamide; albendazole for cysticercosis
Echinococcus granulosus	Eggs in dog feces when ingested can cause cysts in liver; causes anaphylaxis if echinococcal antigens are released from cysts.	Albendazole
Trematodes (flukes)		
Schistosoma	Snails are host; cercariae penetrate skin of humans; causes granulomas, fibrosis, and inflammation of the spleen and liver.	Praziquantel
Clonorchis sinensis	Undercooked fish; causes inflammation of the biliary tract.	Praziquantel
Paragonimus westermani	Undercooked crab meat; causes inflammation and 2° bacterial infection of the lung.	Praziquantel
Nematodes (roundworms)		
Ancylostoma duodenale (hookworm)	Larvae penetrate skin of feet; intestinal infection can cause anemia.	Mebendazole/pyrantel pamoate
Ascaris lumbricoides	Eggs are visible in feces; intestinal infection.	Mebendazole/pyrantel pamoate
Enterobius vermicularis (pinworm)	Food contaminated with eggs; intestinal infection; causes anal pruritus.	Mebendazole/pyrantel pamoate
Strongyloides stercoralis	Larvae in soil penetrate the skin; intestinal infection.	Ivermectin/thiabendazole
Trichinella spiralis	Undercooked meat, usually pork; inflammation of muscle, periorbital edema.	Thiabendazole
Dracunculus medinensis	In drinking water; skin inflammation and ulceration.	Niridazole
Loa loa	Transmitted by deer fly; causes swelling in skin (can see worm crawling in conjunctiva).	Diethylcarbamazine
Onchocerca volvulus	Transmitted by female blackflies; causes river blindness.	Ivermectin
Toxocara canis	Food contaminated with eggs; causes granulomas (if in retina → blindness) and visceral larva migrans.	Diethylcarbamazine
Wuchereria bancrofti	Female mosquito; causes blockage of lymphatic vessels (elephantiasis).	Diethylcarbamazine

Parasite hints

Findings	Organism
Brain cysts, seizures	*Taenia solium*
Liver cysts	*Echinococcus granulosus*
B₁₂ deficiency	*Diphyllobothrium latum*
Biliary tract disease	*Clonorchis sinensis*
Hemoptysis	*Paragonimus westermani*
Portal hypertension	*Schistosoma mansoni*
Hematuria, bladder cancer	*Schistosoma haematobium*
Microcytic anemia	*Ancylostoma, Necator*
Perianal pruritus	*Enterobius*

MICROBIOLOGY—VIROLOGY

DNA viral genomes
All DNA viruses except the Parvoviridae are dsDNA. All are linear except papovaviruses and hepadnaviruses (circular).

All are dsDNA (like our cells), except **"part-of-a-virus"** (**parvovirus**) is ssDNA.

RNA viral genomes
All RNA viruses except Reoviridae are ssRNA.

All are ssRNA (like our mRNA), except **"repeato-virus"** (**reovirus**) is dsRNA.

DNA viruses

Viral Family	Envelope	DNA Structure	Medical Importance

Hepadnavirus	Yes	DS – partial circular	HBV
			  Acute or chronic hepatitis
			  Vaccine available—use has increased tremendously
			  Not a retrovirus but has reverse transcriptase

Herpesviruses	Yes	DS – linear	HSV-1—oral (and some genital) lesions, keratoconjunctivitis HSV-2—genital (and some oral) lesions VZV—chickenpox, zoster, shingles EBV—mononucleosis, Burkitt's lymphoma CMV—infection in immunosuppressed patients, especially transplant recipients HHV-6—roseola (exanthem subitum) HHV-7—monkey bites (fatal in humans) HHV-8—Kaposi's sarcoma–associated herpesvirus (KSHV)
Adenovirus	No	DS – linear	Febrile pharyngitis—sore throat Pneumonia Conjunctivitis—"pink eye"
Parvovirus	No	SS – linear (–) (smallest DNA virus)	B19 virus—aplastic crises in sickle cell disease, "slapped cheeks" rash—erythema infectiosum (fifth disease), hydrops fetalis
Papovavirus	No	DS – circular	HPV—warts, CIN, cervical cancer JC—progressive multifocal leukoencephalopathy (PML) in HIV
Poxvirus	Yes	DS – linear (largest DNA virus)	Smallpox, although eradicated, could be used in germ warfare Vaccinia—cowpox ("milkmaid's blisters") Molluscum contagiosum

DNA virus characteristics

Some general rules—all DNA viruses:

1. Are **HHAPPP**y viruses

   Hepadna, Herpes, Adeno, Pox, Parvo, Papova.

2. Are double stranded

   EXCEPT **Parvo** (single stranded).

3. Are linear

   EXCEPT **Papovavirus** (circular, supercoiled) and **Hepadna** (circular, incomplete).

4. Are icosahedral

   EXCEPT **Pox** (complex).

5. Replicate in the nucleus

   EXCEPT **Pox** (carries own DNA-dependent RNA polymerase).

Naked DNA viruses are **PAP** = **P**arvo, **A**deno, **P**apova; enveloped DNA viruses are **HPH** = **H**epadna, **P**ox, **H**erpes.

You need to be **naked** for a **PAP** smear.

RNA viruses

Viral Family	Envelope	RNA Structure	Capsid Symmetry	Medical Importance

Picornaviruses	No	SS + linear	Icosahedral	**P**oliovirus—polio-Salk/Sabin vaccines—IPV/OPV
				Echovirus—aseptic meningitis
				Rhinovirus—"common cold"
				Coxsackievirus—aseptic meningitis
				   herpangina—febrile pharyngitis
				   hand, foot, and mouth disease
				   myocarditis
				HAV—acute viral hepatitis

Caliciviruses	No	SS + linear	Icosahedral	HEV Norwalk virus—viral gastroenteritis
Reoviruses	No	DS linear Segmented	Icosahedral (double)	Reovirus—Colorado tick fever Rotavirus—#1 cause of fatal diarrhea in children
Flaviviruses	Yes	SS + linear	Icosahedral	HCV Yellow fever Dengue St. Louis encephalitis West Nile virus
Togaviruses	Yes	SS + linear	Icosahedral	Rubella (German measles) Eastern equine encephalitis Western equine encephalitis
Retroviruses	Yes	SS + linear	Icosahedral	Have reverse transcriptase HIV—AIDS HTLV—T-cell leukemia
Orthomyxoviruses	Yes	SS − linear Segmented	Helical	Influenza virus

Paramyxoviruses	Yes	SS − linear
		Nonsegmented
			Helical	**PaRaM**yxovirus:
				   Parainfluenza—croup
				   RSV—bronchiolitis in babies; Rx—ribavirin
				   Measles
				   Mumps

Rhabdoviruses	Yes	SS − linear	Helical	Rabies
Filoviruses	Yes	SS − linear	Helical	Ebola/Marburg hemorrhagic fever—often fatal!
Coronaviruses	Yes	SS + linear	Helical	Coronavirus—"common cold"
Arenaviruses	Yes	SS − circular	Helical	LCV—lymphocytic choriomeningitis Meningitis—spread by mice
Bunyaviruses	Yes	SS − circular	Helical	California encephalitis Sandfly/Rift Valley fevers Crimean-Congo hemorrhagic fever Hantavirus—hemorrhagic fever, pneumonia
Deltavirus	Yes	SS − circular	Helical	HDV

SS, single-stranded; DS, double-stranded; +, + polarity; −, − polarity

(Adapted, with permission, from Levinson W, Jawetz E. *Medical Microbiology and Immunology: Examination and Board Review*, 6th ed. New York: McGraw-Hill, 2000:182.)

HIGH-YIELD FACTS

Microbiology

Naked viral genome infectivity	Naked nucleic acids of most dsDNA (except poxviruses and HBV) and (+) strand ssRNA (≈ mRNA) viruses are infectious. Naked nucleic acids of (–) strand ssRNA and dsRNA viruses are not infectious. **Naked** (nonenveloped) RNA viruses include **C**alicivirus, **P**icornavirus, and **R**eovirus.	Viral nucleic acids with the same structure as host nucleic acids are infective alone; others require special enzymes (contained in intact virion). **Naked CPR.**
Enveloped viruses	Generally, enveloped viruses acquire their envelopes from plasma membrane when they exit from cell. Exceptions are herpesviruses, which acquire envelopes from nuclear membrane.	
Virus ploidy	All viruses are haploid (with 1 copy of DNA or RNA) except retroviruses, which have 2 identical ssRNA molecules (≈ diploid).	

Viral replication

DNA viruses	All replicate in the nucleus (except poxvirus).
RNA viruses	All replicate in the cytoplasm (except influenza virus and retroviruses).

Viral vaccines	Live attenuated vaccines induce humoral and cell-mediated immunity but have reverted to virulence on rare occasions. Killed vaccines induce only humoral immunity but are stable. Live attenuated—measles, mumps, rubella, Sabin polio, VZV, yellow fever, smallpox Killed—rabies, influenza, HAV, and Salk polio vaccines. Recombinant—HBV (antigen = recombinant HBsAg).	Dangerous to give live vaccines to immunocompromised patients or their close contacts. MMR = measles, mumps, rubella. Sal**K** = **K**illed.

Viral genetics

Recombination	Exchange of genes between 2 chromosomes by crossing over within regions of significant base sequence homology.
Reassortment	When viruses with segmented genomes (e.g., influenza virus) exchange segments. High-frequency recombination. Cause of worldwide pandemics.
Complementation	When 1 of 2 viruses that infect the cell has a mutation that results in a nonfunctional protein. The nonmutated virus "complements" the mutated one by making a functional protein that serves both viruses.
Phenotypic mixing	Genome of virus A can be coated with the surface proteins of virus B. Type B protein coat determines the infectivity of the phenotypically mixed virus. However, the progeny from this infection has a type A coat and is encoded by its type A genetic material.

Viral pathogens

Structure	Viruses
DNA enveloped viruses	Herpesviruses (HSV types 1 and 2, VZV, CMV, EBV), HBV, smallpox virus
DNA nucleocapsid viruses	Adenovirus, papillomaviruses, parvovirus
RNA enveloped viruses	Influenza virus, parainfluenza virus, RSV, measles virus, mumps virus, rubella virus, rabies virus, HTLV, HIV
RNA nucleocapsid viruses	Enteroviruses (poliovirus, coxsackievirus, echovirus, HAV), rhinovirus, reovirus

---

Slow virus infections

Virus exists in patient for months to years before it manifests as clinical disease. SSPE (late sequela of measles), PML (reactivation of JC virus) in immunocompromised patients, especially AIDS.

Segmented viruses

All are RNA viruses. They include **B**unyaviruses, **O**rthomyxoviruses (influenza viruses), **A**renaviruses, and **R**eoviruses. Influenza virus consists of 8 segments of negative-stranded RNA. These segments can undergo reassortment, causing antigenic shifts that lead to worldwide epidemics of the flu.

BOAR.

Picornavirus

Includes poliovirus, rhinovirus, coxsackievirus, echovirus, HAV. RNA is translated into 1 large polypeptide that is cleaved by proteases into many small proteins. Can cause aseptic (viral) meningitis (except rhinovirus and HAV).

Pico**RNA**virus = small **RNA** virus.

Rhinovirus

Nonenveloped RNA virus. Cause of common cold— > 100 serologic types.

Rhino has a runny nose.

Rotavirus

Rotavirus, the most important global cause of infantile gastroenteritis, is a segmented dsRNA virus (a reovirus). Major cause of acute diarrhea in the United States during winter.

ROTA = **R**ight **O**ut **T**he **A**nus.

Paramyxoviruses

Paramyxoviruses include those that cause parainfluenza (croup), mumps, and measles as well as RSV, which causes respiratory tract infection (bronchiolitis, pneumonia) in infants. Paramyxoviruses cause disease in children. All paramyxoviruses have 1 serotype except parainfluenza virus, which has 4.

Mumps virus

A paramyxovirus with 1 serotype.

Mumps gives you **b**umps (parotitis).

Symptoms: aseptic **M**eningitis, **O**rchitis (inflammation of testes), and **P**arotitis. Can cause sterility (especially after puberty).

MOP.

Measles virus

A paramyxovirus that causes measles. Koplik spots (bluish-gray spots on buccal mucosa) are diagnostic. SSPE, encephalitis (1:2000), and giant cell pneumonia (rarely, in immunosuppressed) are possible sequelae.

3 C's of measles:
Cough
Coryza
Conjunctivitis
Also look for **K**oplik spots.

Influenza viruses

Enveloped, single-stranded RNA viruses with segmented genome. Contain hemagglutinin and neuraminidase antigens. Responsible for worldwide influenza epidemics; patients at risk for fatal bacterial superinfection. Rapid genetic changes.

Killed viral vaccine is major mode of protection; reformulated vaccine offered each fall to elderly, health-care workers, etc.

Genetic shift — Reassortment of viral genome (such as when human flu A virus recombines with swine flu A virus).

Genetic drift — Minor changes based on random mutation.

Amantadine and rimantadine useful for influenza A (especially prophylaxis).
Zanamivir and oseltamivir (neuraminidase inhibitors) useful for both influenza A and B.

Rabies virus

Negri bodies are characteristic cytoplasmic inclusions in neurons infected by rabies virus. Has bullet-shaped capsid. Rabies has long incubation period (weeks to 3 months). Causes fatal encephalitis with seizures and hydrophobia.
More commonly from bat, raccoon, and skunk bites than from dog bites in the United States.

Travels to the CNS by migrating in a retrograde fashion up nerve axons.

Arboviruses

Transmitted by arthropods (mosquitoes, ticks). Classic examples are dengue fever (also known as break-bone fever) and yellow fever. A variant of dengue fever in Southeast Asia is hemorrhagic shock syndrome.

ARBOvirus—**AR**thropod-**BO**rne virus, including flavivirus, togavirus, and bunyavirus.

Yellow fever

Caused by flavivirus, an arbovirus transmitted by *Aedes* mosquitos. Virus has a monkey or human reservoir.
Symptoms: high fever, black vomitus, and jaundice. Councilman bodies (acidophilic inclusions) may be seen in liver.

Flavi = yellow.

Herpesviruses

Virus	Diseases	Route of transmission	
HSV-1	Gingivostomatitis, keratoconjunctivitis, temporal lobe encephalitis, herpes labialis	Respiratory secretions, saliva	Get herpes in a **CHEV**rolet: **C**MV
HSV-2	Herpes genitalis, neonatal herpes	Sexual contact, perinatal	**H**SV
VZV	Varicella-zoster (shingles), encephalitis, pneumonia	Respiratory secretions	**E**BV **V**ZV
EBV	Infectious mononucleosis, Burkitt's lymphoma	Respiratory secretions, saliva	
CMV	Congenital infection, mononucleosis, pneumonia	Congenital, transfusion, sexual contact, saliva, urine, transplant	
HHV-8	Kaposi's sarcoma (HIV patients)	Sexual contact	

Mononucleosis

Caused by EBV, a herpesvirus. Characterized by fever, hepatosplenomegaly, pharyngitis, and lymphadenopathy (especially posterior auricular nodes).

Peak incidence 15–20 years old. Positive heterophil antibody test. Abnormal circulating cytotoxic T cells (atypical lymphocytes).

Most common during peak kissing years ("kissing disease").

Monospot test—heterophil antibodies detected by agglutination of sheep RBCs.

Tzanck test

A smear of an opened skin vesicle to detect multinucleated giant cells. Used to assay for HSV-1, HSV-2, and VZV.

Tzanck heavens I do not have herpes.

Hepatitis transmission

HAV (RNA picornavirus) is transmitted primarily by fecal-oral route. Short incubation (3 weeks). No carriers.

HBV (DNA hepadnavirus) is transmitted primarily by parenteral, sexual, and maternal-fetal routes. Long incubation (3 months). Carriers. Reverse transcription occurs; however, the virion enzyme is a DNA-dependent DNA polymerase.

HCV (RNA flavivirus) is transmitted primarily via blood and resembles HBV in its course and severity. Carriers. Common cause of IV drug use hepatitis in the United States.

HDV (delta agent) is a defective virus that requires HBsAg as its envelope. Carriers.

HEV (RNA calicivirus) is transmitted enterically and causes water-borne epidemics. Resembles HAV in course, severity, incubation. High mortality rate in pregnant women.

Both HBV and HCV predispose a patient to chronic active hepatitis, cirrhosis, and hepatocellular carcinoma.

Hep **A**: **A**symptomatic (usually).

Hep **B**: **B**lood borne.

Hep **C**: **C**hronic, **C**irrhosis, **C**arcinoma, **C**arriers.

Hep **D**: **D**efective, **D**ependent on HBV.

Hep **E**: **E**nteric, **E**xpectant mothers, **E**pidemics.

A and E by fecal-oral route: "The **vowels** hit your **bowels**."

Hepatitis serologic markers

IgM HAVAb	IgM antibody to HAV; best test to detect active hepatitis A.
HBsAg	Antigen found on surface of HBV; continued presence indicates carrier state.
HBsAb	Antibody to HBsAg; **provides immunity** to hepatitis B.
HBcAg	Antigen associated with core of HBV.
HBcAb	Antibody to HBcAg; positive during **window period.** IgM HBcAb is an indicator of recent disease.
HBeAg	A second, different antigenic determinant in the HBV core. Important indicator of transmissibility. (**BE**ware!)
HBeAb	Antibody to e antigen; indicates low transmissibility.

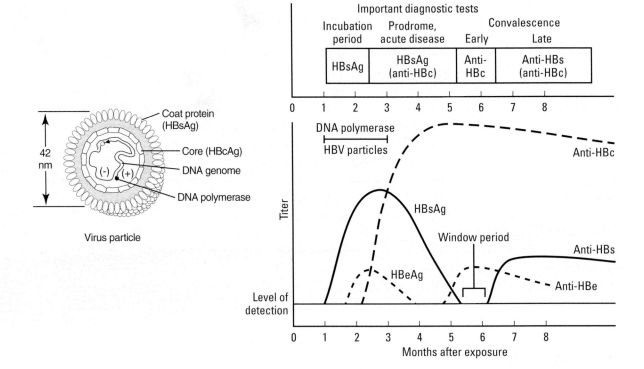

Test	Acute Disease	Window Phase	Complete Recovery	Chronic Carrier
HBsAg	+	–	–	+
HBsAb	–	–	+	–[b]
HBcAb	+[a]	+	+	+

[a]IgM in acute stage; IgG in chronic or recovered stage.

[b]Patient has surface antibody but available antibody is bound to HBsAg.

HIV

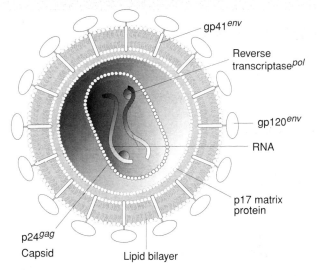

- gp41^{env}
- Reverse transcriptase^{pol}
- gp120^{env}
- RNA
- p17 matrix protein
- p24^{gag}
- Capsid
- Lipid bilayer

Diploid genome (2 molecules of RNA).

p24 = rectangular nucleocapsid protein.

gp41 and gp120 = envelope proteins.

Reverse transcriptase synthesizes dsDNA from RNA; dsDNA integrates into host genome.

(Adapted, with permission, from Levinson W, Jawetz E. *Medical Microbiology and Immunology: Examination and Board Review*, 6th ed. New York: McGraw-Hill, 2000:272.)

HIV diagnosis	Presumptive diagnosis made with ELISA (sensitive, high false-positive rate and low threshold, RULE OUT test); positive results are then confirmed with Western blot assay (specific, high false-negative rate and high threshold, RULE IN test). HIV PCR/viral load tests are increasing in popularity; they allow physician to monitor the effect of drug therapy on viral load.	ELISA/Western blot tests look for antibodies to viral proteins; these tests are often falsely negative in the first 1–2 months of HIV infection.

HIV immunity

CCR5 mutation	Homozygous = immunity.	1% of U.S. Caucasians.
	Heterozygous = slower course.	20% of U.S. Caucasians.
CXCR1 mutation	Rapid progression to AIDS.	

Time course of HIV infection

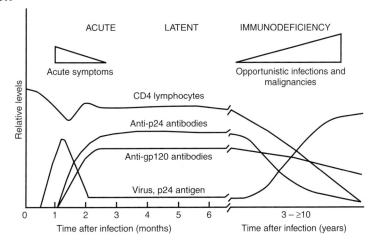

(Adapted, with permission, from Levinson W, Jawetz E. *Medical Microbiology and Immunology: Examination and Board Review*, 6th ed. New York: McGraw-Hill, 2000:276.)

Opportunistic infections in AIDS

Bacterial	Tuberculosis, *Mycobacterium avium–intracellulare* complex.
Viral	HSV, VZV, CMV, PML (JC virus).
Fungal	Thrush (*Candida albicans*), cryptococcosis (cryptococcal meningitis), histoplasmosis, *Pneumocystis* pneumonia.
Protozoan	Toxoplasmosis, cryptosporidiosis.

Prions

Infectious agents that do not contain RNA or DNA (consist only of proteins); encoded by cellular genes. Diseases include Creutzfeldt-Jakob disease (CJD—rapid progressive dementia), kuru, scrapie (sheep), and "mad cow disease." Prions are associated with spongiform encephalopathy. Normal prions have α-helix conformation; pathologic prions (like CJD) are β-pleated sheets.

Normal flora: dominant

Skin—*Staphylococcus epidermidis*.
Nose—*S. aureus*.
Oropharynx—viridans streptococci.
Dental plaque—*Streptococcus mutans*.
Colon—*Bacteroides fragilis* > *E. coli*.
Vagina—*Lactobacillus*, colonized by *E. coli* and group B strep.

Neonates delivered by cesarean section have no flora but are rapidly colonized after birth.

Common causes of pneumonia

Children (6 wks–18 yr) →	Adults (18–40 yr) →	Adults (40–65 yr) →	Elderly
Viruses (RSV)	*Mycoplasma*	*S. pneumoniae*	*S. pneumoniae*
Mycoplasma	*C. pneumoniae*	*H. influenzae*	Viruses
Chlamydia pneumoniae	*S. pneumoniae*	Anaerobes	Anaerobes
Streptococcus pneumoniae		Viruses	*H. influenzae*
		Mycoplasma	Gram-negative rods

Special groups:

Nosocomial (hospital acquired)	*Staphylococcus*, gram-negative rods
Immunocompromised	*Staphylococcus*, gram-negative rods, fungi, viruses, *Pneumocystis carinii*—with HIV
Aspiration	Anaerobes
Alcoholic/IV drug user	*S. pneumoniae*, *Klebsiella*, *Staphylococcus*
Postviral	*Staphylococcus*, *H. influenzae*
Neonate	Group B streptococci, *E. coli*
Atypical	*Mycoplasma*, *Legionella*, *Chlamydia*

Causes of meningitis

Newborn (0–6 mos) →	Children (6 mos–6 yrs) →	6–60 yrs →	60 yrs +
Group B streptococci	Streptococcus pneumoniae	N. meningitidis	S. pneumoniae
E. coli	Neisseria meningitidis	Enteroviruses	Gram-negative rods
Listeria	Haemophilus influenzae type B	S. pneumoniae	Listeria
	Enteroviruses	HSV	

In HIV—*Cryptococcus*, CMV, toxoplasmosis (brain abscess), JC virus (PML).

Note: Incidence of *H. influenzae* meningitis has ↓ greatly with introduction of *H. influenzae* vaccine in last 10–15 years.

CSF findings in meningitis

	Pressure	Cell type	Protein	Sugar
Bacterial	↑	↑ PMNs	↑	↓
Fungal/TB	↑	↑ lymphocytes	↑	↓
Viral	normal/↑	↑ lymphocytes	normal	normal

Osteomyelitis

Most people—*S. aureus.*

Sexually active—*Neisseria gonorrhoeae* (rare), septic arthritis more common.

Drug addicts—*Pseudomonas aeruginosa.*

Sickle cell—*Salmonella.*

Prosthetic replacement—*S. aureus* and *S. epidermidis.*

Vertebral—*Mycobacterium tuberculosis.*

Assume *S. aureus* if no other information.

Most osteomyelitis occurs in children.

Elevated ESR.

Urinary tract infections

Ambulatory—*E. coli* (50–80%), *Klebsiella* (8–10%). *Staphylococcus saprophyticus* (10–30%) is the 2nd most common cause of UTI in young ambulatory women.

Hospital—*E. coli*, *Proteus*, *Klebsiella*, *Serratia*, *Pseudomonas.*

Epidemiology: women to men—10:1 (short urethra colonized by fecal flora).

Predisposing factors: flow obstruction, kidney surgery, catheterization, gynecologic abnormalities, diabetes, and pregnancy.

UTIs mostly caused by ascending infections. In males: babies with congenital defects; elderly with enlarged prostates.

UTI—dysuria, frequency, urgency, suprapubic pain.

Pyelonephritis—fever, chills, flank pain, and CVA tenderness.

UTI bugs

Species	Features of the organism	
Serratia marcescens	Some strains produce a red pigment; often nosocomial and drug resistant.	**SSEEK PP.**
Staphylococcus saprophyticus	2nd leading cause of community-acquired UTI in sexually active women.	
Escherichia coli	Leading cause of UTI. Colonies show metallic sheen on EMB agar.	
Enterobacter cloacae	Often nosocomial and drug resistant.	
Klebsiella pneumoniae	Large mucoid capsule and viscous colonies.	
Proteus mirabilis	Motility causes "swarming" on agar; produces urease; associated with struvite stones.	
Pseudomonas aeruginosa	Blue-green pigment and fruity odor; usually nosocomial and drug resistant.	

Sexually transmitted diseases

Disease	Clinical features	Organism
Gonorrhea	Urethritis, cervicitis, PID, prostatitis, epididymitis, arthritis	*Neisseria gonorrhoeae*
1° syphilis	Painless chancre	*Treponema pallidum*
2° syphilis	Fever, lymphadenopathy, skin rashes, condylomata lata	
3° syphilis	Gummas, tabes dorsalis, general paresis, aortitis, Argyll Robertson pupil	
Genital herpes	Painful penile, vulvar, or cervical ulcers	HSV-2
Chlamydia	Urethritis, cervicitis, conjunctivitis, Reiter's syndrome, PID	*Chlamydia trachomatis* (D–K)
Lymphogranuloma venereum	Ulcers, lymphadenopathy, rectal strictures	*C. trachomatis* (L1–L3)
Trichomoniasis	Vaginitis	*Trichomonas vaginalis*
AIDS	Opportunistic infections, Kaposi's sarcoma, lymphoma	HIV
Condylomata acuminata	Genital warts, koilocytes	HPV 6 and 11
Hepatitis B	Jaundice	HBV
Chancroid	Painful genital ulcer	*Haemophilus ducreyi*

Pelvic inflammatory disease

Top bugs—*Chlamydia trachomatis* (subacute, often undiagnosed), *Neisseria gonorrhoeae* (acute, high fever). *C. trachomatis* is the most common STD in the United States (3–4 million cases per year). Cervical motion tenderness (chandelier sign), purulent cervical discharge. PID may include salpingitis, endometritis, hydrosalpinx, and tubo-ovarian abscess.

Salpingitis is a risk factor for ectopic pregnancy, infertility, chronic pelvic pain, and adhesions.
Other STDs include *Gardnerella* (clue cells) and *Trichomonas* (motile on wet prep).

Nosocomial infections

Risk factor	Pathogen	Notes
Newborn nursery	CMV, RSV	The 2 most common causes
Urinary catheterization	E. coli, Proteus mirabilis	of nosocomial infections are E. coli (UTI) and S. aureus (wound infection).
Respiratory therapy equipment	Pseudomonas aeruginosa	Presume Pseudomonas **AIR**uginosa when **AIR** or
Work in renal dialysis unit	HBV	burns are involved.
Hyperalimentation	Candida albicans	
Water aerosols	Legionella	Legionella when water source is involved.

Infections dangerous in pregnancy

ToRCHeS = Toxoplasma, Rubella, CMV, HSV/HIV, Syphilis.

Bug hints (if all else fails)

Pus, empyema, abscess—S. aureus.

Pediatric infection—Haemophilus influenzae (including epiglottitis).

Pneumonia in cystic fibrosis, burn infection—Pseudomonas aeruginosa.

Branching rods in oral infection—Actinomyces israelii.

Traumatic open wound—Clostridium perfringens.

Surgical wound—S. aureus.

Dog or cat bite—Pasteurella multocida.

Currant jelly sputum—Klebsiella.

Sepsis/meningitis in newborn—group B strep.

HIGH-YIELD FACTS

Microbiology

Antibody structure and function

Variable part of L and H chains recognizes antigens. Constant part of H chain of IgM and IgG fixes complement. Heavy chain contributes to Fc and Fab fractions. Light chain contributes only to Fab fraction.

Fc:

Constant

Carboxy terminal

Complement-binding
(IgG + IgM only)

Carbohydrate
side chains

Opsonization

Antibody promotes phagocytosis

Neutralization

Antibody prevents bacterial adherence

Complement activation

Membrane attack complex (MAC)

C3b

Antibody activates complement, enhancing opsonization and lysis

Immunoglobulin isotypes

IgG	Main antibody in 2° response. Most abundant. Fixes complement, crosses the placenta, opsonizes bacteria, neutralizes bacterial toxins and viruses.
IgA	Prevents attachment of bacteria and viruses to mucous membranes, does not fix complement. Monomer or dimer. Found in secretions. Picks up secretory component from epithelial cells before secretion.
IgM	Produced in the 1° response to an antigen. Fixes complement but does not cross the placenta. Antigen receptor on the surface of B cells. Monomer or pentamer.
IgD	Unclear function. Found on the surface of many B cells and in serum.
IgE	Mediates immediate (type I) hypersensitivity by inducing the release of mediators from mast cells and basophils when exposed to allergen. Mediates immunity to worms. Lowest concentration in serum.

Ig epitopes

Allotype (polymorphism)—Ig epitope that differs among members of same species. Can be on light chain or heavy chain.

Isotype (IgG, IgA, etc.)—Ig epitope common to a single class of Ig (5 classes, determined by heavy chain).

Idiotype (specific for a given antigen)—Ig epitope determined by antigen-binding site.

Isotype = *iso* (same). Common to same class.

Idiotype = *idio* (unique). Hypervariable region is unique.

MHC I and II

MHC—major histocompatibility complex. Consists of 3 class I genes (A, B, C) and 3 class II genes (DP, DQ, DR). All nucleated cells have MHC I proteins.

Antigen-presenting cells (e.g., macrophages and dendritic cells) also have MHC II proteins.

Class II are the main determinants of organ rejection.

MHC I antigen loading occurs in RER (viral antigens).

MHC II antigen loading occurs in acidified endosome.

Class I—1 polypeptide, with β_2-microglobulin.

Class II—2 polypeptides, an α and a β chain.

Differentiation of B and T cells

Th1 cells (produce IL-2 and γ-interferon)—activate macrophages (increase killing efficiency of intracellular bacteria) and Tc cells.

Th2 cells (produce IL-4 and IL-5)—help B cells make antibody (B = 2nd letter of alphabet).

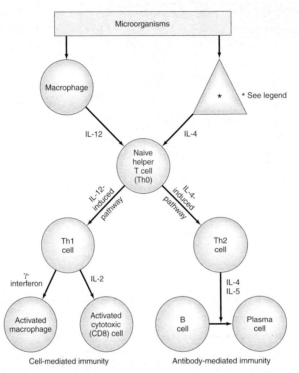

*The human cell that produces the IL-4 that induces naive helper T cells to become Th2 cells has not been identified.

(Adapted, with permission, from Levinson W, Jawetz E. *Medical Microbiology and Immunology: Examination and Board Review*, 6th ed. New York: McGraw-Hill, 2000:349.)

Major function of B cells and T cells

Antibody-mediated immunity (B cells)	Cell-mediated immunity (T cells)
Host defense against infection (opsonize bacteria, neutralize toxins and viruses)	Host defense against infection (especially *Mycobacterium tuberculosis*, viruses, and fungi)
Allergy (e.g., hay fever)	Allergy (e.g., poison oak)
Autoimmunity	Graft and tumor rejection
	Regulation of antibody response (help and suppression)

(Adapted, with permission, from Levinson W, Jawetz E. *Medical Microbiology and Immunology: Examination and Board Review*, 6th ed. New York: McGraw-Hill, 2000:337.)

Adjuvant definition

Adjuvants are nonspecific stimulators of the immune response but are not immunogenic by themselves. Adjuvants are given with a weak immunogen to enhance response. Human vaccines contain aluminum hydroxide or lipid adjuvants.

Adjuvant—that which aids another.

T-cell glycoproteins

Helper T cells have CD4, which binds to MHC II on antigen-presenting cells. Cytotoxic T cells have CD8, which binds to MHC I on virus-infected cells.

Product of CD and MHC = 8. (CD4 × MHC **II** = **8** = CD8 × MHC **I**).

CD3 complex—cluster of polypeptides associated with a T-cell receptor. Important in signal transduction.

Antigen-presenting cells:
1. Macrophage
2. B cell
3. Dendritic cell

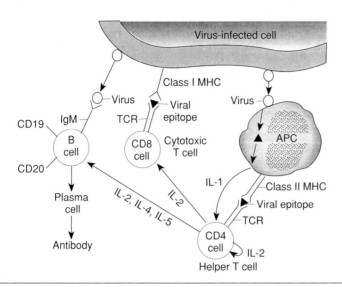

T-cell activation

Th activation:
1. Foreign body is phagocytosed by APC
2. Foreign antigen is presented on MHC II and recognized by TCR on Th cell
3. "Costimulatory signal" is given by interaction of B7 and CD28
4. Th cell activated to produce IL-2 and γ-interferon

Tc activation:
1. Endogenously synthesized (viral or self) proteins are presented on MHC I and recognized by TCR on Tc cell
2. IL-2 from Th cell activates Tc cell to kill virus-infected cell

Anergy
Self-reactive T cells become nonreactive without costimulatory molecule.
B cells also become anergic, but tolerance is less complete than in T cells.

Important cytokines

IL-1	Secreted by macrophages. Stimulates T cells, B cells, neutrophils, fibroblasts, and epithelial cells to grow, differentiate, or synthesize specific products. An endogenous pyrogen.	"**Hot T-bone stEAk**":
		IL-1: fever (**hot**)
		IL-2: stimulates **T** cells
IL-2	Secreted by helper T cells. Stimulates growth of helper and cytotoxic T cells.	IL-3: stimulates **bone** marrow
		IL-4: stimulates Ig**E** production
IL-3	Secreted by activated T cells. Supports the growth and differentiation of bone marrow stem cells. Has a function similar to GM-CSF.	IL-5: stimulates Ig**A** production
IL-4	Secreted by helper T cells. Promotes growth of B cells. Enhances the synthesis of IgE and IgG.	
IL-5	Secreted by helper T cells. Promotes differentiation of B cells. Enhances the synthesis of IgA. Stimulates production and activation of eosinophils.	
IL-8	Major chemotactic factor for neutrophils.	
γ-interferon	Secreted by helper T cells. Stimulates macrophages.	
TNF-α	Secreted by macrophages. ↑ IL-2 receptor synthesis by helper T cells. ↑ B-cell proliferation. Attracts and activates neutrophils.	
TNF-β	Secreted by activated T lymphocytes. Functions similar to those of TNF-α.	

Cell surface proteins

Helper T cells	CD4, TCR, CD3, CD28.
Cytotoxic T cells	CD8, TCR, CD3.
B cells	IgM, B7, CD19, CD20.
Macrophages	MHC II, CD14.
NK cells	Receptors for MHC I, CD16.
All cells except mature red cells	MHC I.

Acute phase response

Complement

Complement defends against gram-negative bacteria. Activated by Ig**G** or Ig**M** in the **classic** pathway, and activated by toxins (including endotoxin), aggregated IgA, or other conditions in the alternate pathway.

GM makes **classic** cars.
C1, C2, C3, C4—viral neutralization.
C3b—opsonization.
C3a, C5a—anaphylaxis.
C5a—neutrophil chemotaxis.
C5b-9—cytolysis by membrane attack complex (MAC).
Deficiency of C1 esterase inhibitor leads to hereditary angioedema (overactive complement).
Deficiency of C3 leads to severe, recurrent pyogenic sinus and respiratory tract infections.
Deficiency of C6–C8 leads to *Neisseria* bacteremia.
Deficiency of decay-accelerating factor (DAF) leads to paroxysmal nocturnal hemoglobinuria (PNH).

(Adapted, with permission, from Levinson W, Jawetz E. *Medical Microbiology and Immunology: Examination and Board Review*, 6th ed. New York: McGraw-Hill, 2000:381.)

Interferon mechanism

Interferons (α, β, γ) are proteins that place uninfected cells in an antiviral state. Interferons induce the production of a 2nd protein that inhibits viral protein synthesis by degrading viral mRNA (but not host mRNA).

Interferes with viral protein synthesis by:
1. α- and β-interferons inhibit viral protein synthesis
2. γ-interferons ↑ MHC I and II expression and antigen presentation in all cells
3. Activates NK cells to kill virus-infected cells

Hypersensitivity

Type I

Mast cell or basophil

Fc receptor

Ag

IgE

Ag

Anaphylactic and atopic—antigen cross-links IgE on presensitized mast cells and basophils, triggering release of vasoactive amines (i.e., histamine). Reaction develops rapidly after antigen exposure due to preformed antibody. Examples include anaphylaxis, asthma, hives, local wheal and flare.

First and **F**ast (anaphylaxis). I, II, and III are all antibody mediated.

Type II

Cell   C*

Cytotoxic—IgM, IgG bind to antigen on "enemy" cell, leading to lysis (by complement) or phagocytosis. Examples include autoimmune hemolytic anemia, Rh disease (erythroblastosis fetalis), Goodpasture's syndrome, rheumatic fever, Graves' disease, bullous pemphigoid.

Cy-**2**-toxic.
Antibody and complement lead to membrane attack complex (MAC).

Type III

Ag   Ag

Ag

Ag

C*

Immune complex—antigen-antibody complexes activate complement, which attracts neutrophils; neutrophils release lysosomal enzymes. Examples include PAN, immune complex GN, SLE, rheumatoid arthritis.

Serum sickness—an immune complex disease (type III) in which antibodies to the foreign proteins are produced (takes 5 days). Immune complexes form and are deposited in membranes, where they fix complement (leads to tissue damage). More common than Arthus reaction.

Arthus reaction—a local subacute antibody-mediated hypersensitivity (type III) reaction. Intradermal injection of antigen induces antibodies, which form antigen-antibody complexes in the skin. Characterized by edema, necrosis, and activation of complement. Examples include hypersensitivity pneumonitis, thermophilic actinomycetes.

Imagine an immune complex as **3** things stuck together: antigen-antibody-complement.

Most serum sickness is now caused by drugs (not serum). Fever, urticaria, arthralgias, proteinuria, lymphadenopathy 5–10 days after antigen exposure.

Antigen-antibody complexes cause the Arthus reaction.

Type IV

Ag   T cell

Ag   T cell

Delayed (cell-mediated) type—sensitized T lymphocytes encounter antigen and then release lymphokines (leads to macrophage activation). Examples include TB skin test, transplant rejection, contact dermatitis (e.g., poison ivy, poison oak).

4th and last—delayed. Cell mediated; therefore, it is not transferable by serum.

ACID:
Anaphylactic and **A**topic (type I)
Cytotoxic (type II)
Immune complex (type III)
Delayed (cell-mediated) (type IV)

C* = complement

Immune deficiencies

B-cell deficiencies

Bruton's agammaglobulinemia	X-linked recessive defect in a tyrosine kinase gene associated with low levels of all classes of immunoglobulins. Associated with recurrent **B**acterial infections after 6 months of age, when levels of maternal IgG antibody decline. Occurs in **B**oys (X-linked).
Selective immunoglobulin deficiency	Deficiency in a specific class of immunoglobulins—possibly due to a defect in isotype switching. Selective IgA deficiency is the most common selective immunoglobulin deficiency. Presents with sinus and lung infections.

T-cell deficiencies

Thymic aplasia (DiGeorge syndrome)	Thymus and parathyroids fail to develop owing to failure of development of the 3rd and 4th pharyngeal pouches. Presents with **T**etany owing to hypocalcemia. Recurrent viral and fungal infections due to T-cell deficiency. Congenital defects of heart and great vessels. 22q11 deletion.
Chronic mucocutaneous candidiasis	T-cell dysfunction specifically against *Candida albicans*. Presents with skin and mucous membrane *Candida* infections.

B- and T-cell deficiencies

Severe combined immunodeficiency (SCID)	Defect in early stem-cell differentiation. Presents with recurrent viral, bacterial, fungal, and protozoal infections. May have multiple causes (e.g., failure to synthesize MHC II antigens, defective IL-2 receptors, or adenosine deaminase deficiency).
Wiskott-Aldrich syndrome	X-linked defect in the ability to mount an IgM response to capsular polysaccharides of bacteria. Associated with elevated IgA levels, normal IgE levels, and low IgM levels. Triad of symptoms includes recurrent pyogenic infections, eczema, and thrombocytopenia.
Ataxia-telangiectasia	Defect in DNA repair enzymes with associated IgA deficiency. Presents with cerebellar problems (ataxia) and spider angiomas (telangiectasia).

Phagocytic deficiencies

Chronic granulomatous disease	Defect in phagocytosis of neutrophils owing to lack of NADPH oxidase activity or similar enzymes. Presents with marked susceptibility to opportunistic infections with bacteria, especially *S. aureus* and *E. coli*, and *Aspergillus*. Diagnosis confirmed with negative nitroblue tetrazolium dye reduction test.
Chédiak-Higashi disease	Autosomal recessive. Defect in microtubular function and lysosomal emptying of phagocytic cells. Presents with recurrent pyogenic infections by staphylococci and streptococci.
Job's syndrome	Failure of γ-interferon production by helper T cells. Neutrophils fail to respond to chemotactic stimuli. Presents with recurrent "cold" (noninflamed) staphylococcal abscesses, eczema, and high levels of IgE.
Leukocyte adhesion deficiency syndrome	Defect in LFA-1 adhesion proteins on phagocytes. Presents early in life with severe pyogenic infections.
Hyper-IgM syndrome	Defect in CD40 ligand on CD4 T helper cells leads to inability to class switch. Presents early in life with severe pyogenic infections. High levels of IgM; very low levels of IgG, IgA, and IgE.
IL-12 receptor deficiency	Presents with disseminated mycobacterial infections.

Passive vs. active immunity

Active	Induced after exposure to foreign antigens. Slow onset. Long-lasting protection (memory).	After exposure to **T**etanus toxin, **B**otulinum toxin, **H**BV, or **R**abies, patients are given preformed antibodies (passive)—**T**o **B**e **H**ealed **R**apidly.
Passive	Based on receiving preformed antibodies from another host. Rapid onset. Short life span of antibodies.	

Antigen variation

	Classic examples:
	  Bacteria—*Salmonella* (two flagellar variants),
	    Borrelia (relapsing fever), *Neisseria gonorrhoeae*
	    (pilus protein).
	  Virus—influenza (major = shift, minor = drift).
	  Parasites—trypanosomes (programmed rearrangement).
		Some mechanisms for variation include DNA rearrangement and RNA segment rearrangement (e.g., influenza major shift).

Autoantibodies

Autoantibody	Associated disorder
Antinuclear antibodies (ANA)	SLE
Anti-dsDNA, anti-Smith	Specific for SLE
Antihistone	Drug-induced lupus
Anti-IgG (rheumatoid factor)	Rheumatoid arthritis
Antineutrophil	Vasculitis
Anticentromere	Scleroderma (CREST)
Anti-Scl-70	Scleroderma (diffuse)
Antimitochondrial	1° biliary cirrhosis
Antigliadin	Celiac disease
Anti–basement membrane	Goodpasture's syndrome
Anti–epithelial cell	Pemphigus vulgaris
Antimicrosomal	Hashimoto's thyroiditis

Transplant rejection

Hyperacute rejection	Antibody mediated due to the presence of preformed anti-donor antibodies in the transplant recipient. Occurs within minutes after transplantation.
Acute rejection	Cell mediated due to cytotoxic T lymphocytes reacting against foreign MHCs. Occurs weeks after transplantation. Reversible with immunosuppressants such as cyclosporin and OKT3.
Chronic rejection	Antibody-mediated vascular damage (fibrinoid necrosis); occurs months to years after transplantation. Irreversible.
Graft-versus-host disease	Grafted immunocompetent T cells proliferate in the irradiated immunocompromised host and reject cells with "foreign" proteins, resulting in severe organ dysfunction. Major symptoms include a maculopapular rash, jaundice, hepatosplenomegaly, and diarrhea.

Pathology

"The beginning of health is to know the disease."
—Spanish proverb

Questions dealing with this discipline are difficult to prepare for because of the sheer volume of material. Review the basic principles and hallmark characteristics of the key diseases. Given the increasingly clinical orientation of Step 1, it is no longer enough to know only the "trigger word" associations of certain diseases (e.g., café-au-lait macules and neurofibromatosis); you must also know the clinical descriptions of these findings.

Given the clinical slant of the USMLE Step 1, it is also important to review the classic presenting signs and symptoms of diseases as well as their associated laboratory findings. Delve into the signs, symptoms, and pathophysiology of the major diseases having a high prevalence in the United States (e.g., alcoholism, diabetes, hypertension, heart failure, ischemic heart disease, infectious disease). Be prepared to think one step beyond the simple diagnosis to treatment or complications.

The examination includes a number of color photomicrographs and photographs of gross specimens that are presented in the setting of a brief clinical history. However, read the question and the choices carefully before looking at the illustration, because the history will help you identify the pathologic process. Flip through an illustrated pathology textbook, color atlases, and appropriate Web sites in order to look at the pictures in the days before the exam. Pay attention to potential clues such as age, sex, ethnicity, occupation, recent activities and exposures, and specialized lab tests.

High-Yield Clinical Vignettes
Congenital
Neoplastic
Hematologic
Gastrointestinal
Respiratory
Neurologic
Rheumatic/Autoimmune
Endocrine
Reproductive
Cardiovascular
Renal
Alcoholism
Findings
Glossy Photos

These abstracted case vignettes are designed to demonstrate the thought processes necessary to answer multistep clinical reasoning questions.

Vignette	Question	Answer
■ Woman with previous cesarean section has a scar in her lower uterus close to the opening of the os.	What is she at ↑ risk for?	Placenta previa.
■ 35-year-old man has high blood pressure in his arms and low pressure in his legs.	What is the diagnosis?	Coarctation of the aorta.
■ Woman presents with diffuse goiter and hyperthyroidism.	What are the expected values of TSH and thyroid hormones?	Low TSH and high thyroid hormones.
■ Patient exhibits an extended expiratory phase.	What is the disease process?	Obstructive lung disease.
■ Woman presents with headache, visual disturbance, galactorrhea, and amenorrhea.	What is the diagnosis?	Prolactinoma.
■ Baby has foul-smelling stool and recurrent pulmonary infections.	What is the diagnosis, and what test is used?	Cystic fibrosis; chloride sweat test.
■ Obese woman presents with hirsutism and ↑ levels of serum testosterone.	What is the diagnosis?	Polycystic ovarian syndrome.
■ Man presents with pain and swelling of the knees, subcutaneous nodules around the joints and Achilles tendon, and exquisite pain in the metatarsophalangeal joint of his right big toe. Biopsy shows needle-like crystals.	What is the diagnosis?	Gouty arthritis.
■ 48-year-old female presents with progressive lethargy and extreme sensitivity to cold temperatures.	What is the diagnosis?	Hypothyroidism.
■ Patient with elevated serum cortisol levels undergoes a dexamethasone suppression test. 1 mg of dexamethasone does not ↓ cortisol levels; 8 mg does.	What is the diagnosis?	Pituitary tumor.
■ During a game, a young football player collapses and dies immediately.	What is the most likely type of cardiac disease?	Hypertrophic cardiomyopathy.

Vignette	Question	Answer
■ Child has been anemic since birth.	Splenectomy would result in increased hematocrit in what disease?	Spherocytosis.
■ 43-year-old man experiences dizziness and tinnitus. CT shows enlarged internal acoustic meatus.	What is the diagnosis?	Schwannoma.
■ Child exhibits weakness and enlarged calves.	What is the disease, and how is it inherited?	Duchenne's muscular dystrophy, X-linked recessive.
■ 25-year-old female presents with sudden uniocular vision loss and slightly slurred speech. She has a history of weakness and paresthesias that have resolved.	What is the diagnosis?	Multiple sclerosis.
■ Teenager presents with nephritic syndrome and hearing loss.	What is his disease?	Alport's syndrome.
■ Tall, thin male teenager has abrupt-onset dyspnea and left-sided chest pain. There is hyperresonant percussion on the affected side, and breath sounds are diminished.	What is the diagnosis?	Pneumothorax.
■ Young man is concerned about his wife's inability to conceive and her recurrent URIs. She has dextrocardia.	Which of her proteins is defective?	Dynein (Kartagener's).
■ 55-year-old man who is a smoker and a heavy drinker presents with a new cough and flu-like symptoms. Gram stain shows no organisms; silver stain of sputum shows gram-negative rods.	What is the diagnosis?	*Legionella* pneumonia.
■ Patient has a stroke after incurring multiple long bone fractures in trauma stemming from a motor vehicle accident.	What caused the infarct?	Fat emboli.
■ 25-year-old woman presents with a low-grade fever, a rash across her nose that gets worse when she is out in the sun, and widespread edema.	You are concerned about what disease?	SLE.

Vignette	Question	Answer
■ 50-year-old man complains of diarrhea; on physical exam his face is plethoric and a heart murmur is detected.	What is the diagnosis?	Carcinoid syndrome.
■ Elderly woman presents with a headache and jaw pain. Labs show elevated ESR.	What is the diagnosis?	Temporal arteritis.
■ Pregnant woman at 16 weeks of gestation presents with an atypically large abdomen.	What abnormality might be seen on blood test, and what is the disorder?	High hCG; hydatidiform mole.
■ 80-year-old man presents with a systolic crescendo-decrescendo murmur.	What is the most likely cause?	Aortic stenosis.
■ Woman of short stature presents with shortened 4th and 5th metacarpals.	What endocrine disorder comes to mind?	Albright's hereditary osteodystrophy, or pseudohypoparathyroidism.
■ After a stressful life event, 30-year-old man has diarrhea and blood per rectum; intestinal biopsy shows transmural inflammation.	What is the diagnosis?	Crohn's.
■ Young man presents with mental deterioration and tremors. He has brown pigmentation in a ring around the periphery of his cornea and altered LFTs.	What treatment should he receive?	Penicillamine for Wilson's disease.
■ Patient presents with fatigue, and blood tests show a macrocytic, megaloblastic anemia.	What is the danger of giving folate alone?	Masks signs of neural damage with vitamin B_{12} deficiency.
■ 10-year-old child "spaces out" in class (e.g., stops talking midsentence and then continues as if nothing had happened). During spells, there is slight quivering of lips.	What is the diagnosis?	Absence seizure.
■ 85-year-old man presents with acute knee pain and swelling. X-ray shows ↑ joint space without erosion.	What is the diagnosis, and what would you find on aspiration?	Pseudogout; rhomboid calcium pyrophosphate crystals.

HIGH-YIELD FACTS

Pathology

Vignette	Question	Answer
■ X-ray shows bilateral hilar lymphadenopathy.	What is the diagnosis?	Sarcoidosis.
■ 5-year-old boy presents with systolic murmur and wide, fixed split S2.	What is the diagnosis?	ASD.

Common congenital malformations

1. Heart defects (congenital rubella)
2. Hypospadias
3. Cleft lip with or without cleft palate
4. Congenital hip dislocation
5. Spina bifida
6. Anencephaly
7. Pyloric stenosis (associated with polyhydramnios); projectile vomiting

Neural tube defects (spina bifida and anencephaly) are associated with ↑ levels of α-fetoprotein (in the amniotic fluid and maternal serum). Their incidence is ↓ with maternal folate ingestion during pregnancy.

Congenital heart disease

Right-to-left shunts (early cyanosis)— "blue babies"

1. **T**etralogy of Fallot (most common cause of early cyanosis)
2. **T**ransposition of great vessels
3. **T**runcus arteriosus

The **3 T's**:
Tetralogy
Transposition
Truncus
Children may squat to ↑ venous return.

Left-to-right shunts (late cyanosis)— "blue kids"

1. VSD (most common congenital cardiac anomaly)
2. ASD (loud S1; wide, fixed split S2)
3. PDA (close with indomethacin)

Frequency—VSD > ASD > PDA.
↑ pulmonary resistance due to arteriolar thickening.
→ progressive pulmonary hypertension; R → L shunt (Eisenmenger's).

Eisenmenger's syndrome

Uncorrected VSD, ASD, or PDA leads to progressive pulmonary hypertension. As pulmonary resistance ↑, the shunt changes from L → R to R → L, which causes late cyanosis (clubbing and polycythemia).

Tetralogy of Fallot

1. **P**ulmonary stenosis
2. **R**VH
3. **O**verriding aorta (overrides the VSD)
4. **V**SD

This leads to **e**arly cyanosis from a right-to-left shunt across the VSD. On x-ray, boot-shaped heart due to RVH. Patients suffer "cyanotic spells."
The cause of tetralogy of Fallot is anterosuperior displacement of the infundibular septum.

PROVe.

(Adapted, with permission, from Chandrasoma P. *Concise Pathology*, 3rd ed. Stamford, CT: Appleton & Lange, 1997:345.)

| **Transposition of great vessels** | Aorta leaves RV (anterior) and pulmonary trunk leaves LV (posterior) → separation of systemic and pulmonary circulations. Not compatible with life unless a shunt is present to allow adequate mixing of blood (e.g., VSD, PDA, or patent foramen ovale). | Due to failure of the aorticopulmonary septum to spiral. Without surgical correction, most infants die within the 1st months of life. Common congenital heart disease in offspring of diabetic mothers. |

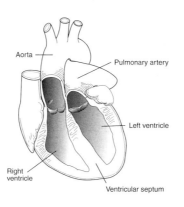

Aorta
Pulmonary artery
Left ventricle
Right ventricle
Ventricular septum

(Adapted, with permission, from Way LW (ed). *Current Surgical Diagnosis and Treatment*, 10th ed. Stamford, CT: Appleton & Lange, 1994:405.)

Coarctation of aorta

Ligamentum arteriosum
Postductal coarctation
Descending aorta

| | Infantile type—aortic stenosis proximal to insertion of ductus arteriosus (preductal). Adult type—stenosis is distal to ductus arteriosus (postductal). Associated with notching of the ribs, hypertension in upper extremities, weak pulses in lower extremities. | Male-to-female ratio 3:1. Check femoral pulses on physical exam. **IN**fantile: **IN** close to the heart. (Associated with Turner's syndrome.) A**D**ult: **D**istal to **D**uctus. |

Patent ductus arteriosus

Aorta
Ductus arteriosus (patent)
Pulmonary artery

| | In fetal period, shunt is right to left (normal). In neonatal period, lung resistance ↓ and shunt becomes left to right with subsequent RVH and failure (abnormal). Associated with a continuous, "machine-like" murmur. Patency is maintained by PGE synthesis and low O_2 tension. | Indomethacin is used to close a PDA. PGE is used to keep a PDA open, which may be necessary to sustain life in conditions such as transposition of the great vessels. |

HIGH-YIELD FACTS

Pathology

Autosomal trisomies

Down syndrome (trisomy 21), 1:700	Most common chromosomal disorder and cause of congenital mental retardation. Findings: mental retardation, flat facial profile, prominent epicanthal folds, simian crease, duodenal atresia, congenital heart disease (most common malformation is septum primum–type ASD due to endocardial cushion defects), Alzheimer's disease in affected individuals > 35 years old, ↑ risk of ALL. 95% of cases due to meiotic nondisjunction of homologous chromosomes; associated with advanced maternal age (from 1:1500 in women < 20 to 1:25 in women > 45). 4% of cases due to robertsonian translocation, and 1% of cases due to Down mosaicism (no maternal association).	Drinking age (21). ↓ levels of α-fetoprotein.
Edwards' syndrome (trisomy 18), 1:8000	Findings: severe mental retardation, rocker bottom feet, low-set ears, micrognathia, congenital heart disease, clenched hands (flexion of fingers), prominent occiput. Death usually occurs within 1 year of birth.	Election age (18).
Patau's syndrome (trisomy 13), 1:6000	Findings: severe mental retardation, microphthalmia, microcephaly, cleft lip/palate, abnormal forebrain structures, polydactyly, congenital heart disease. Death usually occurs within 1 year of birth.	Puberty (13).

Genetic gender disorders

Klinefelter's syndrome [male] (XXY), 1:850	Testicular atrophy, eunuchoid body shape, tall, long extremities, gynecomastia, female hair distribution. Presence of inactivated X chromosome (Barr body).	Common cause of hypogonadism seen in infertility workup.
Turner's syndrome [female] **(XO)**, 1:3000	Short stature, ovarian dysgenesis (streak ovary), webbing of neck, coarctation of the aorta, most common cause of 1° amenorrhea. No Barr body.	"Hugs and kisses" **(XO)** from Tina **Turner** (female).
Double Y males [male] (XYY), 1:1000	Phenotypically normal, very tall, severe acne, antisocial behavior (seen in 1–2% of XYY males).	Observed with ↑ frequency among inmates of penal institutions.

Muscular dystrophies

Duchenne's (X-linked)	Frame-shift mutation → deletion of dystrophin gene → accelerated muscle breakdown. Onset before 5 years of age. Weakness begins in pelvic girdle muscles and progresses superiorly. Pseudohypertrophy of calf muscles due to fibrofatty replacement of muscle; cardiac myopathy. The use of Gowers' maneuver, requiring assistance of the upper extremities to stand up, is characteristic (indicates proximal lower limb weakness).	Duchenne's = Deleted Dystrophin. Diagnose muscular dystrophies by ↑ CPK and muscle biopsy.
Becker's	Mutated dystrophin gene is less severe than Duchenne's.	

Pseudohermaphroditism

	Disagreement between the phenotypic (external genitalia) and gonadal (testes vs. ovaries) sex.	Gender identity is based on external genitalia and sex of upbringing.
Female pseudo-hermaphrodite (XX)	Ovaries present, but external genitalia are virilized or ambiguous. Due to excessive and inappropriate exposure to androgenic steroids during early gestation (i.e., congenital adrenal hyperplasia or exogenous administration of androgens during pregnancy).	
Male pseudo-hermaphrodite (XY)	Testes present, but external genitalia are female or ambiguous. Most common form is testicular feminization (androgen insensitivity), which results from a mutation in the androgen receptor gene (X-linked recessive); blind-end vagina.	

True hermaphrodite (46,XX or 47,XXY)	Both ovary and testicular tissue present; ambiguous genitalia.	
Testicular feminization syndrome (46,XY)	Defect in DHT receptor resulting in normal-appearing female; female external genitalia with rudimentary vagina; uterus and uterine tubes generally absent; develops testes (often found in labia majora; surgically removed to prevent malignancy). Levels of testosterone, estrogen, and LH are all high.	
5α-reductase deficiency	Unable to convert testosterone to DHT. Ambiguous genitalia until puberty, when ↑ testosterone causes masculinization of genitalia. Testosterone/estrogen levels are normal; LH is normal or ↑.	
Cri-du-chat syndrome	Congenital deletion of short arm of chromosome 5 (46,XX or XY, 5p–). Findings: microcephaly, severe mental retardation, high-pitched crying/mewing, epicanthal folds, cardiac abnormalities.	*Cri du chat* = cry of the cat.
Fragile X syndrome	X-linked defect affecting the methylation and expression of the *FMR1* gene. The 2nd most common cause of genetic mental retardation (the most common cause is Down syndrome). Associated with macro-orchidism (enlarged testes), long face with a large jaw, large everted ears, and autism.	Triplet repeat disorder (CGG_n) that may show genetic anticipation. Fragile **X** = e**X**tra-large testes, jaw, ears.

Cystic fibrosis

Autosomal-recessive defect in *CFTR* gene on chromosome 7. Defective Cl⁻ channel → secretion of abnormally thick mucus that plugs lungs, pancreas, and liver → recurrent pulmonary infections (*Pseudomonas* species and *S. aureus*), chronic bronchitis, bronchiectasis, pancreatic insufficiency (malabsorption and steatorrhea), meconium ileus in newborns. ↑ concentration of Cl⁻ ions in sweat test is diagnostic.

Infertility in males due to absent vas deferens. Fat-soluble vitamin deficiencies (A, D, E, K). Can present as failure to thrive in infancy.
Most common lethal genetic disease of Caucasians.
Treatment: *N*-acetylcysteine to loosen mucous plugs.

Autosomal-dominant diseases

Adult polycystic kidney disease	**Always bilateral,** massive enlargement of kidneys due to multiple large cysts. Patients present with pain, hematuria, hypertension, progressive renal failure. 90% of cases are due to mutation in *APKD1* (chromosome 16). Associated with polycystic liver disease, **berry aneurysms,** mitral valve prolapse. Juvenile form is recessive.
Familial hypercholesterolemia (type IIA)	Elevated LDL owing to defective or absent LDL receptor. Heterozygotes (1:500) have cholesterol ≈ 300 mg/dL. Homozygotes (very rare) have cholesterol ≈ 700+ mg/dL, severe atherosclerotic disease early in life, and tendon xanthomas (classically in the Achilles tendon); MI may develop before age 20.
Marfan's syndrome	Fibrillin gene mutation → connective tissue disorders. Skeletal abnormalities—tall with long extremities, hyperextensive joints, and long, tapering fingers and toes. Cardiovascular—cystic medial necrosis of aorta → aortic incompetence and dissecting aortic aneurysms. Floppy mitral valve. Ocular—subluxation of lenses.
Neurofibromatosis type 1 (von Recklinghausen's disease)	Findings: café-au-lait spots, neural tumors, Lisch nodules (pigmented iris hamartomas). Also marked by skeletal disorders (e.g., scoliosis) and ↑ tumor susceptibility. On long arm of chromosome **17**; **17** letters in von Recklinghausen.
Neurofibromatosis type 2	Bilateral acoustic neuroma. *NF***2** gene on chromosome **22**; type **2** = **22.**
Von Hippel–Lindau disease	Findings: hemangioblastomas of retina/cerebellum/medulla; about half of affected individuals develop multiple bilateral renal cell carcinomas and other tumors. Associated with deletion of *VHL* gene (tumor suppressor) on chromosome 3 (3p). Von Hippel–Lindau = **3** words for chromosome **3.**
Huntington's disease	Findings: depression, progressive dementia, choreiform movements, caudate atrophy, and ↓ levels of GABA and ACh in the brain. Symptoms manifest in affected individuals between the ages of 20 and 50. Gene located on chromosome **4**; triplet repeat disorder. "Hunting **4** food."
Familial adenomatous polyposis	Colon becomes covered with adenomatous polyps after puberty. Progresses to colon cancer unless resected. Deletion on chromosome **5**; **5** letters in "polyp."
Hereditary spherocytosis	Spheroid erythrocytes; hemolytic anemia; increased MCHC. Splenectomy is curative.
Achondroplasia	Autosomal-dominant cell-signaling defect of fibroblast growth factor (FGF) receptor 3. Results in dwarfism; short limbs, but head and trunk are normal size.

Autosomal-recessive diseases	Cystic fibrosis, albinism, α_1-antitrypsin deficiency, phenylketonuria, thalassemias, sickle cell anemias, glycogen storage diseases, mucopolysaccharidoses (except Hunter's), sphingolipidoses (except Fabry's), infant polycystic kidney disease, hemochromatosis.
X-linked recessive disorders	Fragile X, Duchenne's muscular dystrophy, hemophilia A and B, Fabry's, G6PD deficiency, Hunter's syndrome, ocular albinism, Lesch-Nyhan syndrome, Bruton's agammaglobulinemia, Wiskott-Aldrich syndrome. Female carriers of X-linked recessive disorders are rarely affected because of random inactivation of X chromosomes in each cell.
Neural tube defects	Associated with low folic acid intake during pregnancy. Elevated α-fetoprotein in amniotic fluid. Spina bifida occulta—failure of bony spinal canal to close, but no structural herniation. Usually seen at lower vertebral levels. Meningocele—meninges herniate through spinal canal defect. Meningomyelocele—meninges and spinal cord herniate through spinal canal defect.

Fetal alcohol syndrome	Newborns of mothers who consumed significant amounts of alcohol (teratogen) during pregnancy (highest risk at 3–8 weeks) have ↑ incidence of congenital abnormalities, including pre- and postnatal developmental retardation, microcephaly, facial abnormalities, limb dislocation, and heart and lung fistulas. Mechanism may include inhibition of cell migration. The number one cause of congenital malformations in the United States.

Neoplastic progression

- Normal cells with basal → apical differentiation

- Cells have increased in number—**hyperplasia**
- Abnormal proliferation of cells with loss of size, shape, and orientation—**dysplasia**

- **In situ carcinoma**
- Neoplastic cells have not invaded basement membrane
- High nuclear/cytoplasmic ratio and clumped chromatin
- Neoplastic cells encompass entire thickness

- Cells have invaded basement membrane using **collagenases** and **hydrolases**
- Will metastasize if they reach a blood or lymphatic vessel

Metastasis—spread to distant organ
- Must survive immune attack
- "Seed and soil" theory of metastasis
  - Seed = tumor embolus
  - Soil = target organ—liver, lungs, bone, brain...

(Adapted, with permission, from McPhee SJ et al. *Pathophysiology of Disease: An Introduction to Clinical Medicine,* 3rd ed. New York: McGraw-Hill, 2000:84.)

-plasia definitions

Hyperplasia— $\uparrow$ in number of cells (reversible).

Metaplasia—1 adult cell type is replaced by another (reversible). Often 2° to irritation and/or environmental exposure (e.g., squamous metaplasia in trachea and bronchi of smokers).

Dysplasia—abnormal growth with loss of cellular orientation, shape, and size in comparison to normal tissue maturation; commonly preneoplastic (reversible).

Anaplasia—abnormal cells lacking differentiation; like primitive cells of same tissue, often equated with undifferentiated malignant neoplasms. Tumor giant cells may be formed.

Neoplasia—a clonal proliferation of cells that is uncontrolled and excessive.

Tumor grade vs. stage

Grade	Histologic appearance of tumor. Usually graded I–IV based on degree of differentiation and number of mitoses per high-power field; character of tumor itself.	Stage has more prognostic value than grade. TNM staging system: T = size of Tumor N = Node involvement M = Metastases
Stage	Based on site and size of 1° lesion, spread to regional lymph nodes, presence of metastases; spread of tumor in a specific patient.	

Tumor nomenclature

Cell type	Benign	Malignant
Epithelium	Adenoma, papilloma	Adenocarcinoma, papillary carcinoma
Mesenchyme		
Blood cells		Leukemia, lymphoma
Blood vessels	Hemangioma	Angiosarcoma
Smooth muscle	Leiomyoma	Leiomyosarcoma
Skeletal muscle	Rhabdomyoma	Rhabdomyosarcoma
Bone	Osteoma	Osteosarcoma
Fat	Lipoma	Liposarcoma
> 1 cell type	Mature teratoma	Immature teratoma

The term **carcinoma** implies epithelial origin, whereas **sarcoma** denotes mesenchymal origin. Both terms imply malignancy.

Diseases associated with neoplasms	Condition	Neoplasm
	1. **Down** syndrome	1. **A**cute **L**ymphoblastic **L**eukemia—"We will **ALL** go **DOWN** together"
	2. Xeroderma pigmentosum	2. Squamous cell and basal cell carcinomas of skin
	3. Chronic atrophic gastritis, pernicious anemia, postsurgical gastric remnants	3. Gastric adenocarcinoma
	4. Tuberous sclerosis (facial angiofibroma, seizures, mental retardation)	4. Astrocytoma and cardiac rhabdomyoma
	5. Actinic keratosis	5. Squamous cell carcinoma of skin
	6. Barrett's esophagus (chronic GI reflux)	6. Esophageal adenocarcinoma
	7. Plummer-Vinson syndrome (atrophic glossitis, esophageal webs, anemia; all due to iron deficiency)	7. Squamous cell carcinoma of esophagus
	8. Cirrhosis (alcoholic, hepatitis B or C)	8. Hepatocellular carcinoma
	9. Ulcerative colitis	9. Colonic adenocarcinoma
	10. Paget's disease of bone	10. 2° osteosarcoma and fibrosarcoma
	11. Immunodeficiency states	11. Malignant lymphomas
	12. AIDS	12. Aggressive malignant lymphomas (non-Hodgkin's) and Kaposi's sarcoma
	13. Autoimmune diseases (e.g., Hashimoto's thyroiditis, myasthenia gravis)	13. Benign and malignant thymomas
	14. Acanthosis nigricans (hyperpigmentation and epidermal thickening)	14. Visceral malignancy (stomach, lung, breast, uterus)
	15. Dysplastic nevus	15. Malignant melanoma

Oncogenes	Gain of function.
Gene	**Associated tumor**
c-myc	Burkitt's lymphoma
bcl-2	Follicular and undifferentiated lymphomas (inhibits apoptosis)
erb B2	Breast, ovarian, and gastric carcinomas
ras	Colon carcinoma
L-myc	Lung tumor
N-myc	Neuroblastoma
ret	Multiple endocrine neoplasia (MEN) types II and III.

Tumor suppressor genes

Loss of function; both alleles must be lost for expression of disease.

Gene	Chromosome	Associated tumor
Rb	13q	Retinoblastoma, osteosarcoma
BRCA1 and *2*	17q, 13q	Breast and ovarian cancer
p53	17p	Most human cancers, Li-Fraumeni syndrome
APC	5q	Colorectal cancer
WT1	11q	Wilms' tumor
NF1	17q	Neurofibromatosis type 1
NF2	22q	Neurofibromotosis type 2

Tumor markers

PSA (prostatic acid phosphatase)	Prostate-specific antigen. Prostatic carcinoma.	Tumor markers should not be used as the primary tool for cancer diagnosis. They may be used to confirm diagnosis, to monitor for tumor recurrence, and to monitor response to therapy.
CEA	Carcinoembryonic antigen. Very nonspecific but produced by ~ 70% of colorectal and pancreatic cancers; also produced by gastric and breast carcinomas.	
α-fetoprotein	Normally made by fetus. Hepatocellular carcinomas. Nonseminomatous germ cell tumors of the testis (e.g., yolk sac tumor).	
β-hCG	**H**ydatidiform moles, **C**horiocarcinomas, and **G**estational trophoblastic tumors.	
CA-125	Ovarian, malignant epithelial tumors.	
S-100	Melanoma, neural tumors, astrocytomas.	
Alkaline phosphatase	Metastases to bone, obstructive biliary disease, Paget's disease of bone.	
Bombesin	Neuroblastoma, lung and gastric cancer.	
TRAP	Tartrate-resistant acid phosphatase. Hairy cell leukemia—a B-cell neoplasm.	

Oncogenic viruses

Virus	Associated cancer
HTLV-1	Adult T-cell leukemia
HBV, HCV	Hepatocellular carcinoma
EBV	Burkitt's lymphoma, nasopharyngeal carcinoma
HPV	Cervical carcinoma (16, 18), penile/anal carcinoma
HHV-8 (Kaposi's sarcoma–associated herpesvirus)	Kaposi's sarcoma, body cavity fluid B cell lymphoma

Chemical carcinogens

Toxin	Affected organ
Aflatoxins, vinyl chloride	Liver
Nitrosamines	Esophagus, stomach
Asbestos	Lung (mesothelioma and bronchogenic carcinoma)
Arsenic	Skin (squamous cell)
CCl_4	Liver (centrilobular necrosis, fatty change)
Naphthalene (aniline) dyes	Bladder (transitional cell carcinoma)

Local effects of tumors

Local effect	Cause
Mass	Tissue lump or tumor.
Nonhealing ulcer	Destruction of epithelial surfaces (e.g., stomach, colon, mouth, bronchus).
Hemorrhage	From ulcerated area or eroded vessel.
Pain	Any site with sensory nerve endings. Tumors in brain are initially painless.
Seizures	Tumor mass in brain.
Obstruction	Of bronchus → pneumonia.
	Of biliary tree → jaundice.
	Of left colon → constipation.
Perforation	Of ulcer in viscera → peritonitis, free air.
Bone destruction	Pathologic fracture, collapse of bone.
Inflammation	Of serosal surface → pleural effusion, pericardial effusion, ascites.
Space-occupying lesion	Raised intracranial pressure with brain neoplasms. Anemia due to bone marrow replacement.
Localized loss of sensory or motor function	Compression or destruction of nerve (e.g., recurrent laryngeal nerve by lung or thyroid cancer, with hoarseness).
Edema	Venous or lymphatic obstruction.

Prostatic adenocarcinoma

Common in men > 50 years of age. Arises most often from the posterior lobe (peripheral zone) of the prostate gland and is most frequently diagnosed by digital rectal examination (hard nodule) and prostate biopsy. Prostatic acid phosphatase and prostate-specific antigen (PSA) are useful tumor markers. Osteoblastic metastases in bone may develop in late stages, as indicated by an ↑ in serum alkaline phosphatase and PSA.

Skin cancer

Squamous cell carcinoma	Very common. Associated with excessive exposure to sunlight and arsenic exposure. Commonly appear on hands and face. Locally invasive, but rarely metastasizes. Histopathology: keratin "pearls."	Actinic keratosis is a precursor to squamous cell carcinoma.
Basal cell carcinoma	Most common in sun-exposed areas of body. Locally invasive, but almost never metastasizes. Gross pathology: pearly papules.	Basal cell tumors have "palisading" nuclei.
Melanoma	Common tumor with significant risk of metastasis. Associated with sunlight exposure; fair-skinned persons are at ↑ risk. Incidence ↑. **Depth** of tumor correlates with risk of metastasis.	Dysplastic nevus is a precursor to melanoma.

Primary bone tumors

Benign

Osteochondroma (exostosis)	Most common benign bone tumor. Usually in men < 25 years of age. Commonly originates from long metaphysis. Malignant transformation to chondrosarcoma is rare.
Giant cell tumor	Occurs most commonly at epiphyseal end of long bones. Peak incidence 20–40 years old. Locally aggressive benign tumor often around the distal femur, proximal tibial region. Characteristic "double bubble" or "soap bubble" appearance on x-ray. Spindle-shaped cells with multinucleated giant cells.

Malignant

Osteosarcoma (osteogenic carcinoma)	Most common 1° malignant tumor of bone. Peak incidence in men 10–20 years old. Commonly found in the metaphysis of long bones. Predisposing factors include Paget's disease of bone, bone infarcts, radiation, and familial retinoblastoma. Codman's triangle (from elevation of periosteum) on x-ray.
Ewing's sarcoma	Anaplastic small blue cell malignant tumor. Most common in boys < 15. Extremely aggressive with early mets, but responsive to chemotherapy. Characteristic "onion-skin" appearance in bone. Commonly appears in diaphysis of long bones, pelvis, scapula, and ribs. 11;22 translocation.
Chondrosarcoma	Malignant cartilaginous tumor. Most common in men aged 30–60. Usually located in pelvis, spine, scapula, humerus, tibia, or femur. May be of 1° origin or from osteochondroma.

Primary brain tumors

Clinical presentation due to mass effects (e.g., seizures, dementia, focal lesions); 1° brain tumors rarely undergo metastasis. The majority of adult tumors are supratentorial, while the majority of childhood tumors are infratentorial.

Adult peak incidence

A. Glioblastoma multiforme (grade IV astrocytoma)

Most common 1° brain tumor. Prognosis grave; < 1 year life expectancy. Found in cerebral hemispheres. Can cross corpus callosum ("butterfly glioma").

"Pseudopalisading" tumor cells border central areas of necrosis and hemorrhage.

B. Meningioma

2nd most common 1° brain tumor. Most often occurs in convexities of hemispheres and parasagittal region. Arises from arachnoid cells external to brain. Resectable.

Psammoma bodies—spindle cells concentrically arranged in a whorled pattern.

C. Schwannoma

3rd most common 1° brain tumor. Schwann cell origin; often localized to 8th nerve → acoustic schwannoma. Bilateral schwannoma found in neurofibromatosis type 2.

Antoni A—compact palisading nuclei. Antoni B—loose pattern.

D. Oligodendroglioma

Relatively rare, slow growing, benign. Most often in frontal lobes.

"Fried egg" cells—round nuclei with clear cytoplasm. Often calcified.

E. Pituitary adenoma

Prolactin secreting is most common form. Bitemporal hemianopia (due to pressure on optic chiasm) and hypopituitarism are sequelae.

Derived from Rathke's pouch.

Childhood peak incidence

F. Low-grade astrocytoma (pilocytic astrocytoma)

Diffusely infiltrating glioma. In children, most often found in posterior fossa. Benign; good prognosis.

Rosenthal fibers.

G. Medulloblastoma

Highly malignant cerebellar tumor. A form of primitive neuroectodermal tumor (PNET). Can compress 4th ventricle, causing hydrocephalus.

Rosettes or perivascular pseudorosette pattern of cells. Radiosensitive.

H. Ependymoma

Ependymal cell tumors most commonly found in 4th ventricle. Can cause hydrocephalus.

Characteristic perivascular rosettes. Rod-shaped blepharoblasts (basal ciliary bodies) found near nucleus.

I. Hemangioblastoma

Most often cerebellar; associated with von Hippel–Lindau syndrome when found with retinoblastoma.

Foamy cells and high vascularity are characteristic. Can produce EPO → 2° polycythemia.

J. Craniopharyngioma

Benign childhood tumor, confused with pituitary adenoma (can also cause bitemporal hemianopia). Calcification is common.

Derived from remnants of Rathke's pouch. Most common childhood supratentorial tumor.

Supratentorial

Infratentorial

Metastasis to brain	1° tumors that metastasize to brain—**L**ung, **B**reast, **S**kin (melanoma), **K**idney (renal cell carcinoma), **G**I. Overall, approximately 50% of brain tumors are from metastases.	**L**ots of **B**ad **S**tuff **K**ills **G**lia.
Metastasis to liver	The liver and lung are the most common sites of metastasis after the regional lymph nodes. 1° tumors that metastasize to the liver—**C**olon > **S**tomach > **P**ancreas > **B**reast > **L**ung.	Metastases >> 1° liver tumors. **C**ancer **S**ometimes **P**enetrates **B**enign **L**iver.
Metastasis to bone	These 1° tumors metastasize to bone—**B**reast, **L**ung, **T**hyroid, **T**estes, **K**idney, **P**rostate. Metastases from breast and prostate are most common. Metastatic bone tumors are far more common than 1° bone tumors.	"**BLT** with a **K**osher **P**ickle." Lung = Lytic. Prostate = blastic. **B**reast = **B**oth lytic and blastic.

Paraneoplastic effects of tumors

Neoplasm	Causes	Effect
Small cell lung carcinoma	ACTH or ACTH-like peptide	Cushing's syndrome
Small cell lung carcinoma and intracranial neoplasms	ADH or ANP	SIADH
Squamous cell lung carcinoma, renal cell carcinoma, breast carcinoma, multiple myeloma, and bone metastasis (lysed bone)	PTH-related peptide, TGF-α, TNF-α, IL-2	Hypercalcemia
Renal cell carcinoma	Erythropoietin	Polycythemia
Thymoma, bronchogenic carcinoma	Antibodies against presynaptic Ca^{2+} channels at neuromuscular junction	Lambert-Eaton syndrome (muscle weakness)
Various neoplasms	Hyperuricemia due to excess nucleic acid turnover (i.e., cytotoxic therapy)	Gout

Cancer epidemiology

	Male	Female	
Incidence	Prostate (32%)	Breast (32%)	Deaths from lung cancer have plateaued in males but continue to ↑ in females.
	Lung (16%)	Lung (13%)	
	Colon and rectum (12%)	Colon and rectum (13%)	Cancer is the 2nd leading
Mortality	Lung (33%)	Lung (23%)	cause of death in the United
	Prostate (13%)	Breast (18%)	States (heart disease is 1st).

Anemia

Type	Etiology	
Microcytic, hypochromic (MCV < 80)	Iron deficiency— ↑ TIBC, ↓ ferritin, ↓ serum iron	Vitamin B_{12} and folate deficiencies are associated with hypersegmented PMNs. Unlike folate deficiency, vitamin B_{12} deficiency is associated with neurologic problems.
	Thalassemias—target cells	
	Lead poisoning	
Macrocytic (MCV > 100)	Megaloblastic—vitamin B_{12}/folate deficiency	
	Drugs that block DNA synthesis (e.g., sulfa drugs, AZT)	
	Marked reticulocytosis	
Normocytic, normochromic	Acute hemorrhage	↓ serum haptoglobin and ↑ serum LDH indicate RBC hemolysis. Direct Coombs' test is used to distinguish between immune- vs. non-immune-mediated RBC hemolysis.
	Enzyme defects (e.g., G6PD deficiency, PK deficiency)	
	RBC membrane defects (e.g., hereditary spherocytosis)	
	Bone marrow disorders (e.g., aplastic anemia, leukemia)	
	Hemoglobinopathies (e.g., sickle cell disease)	
	Autoimmune hemolytic anemia	
	Anemia of chronic disease— ↓ TIBC, ↑ ferritin, ↓ serum iron, ↑ storage iron in marrow macrophages	

	Normal	Iron deficiency	Anemia of chronic disease	Iron overload (hemosiderosis)
TIBC	250–400	↑	↓	Normal
Serum iron	50–150	↓	↓	↑
% sat.	20–50	< 20	20–50	100

Aplastic anemia	Pancytopenia characterized by severe anemia, neutropenia, and thrombocytopenia caused by failure or destruction of multipotent myeloid stem cells, with inadequate production or release of differentiated cell lines.
Causes	Radiation, benzene, chloramphenicol, alkylating agents, antimetabolites, viral agents (HCV, CMV, EBV, herpes zoster-varicella, B19 parvovirus), Fanconi's anemia, idiopathic (immune-mediated, 1° stem-cell defect).
Symptoms	Fatigue, malaise, pallor, purpura, mucosal bleeding, petechiae, infection.
Pathologic features	Pancytopenia with normal cell morphology; hypocellular bone marrow with fatty infiltration. Diagnose with bone marrow biopsy.
Treatment	Withdrawal of offending agent, allogenic bone marrow transplantation, RBC and platelet transfusion, G-CSF or GM-CSF.

Hereditary spherocytosis

Intrinsic, extravascular hemolysis due to spectrin or ankyrin defect. RBCs are small and round with no central pallor → less membrane → ↑ MCHC (normal hemoglobin and MCV). Osmotic fragility test used to confirm. Associated with gallstones, splenomegaly, anemia, and jaundice. Distinguish from warm antibody hemolysis by direct Coombs' test. Hereditary spherocytosis is Coombs' negative.

Blood dyscrasias

Sickle cell anemia	HbS mutation is a single amino acid replacement in β chain (substitution of normal glutamic acid with valine). Low O_2 or dehydration precipitates sickling. Heterozygotes (sickle cell trait) are relatively malaria resistant (balanced polymorphism). Complications in homozygotes (sickle cell disease) include aplastic crisis (due to B19 parvovirus infection), autosplenectomy, ↑ risk of encapsulated organism infection, *Salmonella* osteomyelitis, painful crisis (vaso-occlusive), and splenic sequestration crisis. HbC defect is a different β-chain mutation; patients with HbC or HbSC (1 of each mutant gene) have milder disease than do HbSS patients. New therapies for sickle cell anemia include hydroxyurea (↑ HbF) and bone marrow transplantation.	8% of African-Americans carry the HbS trait; 0.2% have the disease. Sickled cells are crescent-shaped RBCs. "Crew cut" on skull x-ray.
α-thalassemia	There are 4 α-globin genes. In α-thalassemia, the α-globin chain is underproduced (as a function of number of bad genes, 1–4). There is no compensatory ↑ of any other chains. HbH ($β_4$-tetramers, lacks 3 α-globin genes). Hb Barts ($γ_4$-tetramers, lacks all 4 α-globin genes) results in hydrops fetalis and intrauterine fetal death.	α-thalassemia is prevalent in Asia. β-thalassemia is prevalent in Mediterranean populations.
β-thalassemia	In β-thalassemia minor (heterozygote), the β chain is underproduced; in β-thalassemia major (homozygote), the β chain is absent. In both cases, fetal hemoglobin production is compensatorily increased but is inadequate. HbS/β-thalassemia heterozygote has mild to moderate disease.	β-thalassemia major results in severe anemia requiring blood transfusions. Cardiac failure due to 2° hemochromatosis.

HIGH-YIELD FACTS

Pathology

DIC   Activation of coagulation cascade leading to microthrombi and global consumption of platelets, fibrin, and coagulation factors.

Causes   Obstetric complications (most common cause), gram-negative sepsis, transfusion, trauma, malignancy, acute pancreatitis, nephrotic syndrome.

Lab findings   ↑ PT, ↑ PTT, ↑ fibrin split products (D dimers), ↓ platelet count. Helmet-shaped cells and schistocytes on blood smear.

Bleeding disorders

Platelet abnormalities (microhemorrhage)
Mucous membrane bleeding, petechiae, purpura, prolonged bleeding time.
Causes include ITP (antiplatelet antibodies and ↑ megakaryocytes), TTP (schistocytes), drugs, and DIC (↑ fibrin split products).

Coagulation factor defects (macrohemorrhage)
Hemarthroses (bleeding into joints), easy bruising, prolonged PT and/or PTT.
Coagulopathies include hemophilia A (factor VIII deficiency), hemophilia B (factor IX deficiency), and von Willebrand's disease (deficiency of von Willebrand's antigen), the most common bleeding disorder.

PT (extrinsic)   Factors II, V, VII, and X.
PTT (intrinsic)   All factors except VII and XIII.

Hemorrhagic disorders

Disorder	Platelet count[b]	Bleeding time	PT	PTT
Qualitative platelet defects[a]	—	↑	—	—
Vascular bleeding	—	↑	—	—
Thrombocytopenia	↓	↑	—	—
Hemophilia A (factor VIII deficiency)	—	—	—	↑
Hemophilia B (factor IX deficiency)	—	—	—	↑
Von Willebrand's disease	—	↑	—	↑
Disseminated intravascular coagulation	↓	↑	↑	↑

[a]Bernard-Soulier disease = defect of platelet adhesion; Glanzmann's thrombasthenia = defect of platelet aggregation.

[b]Note: platelet count must reach a very low value (15,000–20,000/mm³) before generalized bleeding occurs.

Lymphomas—Hodgkin's and non-Hodgkin's

Hodgkin's

Presence of Reed-Sternberg cells (RS cells are CD30+ and CD15+)

Localized, single group of nodes; extranodal rare; contiguous spread

Constitutional signs/symptoms—low-grade fever, night sweats, weight loss

Mediastinal lymphadenopathy

50% of cases associated with EBV; bimodal distribution: young and old; more common in men except nodular sclerosis type

Good prognosis = ↑ lymphocytes, ↓ RS

Non-Hodgkin's

Non-Hodgkin's associated with HIV and immunosuppression

Multiple, peripheral nodes; extranodal involvement common; noncontiguous spread

Majority involve B cells (except lymphoblastic T-cell origin)

No hypergammaglobulinemia (cf. multiple myeloma, where excess B cells are in resting stage)

Fewer constitutional signs/symptoms

Peak incidence 20–40 years old

Hodgkin's

Type	RS	Lymphocytes	Prognosis	Comments
NS (65–75%)	+	+++	Excellent	Most common; collagen banding; lacunar cells; women > men; primarily young adults
MC (25%)	++++	+++	Intermediate	Numerous RS cells
LP (6%)	+	++++	Excellent	< 35-year-old male
LD (rare)	*	+	Poor	Older males with disseminated disease

*RS high relative to lymphocytes

Ann Arbor Staging

I   Single lymph node or single extralymph organ
II 2 or more sites; on same side of diaphragm
III 2 or more sites; on both sides of diaphragm
IV Disseminated
A   Without constitutional symptoms
B   With constitutional symptoms (fever, night sweats, weight loss)

Non-Hodgkin's

Type	Occurs in	Cell type	Genetics	Comments
Small lymphocytic lymphoma	Adults	B cells		Clinically presents like CLL; low grade
Follicular lymphoma (small cleaved cell)	Adults	B cells	t(14;18) bcl-2 expression	Most common (adult) Difficult to cure; indolent course; bcl-2 is involved in apoptosis
Diffuse large cell	Usually older adults, but 20% occur in children	80% B cells 20% T cells (mature)		Aggressive but up to 50% are curable
Lymphoblastic lymphoma	Children most often	T cells (immature)		Most common in children; commonly presents with ALL and mediastinal mass; very aggressive T-cell lymphoma
Burkitt's lymphoma	Children most often	B cells	t(8;14) c-myc gene moves next to heavy-chain Ig gene(14)	"Starry-sky" appearance (sheets of lymphocytes with interspersed macrophages); associated with EBV; jaw lesion in endemic form in Africa, pelvis or abdomen in sporadic form

Leukemias

General considerations— ↑ number of circulating leukocytes in blood; bone marrow infiltrates of leukemic cells; marrow failure can cause anemia (↓ RBCs), infections (↓ WBCs), and hemorrhage (↓ platelets); leukemic cell infiltrates in liver, spleen, and lymph nodes are common.

ALL — Children; lymphoblasts; most responsive to therapy. Associated with Down syndrome.

AML — Auer rods; myeloblasts; adults.

CLL — Older adults; lymphadenopathy; hepatosplenomegaly; few symptoms; indolent course; ↑ smudge cells in peripheral blood smear; warm antibody autoimmune hemolytic anemia; very similar to SLL (small lymphocytic lymphoma).

CML — Most commonly associated with Philadelphia chromosome (t[9;22], *bcr-abl*); myeloid stem cell proliferation; presents with ↑ neutrophils and metamyelocytes; may accelerate to AML ("blast crisis").

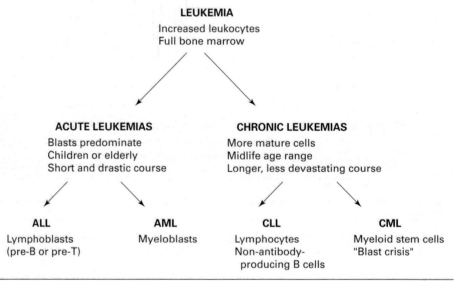

LEUKEMIA
Increased leukocytes
Full bone marrow

ACUTE LEUKEMIAS
Blasts predominate
Children or elderly
Short and drastic course

CHRONIC LEUKEMIAS
More mature cells
Midlife age range
Longer, less devastating course

ALL
Lymphoblasts
(pre-B or pre-T)

AML
Myeloblasts

CLL
Lymphocytes
Non-antibody-
producing B cells

CML
Myeloid stem cells
"Blast crisis"

Chromosomal translocations

Translocation	Associated disorder
t(9;22) (Philadelphia chromosome)	CML (*bcr-abl* hybrid)
t(8;14)	Burkitt's lymphoma (c-*myc* activation)
t(14;18)	Follicular lymphomas (*bcl*-2 activation)
t(15;17)	M3 type of AML (responsive to all-*trans* retinoic acid)
t(11;22)	Ewing's sarcoma
t(11;14)	Mantle cell lymphoma

HIGH-YIELD FACTS

Pathology

Lymphomas and leukemias

Proliferating "undifferentiated" cells		Mature cell types	Acute leukemias	FAB classification	Chronic leukemias	
	T lymphoblast	T lymphocytes	ALL-T	L2	Sézary syndrome CLL-T	Lymphocytic leukemias
Nonmarking lymphoblast			ALL-null ALL-common	L1		
	B lymphoblast	B lymphocytes	ALL-B	L3	CLL-B	
	Monoblast	Monocytes	Acute monocytic	M5	(Chronic monocytic)	
CFU-GM			Acute myelomonocytic	M4	(Chronic myelomonocytic)	
	Myeloblast	Neutrophils and basophils	AML Promyelocytic	M2 M3	CML	
CFU-S (myeloid stem cell)			AML	M1	Polycythemia rubra vera CML Myelofibrosis	Myeloid leukemias
CFU-Eos myeloblast		Eosinophils			(Eosinophilic)	
CFU-E normoblast		Erythrocytes	Acute erythroleukemia	M6	(Chronic erythroid)	
CFU-megakaryoblast		Megakaryocytes and platelets	Acute megakaryocytic leukemia	M7	Idiopathic thrombocythemia	

Lymphoid stem cell

Hematopoietic stem cell

Myeloid stem cell

CFU: Colony-forming unit
GM: Granulocyte-monocyte
E: Erythrocyte
Eos: Eosinophil

AML: Acute myeloblastic leukemia
CML: Chronic myelocytic leukemia
Leukemias in parentheses ( ) are rare

ALL: Acute lymphoblastic leukemia
CLL: Chronic lymphocytic leukemia

(Adapted, with permission, from Chandrasoma P, Taylor CE. *Concise Pathology,* 3rd ed. Stamford, CT: Appleton & Lange, 1998:410.)

Multiple myeloma

M spike

Albumin α_1 α_2 β γ

(Adapted, with permission, from Stobo J et al. *The Principles and Practice of Medicine,* 23rd ed. Stamford, CT: Appleton & Lange, 1996:806.)

Monoclonal plasma cell ("fried-egg" appearance) cancer that arises in the marrow and produces large amounts of IgG (55%) or IgA (25%). Most common 1° tumor arising within bone in adults. Destructive bone lesions and consequent hypercalcemia. Renal insufficiency, ↑ susceptibility to infection, and anemia. Associated with 1° amyloidosis and punched-out lytic bone lesions on x-ray. Characterized by monoclonal immunoglobulin spike (M protein) on serum protein electrophoresis and Ig light chains in urine (Bence Jones protein). Blood smear shows RBCs stacked like poker chips (rouleau formation). Compare with Waldenström's macroglobulinemia → M spike = IgM; no lytic lesions.

Achalasia

Esophagus

Lower esophageal sphincter

Stomach

Failure of relaxation of lower esophageal sphincter due to loss of myenteric (Auerbach's) plexus. Causes progressive dysphagia. Barium swallow shows dilated esophagus with an area of distal stenosis. Associated with an ↑ risk of esophageal carcinoma.

A-chalasia = absence of relaxation.
2° achalasia may arise from Chagas' disease.
"Bird beak" on barium swallow.

Barrett's esophagus

Glandular (columnar epithelial) metaplasia—replacement of nonkeratinized squamous epithelium with gastric (columnar) epithelium in the distal esophagus.

BARRett's = **B**ecomes **A**denocarcinoma, **R**esults from **R**eflux.

Esophagus

Squamocolumnar (epithelial) junction (SCJ)

Lower esophageal sphincter

Stomach

Esophageal cancer

Risk factors for esophageal cancer are:

    Achalasia
    Barrett's esophagus
    Corrosive esophagitis/**C**igarettes
    Diverticuli (e.g., Zenker's diverticulum)
    Esophageal web/**E**tOH
    Familial

ABCDEF.
Usually squamous cell carcinoma (Barrett's is an exception).

Congenital pyloric stenosis

Hypertrophy of the pylorus causes obstruction. Palpable mass in epigastric region and projectile vomiting at ≈ 2 weeks of age. Treatment is surgical incision.

Malabsorption syndromes

Celiac sprue	Autoantibodies to gluten (gliadin) in wheat and other grains. Villus flattening and lymphocytic infiltrate.
Tropical sprue	Probably infectious; responds to antibiotics.
Whipple's disease	Infection with *Tropheryma whippelii*; PAS-positive macrophages.
Disaccharidase deficiency	Most common is lactase deficiency → milk intolerance.

Chronic gastritis

Type A (fundal)	Autoimmune disorder characterized by **A**utoantibodies to parietal cells, pernicious **A**nemia, and **A**chlorhydria.	Type **A** = 4 **A**'s.
Type B (antral)	Caused by *H. pylori* infection.	Type **B** = a **B**ug, *H. pylori*. Both carry ↑ risk of gastric carcinoma.

Peptic ulcer disease

Gastric ulcer	Pain **G**reater with meals—weight loss.
	H. pylori infection in 70%; NSAID use also implicated.
	Due to ↓ mucosal protection against gastric acid.
Duodenal ulcer	Pain **D**ecreases with meals—weight gain.
	Almost 100% have *H. pylori* infection.
	Due to ↑ gastric acid secretion or ↓ mucosal protection.
	Hypertrophy of Brunner's glands.
	Tend to have clean, "punched-out" margins unlike the raised/irregular margins of carcinoma. Potential complications include bleeding, penetration, perforation, and obstruction (not intrinsically precancerous). *H. pylori* infection can be treated with "triple therapy" (metronidazole, bismuth salicylate, and either amoxicillin or tetracycline) with or without a proton pump inhibitor. Incidence of peptic ulcer disease is twice as great in smokers.

Inflammatory bowel disease

	Crohn's disease	Ulcerative colitis
Possible etiology	Infectious.	Autoimmune.
Location	May involve any portion of the GI tract, usually the terminal ileum, small intestine, and colon. **Skip** lesions, rectal sparing.	*Colitis* = colon inflammation. Continuous lesions with rectal involvement.
Gross morphology	Transmural inflammation. **Cobblestone** mucosa, creeping **fat,** bowel wall thickening ("string sign" on x-ray), linear ulcers, fissures.	Mucosal inflammation. Friable mucosal pseudopolyps with freely hanging mesentery.
Microscopic morphology	Noncaseating granulomas.	Crypt abscesses and ulcers.
Complications	Strictures, fistulas, perianal disease, malabsorption–nutritional depletion.	Severe stenosis, toxic megacolon, **colorectal carcinoma.**
Extraintestinal manifestations	Migratory polyarthritis, erythema nodosum.	Pyoderma gangrenosum, sclerosing cholangitis.

For **Crohn's,** think of a **fat** old **crone skipping** down a **cobblestone** road.

Diverticular disease

Diverticulum	Blind pouch leading off the alimentary tract, lined by mucosa, muscularis, and serosa, that communicates with the lumen of the gut. Most diverticula (esophagus, stomach, duodenum, colon) are acquired and are termed "false" in that they lack or have an attenuated muscularis propria.
Diverticulosis	The prevalence of diverticulosis (many diverticula) in patients > 60 years of age approaches 50%. Caused by ↑ intraluminal pressure and focal weakness in the colonic wall. Most frequently involves the sigmoid colon. Associated with low-fiber diets. Most often asymptomatic or associated with vague discomfort.
Diverticulitis	Inflammation of diverticula classically causing LLQ pain. May be complicated by perforation, peritonitis, abscess formation, or bowel stenosis.

Intussusception and volvulus

Intussusception—"telescoping" of 1 bowel segment into distal segment; can compromise blood supply.

Volvulus—twisting of portion of bowel around its mesentery; can lead to obstruction.

Stomach cancer

Almost always adenocarcinoma. Early aggressive local spread and node/liver mets. Associated with dietary nitrosamines, achlorhydria, chronic gastritis. Termed linitis plastica when diffusely infiltrative (thickened, rigid appearance).

Virchow's node—involvement of supraclavicular node by mets from stomach.

Krukenberg's tumor—bilateral mets to ovaries. Abundant mucus, "signet-ring" cells.

Hirschsprung's disease

Congenital megacolon characterized by lack of enteric nervous plexus in segment (Auerbach's and Meissner's plexuses) on intestinal biopsy. Due to failure of neural crest cell migration. Presents as chronic constipation early in life. Dilated portion of the colon proximal to the aganglionic segment, resulting in a "transition zone."

Think of a giant spring that has **sprung** in the colon.

Colorectal cancer risk factors

Risk factors for carcinoma of colon—colorectal villous adenomas, chronic inflammatory bowel disease, low-fiber diet, ↑ age, familial adenomatous polyposis (FAP), hereditary nonpolyposis colorectal cancer (HNPCC), personal and family history of colon cancer. Peutz-Jeghers, a benign polyposis syndrome, is not a risk factor. Screen patients > 50 years old with stool occult blood test.

Cirrhosis/portal hypertension

Effects of portal hypertension
- Esophageal varices
  - ↓ Hematemesis
- Peptic ulcer
- Melena
- Splenomegaly
- Caput medusae
- Ascites
- Testicular atrophy
- Hemorrhoids

Effects of liver cell failure
- Coma
- Scleral icterus
- Fetor hepaticus (breath smells like a freshly opened corpse)
- Spider nevi
- Gynecomastia
- Jaundice
- Loss of sexual hair
- Liver "flap" = asterixis (coarse hand tremor)
- Bleeding tendency (decreased prothrombin)
- Anemia
- Ankle edema

(Adapted, with permission, from Chandrasoma P, Taylor CE. *Concise Pathology*, 3rd ed. Stamford, CT: Appleton & Lange, 1998:654.)

Cirrho (Greek) = tawny yellow. Diffuse fibrosis of liver, destroys normal architecture.
Nodular regeneration.
Micronodular—nodules < 3 mm, uniform size. Due to metabolic insult (e.g., alcohol).
Macronodular—nodules > 3 mm, varied size. Usually due to significant liver injury leading to hepatic necrosis (e.g., postinfectious or drug-induced hepatitis).
↑ risk of hepatocellular carcinoma.
Portacaval shunt between splenic vein and left renal vein may relieve portal hypertension.

Alcoholic hepatitis	Swollen and necrotic hepatocytes, neutrophil infiltration, Mallory bodies (hyaline), fatty change, and sclerosis around central vein. SGOT (AST) to SGPT (ALT) ratio is usually > 1.5.	**A** **S**cotch and **T**onic: **AST** elevated (> ALT) with alcoholic hepatitis.
Budd-Chiari syndrome	Occlusion of IVC or hepatic veins with centrilobular congestion and necrosis, leading to congestive liver disease (hepatomegaly, ascites, abdominal pain, and eventual liver failure). Associated with polycythemia vera, pregnancy, hepatocellular carcinoma.	
Wilson's disease	Due to failure of copper to enter circulation in the form of ceruloplasmin. Leads to copper accumulation, especially in liver, brain, cornea. Also known as hepatolenticular degeneration. Wilson's disease is characterized by: **A**sterixis **B**asal ganglia degeneration (parkinsonian symptoms) **C**eruloplasmin ↓, **C**irrhosis, **C**orneal deposits (Kayser-Fleischer rings), **C**opper accumulation, **C**arcinoma (hepatocellular), **C**horeiform movements **D**ementia	Treat with penicillamine. **ABCD.**
Hemochromatosis	Hemosiderosis is the deposition of hemosiderin (iron); hemochromatosis is the disease caused by this iron deposition. Classic triad of micronodular cirrhosis, pancreatic fibrosis, and skin pigmentation → "bronze" diabetes. Results in CHF and ↑ risk of hepatocellular carcinoma. Disease may be 1° (autosomal recessive) or 2° to chronic transfusion therapy. ↑ ferritin, ↑ iron, ↓ TIBC → ↑ transferrin saturation.	Total body iron may reach 50 g, enough to set off metal detectors at airports. Treat with repeated phlebotomy, deferoxamine.

Jaundice

Normally, liver cells conjugate bilirubin and excrete it into bile, where it is converted by bacteria to urobilinogen (some of which is reabsorbed). Some urobilinogen is also formed directly from heme metabolism. Termed unconjugated (indirect) bilirubin before conjugation and conjugated (direct) after. Conjugated is soluble (can enter urine).

Jaundice type	Hyperbilirubinemia	Urine bilirubin	Urine urobilinogen
Hepatocellular	Conjugated/unconjugated	↑	Normal/↓
Obstructive	Conjugated	↑	↓
Hemolytic	Unconjugated	Absent (acholuria)	↑

Hereditary hyperbilirubinemias

Gilbert's syndrome	Mildly ↓ UDP-glucuronyl transferase. Asymptomatic, but unconjugated bilirubin is elevated without overt hemolysis. Associated with stress.	Gilbert's may represent a milder form.
Crigler-Najjar syndrome, type I	Absent UDP-glucuronyl transferase. Presents early in life; patients die within a few years. Findings: jaundice, kernicterus (bilirubin deposition in brain), ↑ unconjugated bilirubin. Treatment: plasmapheresis and phototherapy.	Crigler-Najjar type I is a severe disease. Type II is less severe and responds to phenobarbital.
Dubin-Johnson syndrome	Conjugated hyperbilirubinemia due to defective liver excretion. Grossly black liver.	Rotor's syndrome is similar but less severe and does not cause black liver.

(Adapted, with permission, from Junqueira LC, Carneiro J, Kelley RO. *Basic Histology,* 9th ed. Stamford, CT: Appleton & Lange, 1999.)

Primaly sclerosing cholangitis	Inflammation and fibrosis of bile ducts → alternating strictures and dilation with "beading" on ERCP. Associated with ulcerative colitis. Can lead to 2° biliary cirrhosis.

Biliary cirrhosis

Primary	Autoimmune disorder with antimitochondrial antibodies; severe obstructive jaundice, itching, hypercholesterolemia (xanthoma).
Secondary	Due to extrahepatic biliary obstruction. ↑ in pressure in intrahepatic ducts → injury/ fibrosis. Often complicated by ascending cholangitis (bacterial infection), bile stasis, and "bile lakes."

Hepatocellular carcinoma	Also called hepatoma. Most common 1° malignant tumor of the liver in adults. ↑ incidence of hepatocellular carcinoma is associated with hepatitis B and C, Wilson's disease, hemochromatosis, α_1-antitrypsin deficiency, alcoholic cirrhosis, and carcinogens (e.g., aflatoxin B1).	Hepatocellular carcinoma, like renal cell carcinoma, is commonly spread by hematogenous dissemination. Elevated α-fetoprotein.

Reye's syndrome	Rare, often fatal childhood hepatoencephalopathy. Findings: fatty liver (microvesicular fatty change), hypoglycemia, coma. Associated with viral infection (especially VZV and influenza B) and salicylates; thus, aspirin is no longer recommended for children (use acetaminophen, with caution).

Gallstones	Form when solubilizing bile acids and lecithin are overwhelmed by ↑ cholesterol and/or bilirubin. Three types of stones:	Risk factors (**4 F's**): 1. **F**emale 2. **F**at 3. **F**ertile 4. **F**orty
Cystic duct Hepatic duct Stone in the common bile duct Fibrosed gallbladder with gallstones Pancreatic duct	1. Cholesterol stones (radiolucent with 10–20% opaque due to calcifications)—associated with obesity, Crohn's disease, cystic fibrosis, advanced age, clofibrate, estrogens, multiparity, rapid weight loss, and Native American origin. 2. Mixed stones (radiolucent)—have both cholesterol and pigment components. Most common type. 3. Pigment stones (radiopaque)—seen in patients with chronic RBC hemolysis, alcoholic cirrhosis, advanced age, and biliary infection. Diagnose with ultrasound. Treat with cholecystectomy.	May present with Charcot's triad of epigastric/RUQ pain, fever, jaundice.

Acute pancreatitis	Caused by activation of pancreatic enzymes → autodigestion. Causes: **G**allstones, **E**thanol, **T**rauma, **S**teroids, **M**umps, **A**utoimmune disease, **S**corpion sting, **H**yperlipidemia, **D**rugs. Clinical presentation: epigastric abdominal pain radiating to back. Labs: elevated amylase, lipase (higher specificity). Can lead to DIC, ARDS, diffuse fat necrosis, hypocalcemia, and pseudocyst formation. Chronic pancreatitis is strongly associated with alcoholism.	**GET SMASHeD.** ddI can cause a fatal pancreatitis!

Pancreatic adenocarcinoma

Prognosis averages 6 months or less; very aggressive; usually already metastasized at presentation; tumors more common in pancreatic head (obstructive jaundice).

Often presents with:

1. Abdominal pain radiating to back
2. Weight loss
3. Anorexia
4. Migratory thrombophlebitis (Trousseau's syndrome)
5. Pancreatic duct obstruction (malabsorption with palpable gallbladder)

Obstructive lung disease (COPD)

Obstruction of air flow, resulting in air trapping in the lungs. PFTs— $\downarrow$ FEV_1/FVC ratio (hallmark).

Types:

1. Chronic **B**ronchitis ("**B**lue **B**loater")—productive cough for > 3 consecutive months in 2 or more years. Hypertrophy of mucus-secreting glands in the bronchioles (Reid index > 50%). Leading cause is smoking. Findings: wheezing, crackles, cyanosis.
2. Emphysema ("pink puffer")—enlargement of air spaces and $\downarrow$ recoil resulting from destruction of alveolar walls. Caused by smoking (centriacinar emphysema) and α_1-antitrypsin deficiency (panacinar emphysema and liver cirrhosis) → $\uparrow$ elastase activity. Findings: dyspnea, $\downarrow$ breath sounds, tachycardia, $\downarrow$ I/E ratio.
3. Asthma—bronchial hyperresponsiveness causes reversible bronchoconstriction. Can be triggered by viral URIs, allergens, and stress. Findings: cough, wheezing, dyspnea, tachypnea, hypoxemia, $\downarrow$ I/E ratio, pulsus paradoxus.
4. Bronchiectasis—chronic necrotizing infection of bronchi → dilated airways, purulent sputum, recurrent infections, hemoptysis. Associated with bronchial obstruction, cystic fibrosis, poor ciliary motility.

Restrictive lung disease

Restricted lung expansion causes $\downarrow$ lung volumes ($\downarrow$ VC and TLC). PFTs—FEV_1/FVC ratio > 80%.

Types:

1. Poor breathing mechanics (extrapulmonary):
   a. Poor muscular effort—polio, myasthenia gravis
   b. Poor apparatus—scoliosis
2. Interstitial lung diseases (pulmonary):
   a. Adult respiratory distress syndrome (ARDS)
   b. Neonatal respiratory distress syndrome (hyaline membrane disease)
   c. Pneumoconioses (anthracosis, silicosis, asbestosis)
   d. Sarcoidosis
   e. Idiopathic pulmonary fibrosis
   f. Goodpasture's syndrome
   g. Wegener's granulomatosis
   h. Eosinophilic granuloma

HIGH-YIELD FACTS

Pathology

Lung—physical findings

Abnormality	Breath Sounds	Resonance	Fremitus	Tracheal Deviation
Bronchial obstruction	Absent over area	↓	↓	Toward side of lesion
Pleural effusion	↓ over effusion	Dullness	↓	—
Pneumonia (lobar)	May have bronchial breath sounds over lesion	Dullness	↑	—
Pneumothorax	↓	Hyperresonant	Absent	Away from side of lesion

Obstructive vs. restrictive lung disease

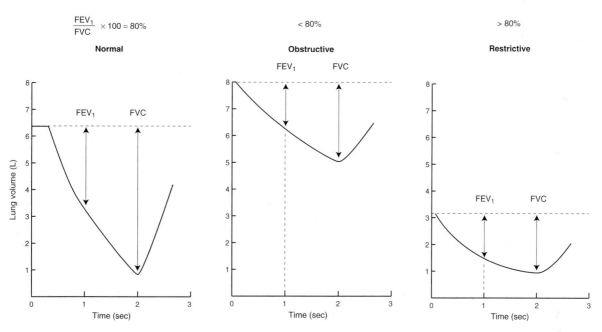

$$\frac{FEV_1}{FVC} \times 100 = 80\%$$

Normal   < 80%   **Obstructive**   > 80%   **Restrictive**

Note: Obstructive lung volumes > normal (↑ TLC, ↑ FRC, ↑ RV); restrictive lung volumes < normal. In both obstructive and restrictive, FEV_1 and FVC are reduced, but in obstructive, FEV_1 is more dramatically reduced, resulting in a ↓ FEV_1/FVC ratio.

Asbestosis

Diffuse pulmonary interstitial fibrosis caused by inhaled asbestos fibers. ↑ risk of pleural mesothelioma and bronchogenic carcinoma. Long latency.
Ferruginous bodies in lung (asbestos fibers coated with hemosiderin). Ivory-white pleural plaques.

Asbestosis and smoking greatly ↑ risk of bronchogenic cancer (smoking not additive with mesothelioma). Seen in shipbuilders and plumbers.

HIGH-YIELD FACTS

Pathology

Neonatal respiratory distress syndrome	Surfactant deficiency leading to ↑ surface tension, resulting in alveolar collapse. Surfactant is made by type II pneumocytes most abundantly after 35th week of gestation. The lecithin-to-sphingomyelin ratio in the amniotic fluid, a measure of lung maturity, is usually < 1.5 in neonatal respiratory distress syndrome. Surfactant—dipalmitoyl phosphatidylcholine. Treatment: maternal steroids before birth; artificial surfactant for infant.
Kartagener's syndrome	Immotile cilia due to a dynein arm defect. Results in sterility (sperm also immotile), bronchiectasis, and recurrent sinusitis (bacteria and particles not pushed out); associated with situs inversus (e.g., dextrocardia).

Lung cancer

Bronchogenic carcinoma	Tumors that arise centrally: 1. Squamous cell carcinoma—clear link to **S**moking; ectopic PTH-related peptide production 2. **S**mall cell carcinoma—clear link to **S**moking; associated with ectopic hormone production (ADH, ACTH); may lead to Lambert-Eaton syndrome. Tumors that arise peripherally: 1. Adenocarcinoma (most common) 2. Bronchioalveolar carcinoma (thought not to be related to smoking) 3. Large cell carcinoma—undifferentiated	Lung cancer is the leading cause of cancer death. Presentation: cough, hemoptysis, bronchial obstruction, wheezing, pneumonic "coin" lesion on x-ray. **SPHERE** of complications: **S**uperior vena cava syndrome **P**ancoast's tumor **H**orner's syndrome **E**ndocrine (paraneoplastic) **R**ecurrent laryngeal symptoms (hoarseness) **E**ffusions (pleural or pericardial)
Carcinoid tumor	Can cause carcinoid syndrome (flushing, diarrhea, wheezing, and salivation).	
Metastases	Very common. Brain (epilepsy), bone (pathologic fracture), and liver (jaundice, hepatomegaly).	

Pancoast's tumor	Carcinoma that occurs in apex of lung and may affect cervical sympathetic plexus, causing Horner's syndrome.	Horner's syndrome—ptosis, miosis, anhidrosis.

Pneumonia

Type	Organism(s)	Characteristics
Lobar	Pneumococcus most frequently	Intra-alveolar exudate → consolidation; may involve entire lung.
Bronchopneumonia	*S. aureus, H. flu, Klebsiella, S. pyogenes*	Acute inflammatory infiltrates from bronchioles into adjacent alveoli; patchy distribution involving ≥ 1 lobes.
Interstitial (atypical) pneumonia	Viruses (RSV, adenoviruses), *Mycoplasma, Legionella, Chlamydia*	Diffuse patchy inflammation localized to interstitial areas at alveolar walls; distribution involving ≥ 1 lobes.

Degenerative diseases

Cerebral cortex	**Alzheimer's disease**—most common cause of dementia in the elderly. Associated with senile plaques (β-amyloid core) and neurofibrillary tangles (abnormally phosphorylated tau protein). Familial form (10%) associated with genes on chromosomes 1, 14, 19 (*APOE4* allele), and 21 (p-*App* gene).	Multi-infarct dementia is the 2nd most common cause of dementia in the elderly. May cause amyloid angiopathy → intracranial hemorrhage.
	Pick's disease—associated with Pick bodies (intracytoplasmic inclusion bodies) and is specific for the frontal and temporal lobes.	
Basal ganglia and brain stem	**Huntington's disease**—autosomal-dominant inheritance, chorea, dementia. Atrophy of caudate nucleus (loss of GABAergic neurons).	Chromosome 4—expansion of CAG repeats.
	Parkinson's disease—associated with Lewy bodies and depigmentation of the substantia nigra (loss of dopaminergic neurons). Rare cases have been linked to exposure to MPTP, a contaminant in illicit street drugs.	**TRAP** = **T**remor (at rest), cogwheel **R**igidity, **A**kinesia, and **P**ostural instability (you are **TRAP**ped in your body).
Spinocerebellar	**Olivopontocerebellar atrophy; Friedreich's ataxia.**	
Motor neuron	**Amyotrophic lateral sclerosis (ALS)**—associated with **both** LMN and UMN signs.	Commonly known as Lou Gehrig's disease.
	Werdnig-Hoffmann disease—presents at birth as a "floppy baby"; tongue fasciculations.	
	Polio—LMN signs.	

Intracranial hemorrhage

Epidural hematoma	Rupture of middle meningeal artery, often 2° to fracture of temporal bone. Lucid interval.	CT shows "biconcave disk" not crossing suture lines.
Subdural hematoma	Rupture of bridging veins. Venous bleeding (less pressure) with delayed onset of symptoms. Seen in elderly individuals, alcoholics, blunt trauma.	Crescent-shaped hemorrhage that crosses suture lines.
Subarachnoid hemorrhage	Rupture of an aneurysm (usually berry aneurysm) or an AVM. Patients complain of "worst headache of my life." Bloody or xanthochromic spinal tap.	
Parenchymal hematoma	Caused by hypertension, amyloid angiopathy, diabetes mellitus, and tumor.	

HIGH-YIELD FACTS

Pathology

HIGH-YIELD FACTS

Pathology

Berry aneurysms

Berry aneurysms occur at the bifurcations in the circle of Willis. Most common site is bifurcation of the anterior communicating artery. Rupture (most common complication) leads to hemorrhagic stroke/subarachnoid hemorrhage. Associated with adult polycystic kidney disease, Ehlers-Danlos syndrome, and Marfan's syndrome.

Demyelinating and dysmyelinating diseases

1. Multiple sclerosis (MS)—↑ prevalence with ↑ distance from the equator; periventricular plaques, preservation of axons, loss of oligodendrocytes, reactive astrocytic gliosis; ↑ protein (IgG) in CSF. Many patients have a relapsing-remitting course. Patients can present with optic neuritis (sudden loss of vision), MLF syndrome (internuclear ophthalmoplegia), hemiparesis, hemisensory symptoms, or bladder/bowel incontinence.
2. Progressive multifocal leukoencephalopathy (PML)—associated with JC virus and seen in 2–4% of AIDS patients (reactivation of latent viral infection).
3. Postinfectious encephalomyelitis.
4. Metachromatic leukodystrophy (a sphingolipidosis).
5. Guillain-Barré syndrome (see below).

Classic triad of **MS** is a **SIN**:
   Scanning speech
   Intention tremor
   Nystagmus
Most often affects women in their 20s and 30s.

Guillain-Barré syndrome (acute idiopathic polyneuritis)

Inflammation and demyelination of peripheral nerves and motor fibers of ventral roots (sensory effect less severe than motor), causing symmetric ascending muscle weakness beginning in distal lower extremities. Facial diplegia in 50% of cases. Autonomic function may be severely affected (e.g., cardiac irregularities, hypertension, or hypotension). Findings: elevated CSF protein with normal cell count ("albumino-cytologic dissociation"). Elevated protein → papilledema.

Associated with infections (e.g., herpesvirus or *Campylobacter jejuni* infection), inoculations, and stress, but no definitive link to pathogens.

Poliomyelitis

Caused by poliovirus, which is transmitted by the fecal-oral route. Replicates in the oropharynx and small intestine before spreading through the bloodstream to the CNS, where it leads to the destruction of cells in the anterior horn of the spinal cord, leading in turn to LMN destruction.

Symptoms
Malaise, headache, fever, nausea, abdominal pain, sore throat. Signs of LMN lesions—muscle weakness and atrophy, fasciculations, fibrillation, and hyporeflexia.

Findings
CSF with lymphocytic pleocytosis with slight elevation of protein. Virus recovered from stool or throat.

Seizures

Partial seizures—1 area of the brain.
1. Simple partial (awareness intact)—motor, sensory, autonomic, psychic
2. Complex partial (impaired awareness)

Generalized seizures—diffuse.
1. Absence—blank stare (petit mal)
2. Myoclonic—quick, repetitive jerks
3. Tonic-clonic—alternating stiffening and movement (grand mal)
4. Tonic—stiffening
5. Atonic—"drop" seizures

Epilepsy is a disorder of recurrent seizures (febrile seizures are not epilepsy).

Partial seizures can secondarily generalize.

Causes of seizures by age:
Children—genetic, infection, trauma, congenital, metabolic.
Adults—tumors, trauma, stroke, infection.
Elderly—stroke, tumor, trauma, metabolic, infection.

Aphasia

Broca's (expressive)

Wernicke's (receptive)

Nonfluent aphasia with intact comprehension.
Broca's area—inferior frontal gyrus.
Fluent aphasia with impaired comprehension.
Wernicke's area—superior temporal gyrus.

Broca's is **Bro**ken speech;
Wernicke's is **W**ordy but makes no sense.
Wernicke's = "**What?**"

Horner's syndrome

Sympathectomy of face (lesion above T1):
1. **P**tosis (slight drooping of eyelid)
2. **A**nhidrosis (absence of sweating) and flushing (rubor) of affected side of face
3. **M**iosis (pupil constriction)

Associated with Pancoast's tumor.

PAM is horny.

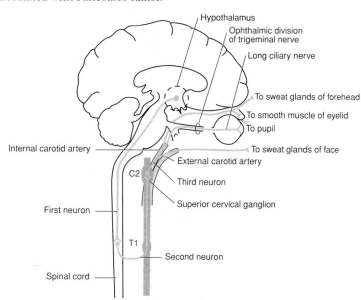

Hypothalamus
Ophthalmic division of trigeminal nerve
Long ciliary nerve
To sweat glands of forehead
To smooth muscle of eyelid
To pupil
Internal carotid artery
To sweat glands of face
External carotid artery
C2
Third neuron
Superior cervical ganglion
First neuron
T1
Second neuron
Spinal cord

(Adapted, with permission, from Simon RP et al. *Clinical Neurology,* 4th ed. Stamford, CT: Appleton & Lange, 1999:146.)

The 3-neuron oculosympathetic pathway above projects from the hypothalamus to the intermediolateral column of the spinal cord, then to the superior cervical (sympathetic) ganglion, and finally to the pupil, the smooth muscle of the eyelids, and the sweat glands of the forehead and face. Interruption of these pathways results in Horner's syndrome.

Syringomyelia

Enlargement of the central canal of spinal cord. Crossing fibers of spinothalamic tract are damaged. Bilateral loss of pain and temperature sensation in upper extremities with preservation of touch sensation.

Syrinx (Greek) = tube, as in syringe.

Often presents in patients with Arnold-Chiari malformation.

Most common at C8–T1.

Tabes dorsalis

Degeneration of dorsal columns and dorsal roots due to 3° syphilis, resulting in impaired proprioception and locomotor ataxia. Associated with Charcot's joints, shooting (lightning) pain, Argyll Robertson pupils, and absence of DTRs.

Osteoarthritis

Mechanical—wear and tear of joints leads to destruction of articular cartilage, subchondral bone formation, sclerosis, osteophytes, eburnation, Heberden's nodes (DIP), and Bouchard's nodes (PIP).

Common in older patients.

Classic presentation: pain in weight-bearing joints after use (e.g., at the end of the day), improving with rest. No systemic symptoms.

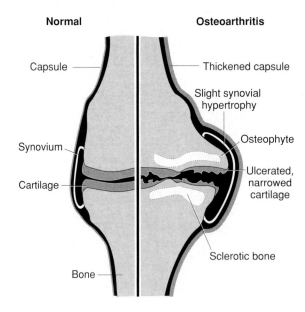

(Adapted, with permission, from Stobo J et al. *The Principles and Practice of Medicine*, 23rd ed. Stamford, CT: Appleton & Lange, 1996:241.)

Rheumatoid arthritis

Autoimmune—inflammatory disorder affecting synovial joints, with pannus formation in joints (MCP, PIP), subcutaneous rheumatoid nodules, ulnar deviation, subluxation.

Common in females. 80% of RA patients have positive rheumatoid factor (anti-IgG antibody).

Classic presentation: morning stiffness improving with use, symmetric joint involvement, and systemic symptoms (fever, fatigue, pleuritis, pericarditis).

Sjögren's syndrome

Classic triad—dry eyes (conjunctivitis, xerophthalmia), dry mouth (dysphagia, xerostomia), arthritis. Parotid enlargement, increased risk of B-cell lymphoma. Predominantly affects **females** between 40 and 60 years of age.

Associated with rheumatoid arthritis.

Sicca syndrome—dry eyes, dry mouth, nasal and vaginal dryness, chronic bronchitis, reflux esophagitis.

Gout

Uric acid crystals

Precipitation of monosodium urate crystals into joints due to hyperuricemia, which can be caused by Lesch-Nyhan syndrome, PRPP excess, ↓ excretion of uric acid, or glucose-6-phosphatase deficiency. Also associated with the use of thiazide diuretics, which competitively inhibit the secretion of uric acid. Asymmetric joint distribution. Favored manifestation is painful MTP joint in the big toe (podagra). Tophus formation (often on external ear or Achilles tendon). Crystals are needle shaped and negatively birefringent. Treatment is allopurinol, probenecid, colchicine, and NSAIDs. More common in men. Acute attack tends to occur after alcohol consumption or a large meal.

Pseudogout

Caused by deposition of calcium pyrophosphate crystals within the joint space. Forms basophilic, rhomboid crystals (as opposed to the negatively birefringent, needle-shaped crystals in gout). Usually affects large joints (classically the knee). > 50 years old; both sexes affected equally. No treatment.

Celiac sprue

Autoimmune-mediated intolerance of gliadin (wheat) leading to steatorrhea. Associated with people of northern European descent. Findings include blunting of villi, lymphocytes in the lamina propria, and abnormal D-xylose test. Tends to affect jejunum. Associated with dermatitis herpetiformis. 10–15% lead to malignancy (most often T-cell lymphoma).

Systemic lupus erythematosus

90% are female and between ages 14 and 45. Symptoms are fever, fatigue, weight loss, joint pain, malar rash, and photosensitivity. May also occur with pleuritis, pericarditis, nonbacterial verrucous endocarditis, Raynaud's phenomenon. **Wire loop** lesions in kidney with immune complex deposition (with nephrotic syndrome); death from renal failure and infections. False positives on syphilis tests (RPR/VDRL). Lab tests detect presence of:

1. Antinuclear antibodies (ANA)—sensitive, but not specific for SLE
2. Antibodies to double-stranded DNA (anti-dsDNA)—very specific, poor prognosis
3. Anti-Smith antibodies (anti-Sm)—very specific, but not prognostic
4. Antihistone antibodies—drug-induced lupus

SLE causes **LSE** (Libman-Sacks Endocarditis)—valvular vegetations found on **both** sides of valve (mitral valve stenosis) and do not embolize.

Most common and severe in black females.

Drugs that can produce an SLE-like syndrome that is commonly reversible—**HIPP**: **H**ydralazine, **I**NH, **P**henytoin, **P**rocainamide.

Associated with thymoma.

Sarcoidosis

Characterized by immune-mediated, widespread noncaseating granulomas and elevated serum ACE levels. Common in black females.

Associated with restrictive lung disease, bilateral hilar lymphadenopathy, erythema nodosum, Bell's palsy, epithelial granulomas containing microscopic Schaumann and asteroid bodies, uveoparotitis, and hypercalcemia (due to elevated conversion of vitamin D to its active form in epithelioid macrophages).

GRAIN:
Gammaglobulinemia
Rheumatoid arthritis
ACE increase
Interstitial fibrosis
Noncaseating granulomas

Seronegative spondylo-arthropathies

Arthritis without rheumatoid factor (no anti-IgG antibody). Strong association with HLA-B27 (gene that codes for HLA MHC I). Occurs more often in males.

Ankylosing spondylitis

Chronic inflammatory disease of spine and sacroiliac joints → ankylosis (stiff spine), uveitis, and aortic regurgitation.

Reiter's syndrome

Classic triad:
1. Urethritis
2. Conjunctivitis and anterior uveitis
3. Arthritis

"Can't **see** (anterior uveitis/ conjunctivitis), can't **pee** (urethritis), can't climb a **tree** (arthritis)."
Post-GI or chlamydia infections.

Scleroderma (progressive systemic sclerosis—PSS)

Excessive fibrosis and collagen deposition throughout the body. 75% female. Commonly sclerosis of skin but also of cardiovascular and GI systems and kidney. 2 major categories:
1. Diffuse scleroderma—widespread skin involvement, rapid progression, early visceral involvement. Associated with anti-Scl-70 antibody.
2. **CREST** syndrome—**C**alcinosis, **R**aynaud's phenomenon, **E**sophageal dysmotility, **S**clerodactyly, and **T**elangiectasia. Limited skin involvement, often confined to fingers and face. More benign clinical course. Associated with anticentromere antibody.

Skin disorders

Dermatitis

A group of inflammatory pruritic skin disorders. Etiology: allergy (usually type IV hypersensitivity), chemical injury, or infection.

Psoriasis

Nonpruritic chronic inflammation of the skin, particularly on the knees and elbows. Associated with HLA-B27, HLA-13, and HLA-17.

Bullous pemphigoid

Autoimmune disorder with IgG antibody against epidural basement membrane (linear immunofluorescence). Similar to but less severe than pemphigus vulgaris—affects skin but spares oral mucosa.

Pemphigus vulgaris

Potentially fatal autoimmune skin disorder. Intradermal bullae involving the oral mucosa and skin. Findings: acantholysis (breakdown of epithelial cell-to-cell junctions), IgG antibody against epidermal cell surface.

| Goodpasture's syndrome | Findings: pulmonary hemorrhages → hemoptysis; renal lesions → hematuria, anemia, crescentic glomerulonephritis.
Anti–glomerular basement membrane antibodies produce linear staining on immunofluorescence. | There are **2 Good Pastures** for this disease: **G**lomerulus and **P**ulmonary. A type **II** hypersensitivity disease. Most common in men 20–40 years. |

PATHOLOGY—ENDOCRINE

| Cushing's syndrome | ↑ cortisol due to a variety of causes.
Etiologies include:
  1. Cushing's disease (1° pituitary adenoma); ↑ ACTH
  2. 1° adrenal (hyperplasia/neoplasia); ↓ ACTH
  3. Ectopic ACTH production (e.g., small cell lung cancer); ↑ ACTH
  4. Iatrogenic; ↓ ACTH
The clinical picture includes hypertension, weight gain, moon facies, truncal obesity, buffalo hump, hyperglycemia (insulin resistance), skin changes (thinning, striae), osteoporosis, and immune suppression. |

Hyperaldosteronism

| Primary (Conn's syndrome) | Caused by an aldosterone-secreting tumor, resulting in hypertension, hypokalemia, metabolic alkalosis, and **low** plasma renin. | Treatment includes spironolactone, a diuretic that works by acting as an aldosterone antagonist. |
| Secondary | Due to renal artery stenosis, chronic renal failure, CHF, cirrhosis, or nephrotic syndrome. Kidney perception of low intravascular volume results in an overactive renin-angiotensin system. Therefore, it is associated with **high** plasma renin. | |

| Addison's disease | 1° deficiency of aldosterone and cortisol due to adrenal atrophy, causing hypotension (hyponatremic volume contraction) and skin hyperpigmentation (↑ ACTH → MSH activity). Characterized by **A**drenal **A**trophy and **A**bsence of hormone production; involves **A**ll 3 cortical divisions. Distinguish from 2° insufficiency, which has no skin hyperpigmentation (↓ pituitary ACTH production). |

Tumors of the adrenal medulla

| Pheochromocytoma | The most common tumor of the adrenal medulla in adults. Derived from chromaffin cells (arise from neural crest). | Pheochromocytomas may be associated with neurofibromatosis, MEN types II and III. |
| Neuroblastoma | The most common tumor of the adrenal medulla in children, but it can occur anywhere along the sympathetic chain. | |

Pheochromocytoma

Most of these neoplasms secrete a combination of NE and epinephrine. Urinary VMA levels and plasma catecholamines are elevated. Associated with MEN types II and III. Treated with α-antagonists, especially phenoxybenzamine, a nonselective, **irreversible** α-blocker.

Episodic hyperadrenergic symptoms **(5 P's)**:

- **P**ressure (elevated blood pressure)
- **P**ain (headache)
- **P**erspiration
- **P**alpitations
- **P**allor/diaphoresis

Rule of 10's:

- **10%** malignant
- **10%** bilateral
- **10%** extra-adrenal
- **10%** calcify
- **10%** kids
- **10%** familial

Symptoms occur in "spells"—relapse and remit.

Multiple endocrine neoplasias (MEN)

MEN type I (Wermer's syndrome)—pancreas (e.g., Zollinger-Ellison syndrome, insulinomas, VIPomas), parathyroid, and pituitary tumors. Presents with kidney stones and stomach ulcers.

MEN type II (Sipple's syndrome)—medullary carcinoma of the thyroid, pheochromocytoma, parathyroid tumor, or adenoma.

MEN type III (formerly MEN IIb)—medullary carcinoma of the thyroid, pheochromocytoma, and oral and intestinal ganglioneuromatosis (mucosal neuromas).

MEN I = 3 "P" organs (**P**ancreas, **P**ituitary, and **P**arathyroid).

All MEN syndromes have autosomal-dominant inheritance.

Associated with *ret* gene in MEN types II and III.

Hypothyroidism and hyperthyroidism

Hypothyroidism — Cold intolerance, hypoactivity, weight gain, fatigue, lethargy, ↓ appetite, constipation, weakness, ↓ reflexes, myxedema (facial/periorbital), dry, cool skin, and coarse, brittle hair.

Hyperthyroidism — Heat intolerance, hyperactivity, weight loss, chest pain/palpitations, arrhythmias, diarrhea, ↑ reflexes, warm, moist skin, and fine hair.

Graves' disease — An autoimmune hyperthyroidism with thyroid-stimulating/TSH receptor antibodies. Ophthalmopathy (proptosis, EOM swelling), pretibial myxedema, diffuse goiter. Often presents during stress (e.g., childbirth).

↑ TSH (sensitive test for 1° hypothyroidism), ↓ total T_4, ↓ free T_4, ↓ T_3 uptake.

Riedel's thyroiditis—thyroid replaced by fibrous tissue (hypothyroid).

↓ TSH (if 1°), ↑ total T_4, ↑ free T_4, ↑ T_3 uptake.

Graves' is a type II hypersensitivity.

Hashimoto's thyroiditis	Autoimmune disorder resulting in hypothyroidism. Slow course; moderately enlarged, nontender thyroid. Lymphocytic infiltrate with germinal centers. Antimicrosomal antibodies.	
Subacute thyroiditis (de Quervain's)	Self-limited hypothyroidism often following a flu-like illness. Elevated ESR, jaw pain, early inflammation, and very tender thyroid gland.	May be hyperthyroid early in course.
Thyroid cancer	1. Papillary carcinoma—most common, good prognosis, "ground-glass" nuclei, psammoma bodies. 2. Follicular carcinoma—poor prognosis, uniform follicles. 3. Medullary carcinoma—from parafollicular "C cells"; produces calcitonin, sheets of cells in amyloid stroma. MEN types II and III. 4. Undifferentiated/anaplastic—older patients, horrible prognosis.	
Cretinism	Endemic cretinism occurs wherever endemic goiter is prevalent (lack of dietary iodine); sporadic cretinism is caused by defect in T_4 formation or developmental failure in thyroid formation. Findings: pot-bellied, pale, puffy-faced child with protruding umbilicus and protuberant tongue.	Cretin means Christlike (French *chrétien*). Those affected were considered so mentally retarded as to be incapable of sinning. Still common in China.
Acromegaly	Excess GH in adults. Findings: large tongue with deep furrows, deep voice, large hands and feet, coarse facial features. $\uparrow$ GH in children $\rightarrow$ gigantism.	

Diabetes mellitus

Acute manifestations

Polydipsia, polyuria, polyphagia, weight loss, DKA (type 1), hyperosmolar coma (type 2), unopposed secretion of GH and epinephrine (exacerbating hyperglycemia).

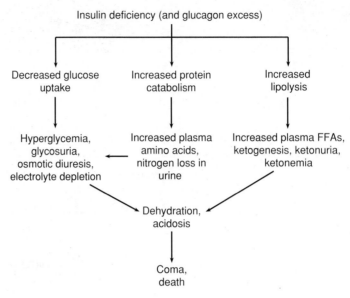

Chronic manifestations

Nonenzymatic glycosylation:

1. Small vessel disease (diffuse thickening of basement membrane), retinopathy (hemorrhage, exudates, microaneurysms), nephropathy (nodular sclerosis, progressive proteinuria, chronic renal failure, arteriosclerosis leading to hypertension)
2. Large vessel atherosclerosis, CAD, peripheral vascular occlusive disease and gangrene, cerebrovascular disease
3. Neuropathy (motor, sensory, and autonomic degeneration)
4. Cataracts, glaucoma (sorbitol accumulation)

Tests

Fasting serum glucose, glucose tolerance test, HbA_{1c} (measures long-term diabetic control)

(Adapted, with permission, from Wyngaarden JB, Smith LH Jr, Bennett JC (eds). *Cecil Textbook of Medicine*, 19th ed. Philadelphia: W. B. Saunders, 1992.)

In the sorbitol pathway shown above, hyperglycemia ↑ intracellular sorbitol, which in turn is associated with depletion of intracellular myoinositol levels. Hyperglycemia may also ↓ myoinositol directly by inhibiting its uptake.

Streptococcus pneumoniae. Sputum sample from a patient with pneumonia shows gram-positive diplococci.

A

Acute bacterial endocarditis. Virulent organisms (e.g., *Staphylococcus aureus*) infect previously normal valves, causing marked damage (here, in the aortic valve) and potentially giving rise to septic emboli.

B

C

Microscopically, **tuberculosis (A)** is characterized by caseating granulomas containing Langhans' giant cells, which have a "horseshoe" pattern of nuclei (see arrow). Organisms **(B)** are identified by their red color on acid-fast staining ("red snappers"). **Miliary tuberculosis (C)** is seen here with large caseous lesions at the left medial upper lobe and miliary lesions in the surrounding hilar node. This life-threatening infection is caused by blood-borne dissemination of *Mycobacterium tuberculosis* to many organs from a quiescent site of infection.*

Staphylococcus aureus. Sputum sample from another patient with pneumonia shows gram-positive cocci in clusters.

*Reproduced courtesy of the Pathology Education Instructional Resource Digital Library (http://peir.net) at the University of Alabama, Birmingham.

Neisseria meningitidis. Gram-negative diplococci are seen within neutrophils from CSF.*

Cytomegalovirus (CMV) giant cell with multiple hyaline inclusions in a renal tubule. Of special concern in HIV patients (CMV retinitis) and organ transplant patients (as here, in a transplanted kidney); however, CMV can infect almost anything. Treatment is ganciclovir or foscarnet.

Coccidioidomycosis. Endospores within a spherule in infected lung parenchyma. Initial infection usually resolves spontaneously, but when immunity is compromised, dissemination to almost any organ can occur. Endemic in the southwestern United States.

Cryptococcus neoformans. The polysaccharide capsule is visible by India ink preparation in CSF from an AIDS patient with meningoencephalitis.*

Giardia lamblia, small intestine, microscopic. The trophozoite has a classic pear shape, with double nuclei giving an "owl's-eye" appearance.

Trichomonas vaginalis demonstrating trophozoites with flagellae.*

Taenia solium, the pig tapeworm, infesting porcine myocardium. When humans ingest this meat, the larvae attach to the wall of the small intestine and mature to adult worms.

Infectious granuloma in bone marrow, with intracytoplasmic inclusions. Cultures grew *Cryptococcus neoformans.**

Herpes zoster. Reactivation of virus spreads along the dermatomal distribution of infected nerves and can occur many years after initial infection. It is considered benign unless it affects an immunocompromised host or is a reinfection of the V_1 branch of the trigeminal nerve with eye/cornea involvement.*

A

B

C

Syphilis. (A) Chancre associated with primary syphilis. These ulcerative lesions are painless. **(B) Primary syphilis.** A dense infiltrate of plasma cells and dilated blood vessels can be seen. There is epidermal ulceration with crust; neutrophils are present within the predominantly plasmocytic infiltrate. **(C) Tabes dorsalis** resulting from progressive syphilis infection, thoracic spinal cord. Note degeneration of the dorsal columns and dorsal roots.* (Second image reproduced, with permission, from Hurwitz RM et al. *Pathology of the Skin: Atlas of Clinical-Pathological Correlation,* 2nd ed. Stamford, CT: Appleton & Lange, 1998.)

Clostridium **cellulitis.** Gross buttock and thigh are shown with severe cellulitis and desquamation.*

Coxsackie exanthem. Diffuse eruptive vesiculopapules are seen on the hand of a three-year-old child. (Reproduced, with permission, from Hurwitz RM et al. *Pathology of the Skin: Atlas of Clinical-Pathological Correlation*, 2nd ed., Stamford, CT: Appleton & Lange, 1998.)

Pneumocystis carinii. Special silver stain of lung epithelium reveals the presence of organisms.*

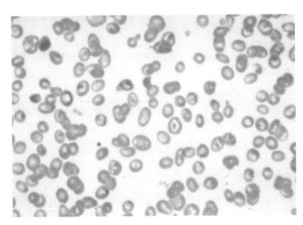

Target cells. Due to an increase in surface area–to-volume ratio from iron deficiency anemia (decreased cell volume) or in obstructive liver disease (increased cell membrane).*

Thalassemia major. A blood dyscrasia caused by a defect in β-chain synthesis in hemoglobin. Note the presence of target cells.*

Iron deficiency anemia. Microcytosis and hypochromia can be seen.

A

B

Sickle cell anemia. (A) Sickle cell peripheral blood smear. Note the sickled cells as well as anisocytosis, poikilocytosis, and nucleated RBCs. **(B) Splenic infarction.** The splenic artery lacks collateral supply, making the spleen particularly susceptible to ischemic damage. Coagulative necrosis has occurred in a wedge shape along the pattern of vascular supply. Individual sickle cells cause generalized splenic infarcts that result in autosplenectomy by adolescence.*

A

B

C

D

Leukemia. (A) Acute lymphocytic leukemia, peripheral blood smear. Affects children less than 10 years old. **(B) Acute myelocytic leukemia** with Auer rods, peripheral blood smear. Affects adolescents to young adults. **(C) Chronic lymphocytic leukemia,** peripheral blood smear. In CLL, the lymphocytes are excessively fragile. These lymphocytes are easily destroyed during slide preparation, forming "smudge cells." Affects individuals older than 60 years of age. **(D) Chronic myeloid leukemia,** peripheral blood smear. Promyelocytes and myelocytes are seen adjacent to a vascular structure. Affects individuals from 30 to 60 years of age.*

A

B

C

Multiple myeloma. (A) X-ray shows numerous punched-out lytic lesions (lucent areas) typical of multiple myeloma. Note the generalized osteopenia and multiple compression fractures (arrow). **(B)** Classic bone lytic lesions seen in multiple myeloma. **(C)** Smears from a patient with multiple myeloma display an abundance of plasma cells. RBCs will often be seen in rouleaux formation, stacked like poker chips. Multiple myeloma is associated with hypercalcemia, lytic bone lesions, and renal insufficiency due to Bence Jones (light-chain) proteinuria.*

Burkitt's lymphoma. The classic "starry-sky" appearance from macrophage ingestion of tumor cells can be seen.*

Hodgkin's disease (Reed-Sternberg cells). Binucleate RS cells displaying prominent inclusion-like nucleoli surrounded by lymphocytes and other reacting inflammatory cells. The RS cell is a necessary but insufficient pathologic finding for the diagnosis of Hodgkin's disease.

Hemochromatosis with cirrhosis. Prussian blue iron stain shows hemosiderin in the liver parenchyma. Such deposition occurs throughout the body, causing organ damage and the characteristic darkening of the skin.*

Metastatic carcinoma to the liver. The most common primary sites are the breast, colon, and lung.*

Fatty metamorphosis (macrovesicular steatosis) of the liver, microscopic. Early reversible change associated with alcohol consumption; there are abundant fat-filled vacuoles but no inflammation due to fibrosis of more serious alcoholic liver damage (yet).*

A

B

C

D

Cirrhosis. (A) Micronodular cirrhosis of the liver, gross, from an alcoholic patient. The liver is approximately normal in size with a fine, granular appearance. Later stages of disease result in an irregularly shrunken liver with larger nodules. **(B) Cirrhosis,** microscopic. Regenerative lesions are surrounded by fibrotic bands of collagen ("bridging fibrosis"), forming the characteristic nodularity. **(C)** Gross natural color with macronodularity that is difficult to see. Hepatitis B surface antigen and core antigen negative. **(D)** Chronic passive biliary congestion gives the liver a "nutmeg" appearance.*

A

B

Colonic polyps. Tubular adenomas (A) are smaller and rounded in morphology and have less malignant potential than do **villous adenomas (B),** which are composed of long, fingerlike projections.

Diverticulitis. Inflammation of the diverticula typically causes LLQ pain and can progress to perforation, peritonitis, abscess formation, or bowel stenosis. Note the presence of macrophages. Gut lumen is seen at the top of the photo.*

Celiac sprue (gluten-sensitive enteropathy). Histology shows blunting of villi and crypt hyperplasia.

Sclerosed esophageal varix. Overlying esophageal mucosa is generally normal.*

Intussusception of infant gut, gross.*

A

Squamous cell carcinoma of the lung, gross, from a patient with a long smoking history. This tumor arises from the bronchial epithelium and is centrally located.*

B

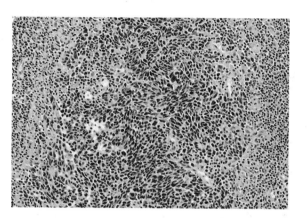

Small (oat) cell carcinoma in a pulmonary hilar lymph node. Almost all of these tumors are related to tobacco smoking. They can arise anywhere in the lung, most often near the hilum, and quickly spread along the bronchi.*

C

Pulmonary emboli. (A) Pulmonary thromboembolus, gross. Most often arises from deep venous thrombosis. **(B) Pulmonary thromboembolus** in a small muscular pulmonary artery. The interdigitating areas of pale pink and red within the organizing embolus form the "lines of Zahn" characteristic of a thrombus. These lines represent layers of red cells, platelets, and fibrin that are laid down in the vessel as the thrombus forms. **(C) Air embolism** showing multiple petechial hemorrhages in the pons and cerebellum.*

Acute respiratory distress syndrome (ARDS). Persistent inflammation leads to poor pulmonary compliance and edema; note both alveolar fluid and hyaline membranes.

Tension pneumothorax. Note these features:

1—Hyperlucent lung field
2—Hyperexpansion lowers diaphragm
3—Collapsed lung
4—Deviation of trachea
5—Mediastinal shift
6—Compression of opposite lung

Asbestosis. Ferruginous bodies (asbestos bodies with Prussian blue iron stain) in the lung, microscopic. Inhaled asbestos fibers are ingested by macrophages.*

Pneumonia. An example of consolidation with acute peribronchial localization surrounding edema (H&E, low magnification).*

A

B

C

Alzheimer's disease. Key histologic features include "senile plaques" **(A)**, a coronal section showing atrophy, especially of the temporal lobes **(B)**, and focal masses of interwoven neuronal processes around an amyloid core. The remnants of neuronal degeneration **(C)** are also associated with Alzheimer's disease, the most common cause of dementia in older persons.*

Epidural hematoma from skull fracture. Note the lens-shaped (biconcave) dense blood next to the fracture. 1—skull fracture; 2—hematoma in epidural space; 3—temporalis muscle; 4—Sylvian fissure; 5—frontal sinus.

Brain with **hypertensive hemorrhage** in the region of the basal ganglia, gross.*

Subdural hemorrhage. Note the hyperdense extra-axial blood on the left side. Concomitant subarachnoid hemorrhage. 1—subdural blood, layering; 2—skull; 3—falx; 4—subarachnoid blood; 5—shunt catheter; 6—frontal sinus.

A

B

Berry aneurysm (A) located on the anterior cerebral artery. The small, saclike structure can easily rupture during periods of hypertension or stress. The histologic section **(B)** at the origin of the aneurysm shows lack of internal elastic lamina.*

A

B

Glioblastoma multiforme (A) extending across the midline of the cerebral cortex, gross. **(B)** Small cells with elongated nuclei and bipolar processes are characteristic. The chromatin is generally not markedly dense, nor are nucleoli usually prominent.*

A

B

Multiple sclerosis. (A) Lumbar spinal cord with mostly random and asymmetric white-matter lesions. **(B)** Brain with periventricular white-matter plaques of demyelination, gross. Demyelination occurs in a bilateral asymmetric distribution. Classic clinical findings are nystagmus, scanning speech, and intention tremor.*

A

B

Oligodendroglioma. (A) Gross natural-color coronal section of cerebral hemisphere with a large lesion of the left parieto-occipital white matter. **(B)** Classic "fried egg" appearance with perinuclear halos and "chicken-wire" capillary pattern.*

Left middle cerebral artery stroke. Large left MCA territory stroke with edema and mass effect but no visible hemorrhage. The patient experienced deficits in speech and in the right side of the face and upper extremities. 1—ischemic brain parenchyma; 2—subtle midline shift to the right; 3—the right frontal horn of the lateral ventricle; 4—the left lateral ventricles obliterated by edema.

Scleroderma. The progressive "tightening" of the skin has contracted the fingers and eliminated creases over the knuckles. Fibrosis is widespread and may also involve the esophagus (dysphagia), lung (restrictive disease), and small vessels of the kidney (hypertension).

A

B

Gout. (A) Monosodium urate crystal deposition in joints with negative birefringence and an apple-green color under polarized light, causing tophi **(B)** that affect the proximal interphalangeal (PIP) joints, knees, and elbows, growing like tubers from the bones.*

Erythema multiforme/toxic epidermal necrolysis/ Stevens-Johnson syndrome, captopril induced. Erythematous macules, papules, vesicles, bullae, and erosions are seen. (Reproduced, with permission, from Hurwitz RM et al. *Pathology of the Skin: Atlas of Clinical-Pathological Correlation,* 2nd ed. Stamford, CT: Appleton & Lange, 1998.)

Rheumatoid arthritis. Note the swan-neck deformities of the digits and severe, symmetric involvement of the PIP joints.

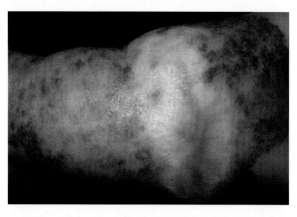

Arteriovenous malformation. The markedly enlarged and distorted arm of a six-month-old boy with confluent erythematous papules and nodules. (Reproduced, with permission, from Hurwitz RM et al. *Pathology of the Skin: Atlas of Clinical-Pathological Correlation*, 2nd ed. Stamford, CT: Appleton & Lange, 1998.)

Capillary malformation, port-wine type. Irregular purple patches and plaques are seen on the neck and chest of the mother, and pink patches are seen on the cheek, lip, chin, neck, and chest of the daughter. Both lesions were present at birth. (Reproduced, with permission, from Hurwitz RM et al. *Pathology of the Skin: Atlas of Clinical-Pathological Correlation*, 2nd ed. Stamford, CT: Appleton & Lange, 1998.)

Scabies. Adult female mite with egg containing embryo within the epidermis. (Reproduced, with permission, from Hurwitz RM et al. *Pathology of the Skin: Atlas of Clinical-Pathological Correlation*, 2nd ed. Stamford, CT: Appleton & Lange, 1998.)

Squamous cell carcinoma. Malignant skin tumor involving the epidermal skin layer. Note the presence of keratin pearls.*

A

B

Malignant melanoma. (A) Lesion just beneath the epidermis with pigmented and nonpigmented cells. The tumor cells are usually polyhedral but may be spindle shaped, dendritic, or ballooned or may resemble oat cells. Many but by no means all melanomas make melanin. Big nucleoli are common.* **(B)** A multicolored tan, red, and dark brown irregular plaque on the abdomen. (Second image reproduced, with permission, from Hurwitz RM et al. *Pathology of the Skin: Atlas of Clinical-Pathological Correlation*, 2nd ed. Stamford, CT: Appleton & Lange, 1998.)

A

B

Basal cell carcinoma. Cytologic details show that islands of tumor within a mucinous dermis **(A)** are composed of small, round-to-fusiform cells with inconspicuous cytoplasm and densely hyperchromatic nuclei. Also evident is an early **(A)** and well-developed **(B)** separation artifact.*

A

B

Pemphigus vulgaris. (A) Numerous crusted, denuded, and weepy erythematous plaques are seen on the chest, breast, abdomen, and arms. **(B)** Vesicles on the gingiva. (Reproduced, with permission, from Hurwitz RM et al. *Pathology of the Skin: Atlas of Clinical-Pathological Correlation,* 2nd ed. Stamford, CT: Appleton & Lange, 1998.)

Bullous pemphigoid. Erythematous plaques contiguous with small large bullae. (Reproduced, with permission, from Hurwitz RM et al. *Pathology of the Skin: Atlas of Clinical-Pathological Correlation,* 2nd ed. Stamford, CT: Appleton & Lange, 1998.)

Psoriasis, fully developed plaque. (Reproduced, with permission, from Hurwitz RM et al. *Pathology of the Skin: Atlas of Clinical-Pathological Correlation,* 2nd ed. Stamford, CT: Appleton & Lange, 1998.)

A

B

Acanthosis nigricans. (A) Extensive hyperpigmented plaques on the arms in a patient with congenital lipodystrophy. This is an unusual distribution for acanthosis nigricans. **(B)** Hyperkeratosis and papillomatosis. (Reproduced, with permission, from Hurwitz RM et al. *Pathology of the Skin: Atlas of Clinical-Pathological Correlation,* 2nd ed. Stamford, CT: Appleton & Lange, 1998.)

A

B

Pancreas. (A) Pancreatic acinar cell (EM). A condensing vacuole (C) is receiving secretory product (arrow) from the Golgi complex (G). M—mitochondrion; RER—rough endoplasmic reticulum; S—mature condensed secretory zymogen granules. **(B)** Pancreatic islet cells in **diabetes mellitus type 1.** In patients with diabetes mellitus type 1, autoantibodies against β cells cause a chronic inflammation until, over time, islet cells are entirely replaced by amyloid.

Adrenocortical adenoma, gross. Cause of hypercortisolism (Cushing's syndrome) or hyperaldosteronism (Conn's syndrome)*

Pheochromocytoma. The tumor cells have numerous vacuolar spaces within the cytoplasm (pseudoacini). Most of the punctate blue-black granules of variable density are dense-core neurosecretory granules.*

A

B

Cushing's disease. The clinical picture includes **(A)** moon facies and buffalo hump and **(B)** truncal obesity and abdominal striae.

Arteriolar sclerosis showing masses of hyaline material in glomerular afferent and efferent arterioles and in the glomerulus. From a type 1 diabetic patient.*

A

B

C

Graves' disease. (A) Exophthalmos in a patient with proptosis and periorbital edema. **(B)** CT shows extraocular muscle enlargement at the orbital apex. **(C)** Stimulation of follicular cells by TSH causes the normal uniform architecture to be replaced by hyperplastic papillary, involuted borders, and decreased colloid. Typical medical therapy is propylthiouracil, which inhibits the production of thyroid hormone as well as peripheral conversion of T_4 to T_3.*

Papillary intraductal adenocarcinoma of the breast. Invasive tumor with marked desmoplastic reaction. Intraductal lesions are also seen.*

Hydatidiform mole. The characteristic gross appearance is a "bunch of grapes." Hydatidiform moles are the most common precursors of choriocarcinoma. Complete moles usually display a 46,XX diploid pattern with all the chromosomes derived from the sperm. In partial moles, the karyotype is triploid or tetraploid, and fetal parts may be present.

Metastatic prostatic adenocarcinoma in a supraclavicular lymph node. Despite the relatively solid growth, the nuclei do not show great variation in size. Note the typical prominent nucleoli. Some cells have eosinophilic cytoplasm, whereas others have pale cytoplasm.*

Seminiferous tubules. Sertoli cells play a supportive and protective role in spermatogenesis. Note cells in various stages of differentiation, with spermatogonia near the basal lamina and more mature forms near the lumen.

A

B

Histologic appearance of endometriosis. (A) Endometriosis of the ovary. **(B)** Endometriosis of the cervix. (Reproduced, with permission, from DeCherney A et al. *Current Obstetric and Gynecologic Diagnosis and Treatment,* 9th ed. New York: McGraw-Hill, 2002.)

Endocardial chronic ischemia. Microscopic example of myocytolysis and coagulation necrosis beneath the endocardium.*

Atherosclerosis. Aorta with fibrous intimal thickening and foam cells dispersed throughout smooth muscle cells, micro.*

A

B

C

D

Evolution of a **myocardial infarction.** Contraction band necrosis (arrow) is the first visible change, occurring in one to two hours **(A).** In the first three days, neutrophilic infiltration and coagulation necrosis occur **(B).** By three to seven days, neutrophils have been replaced by macrophages, and clearing of myocyte debris has begun **(C).** Within weeks, granulation and scarring occur **(D).**

Heart with marked concentric **left ventricular hypertrophy** from hypertension, gross.*

Pulmonary edema. Posteroanterior chest x-ray in a man with acute pulmonary edema due to left ventricular failure. Note the bat's-wing density, cardiac enlargement, increased size of upper lobe vessels, and pulmonary venous congestion. (Reproduced, with permission, from McPhee SJ et al. *Pathophysiology of Disease: An Introduction to Clinical Medicine*, 4th ed. New York: McGraw-Hill, 2002.)

Calcified **bicuspid aortic valve** showing false raphe. The abnormal architecture of the valve makes its leaflets susceptible to otherwise ordinary hemodynamic stresses, which ultimately leads to valvular thickening, calcification, increased rigidity, and stenosis.*

Aortic dissection with a blood clot compressing the aortic lumen. A tear in the intima allowed blood to surge through the muscular layer to the adventitia (may lead to sudden death from hemothorax). Risk factors are hypertension, Marfan's syndrome, pregnancy, Ehlers-Danlos syndrome, and trauma.*

The **Aschoff body,** an area of fibrinoid necrosis surrounded by mononuclear and multinucleated giant cells, is pathognomonic for **rheumatic heart disease.** The mitral valve is most commonly affected.*

Carotid angiogram showing aneurysm. Note the path of the internal carotid artery through the neck and its major branches (ophthalmic artery, anterior cerebral artery, middle cerebral artery). The aneurysm is inferior to the terminal branches in this angiogram.*

Bacterial endocarditis of the mitral valve. Vegetations can embolize and infect distant organ systems.*

Left atrial myxoma. The most common primary cardiac tumor; known to produce VEGF (vascular endothelial growth factor).*

A

B

Acute pyelonephritis (A) is characterized by neutrophilic infiltration and abscess formation within the renal interstitium. Abscesses may rupture, introducing collections of white cells to the tubular lumen. In contrast, **chronic pyelonephritis (B)** has a lymphocytic invasion with fibrosis.

Transitional cell carcinoma of the urinary bladder, microscopic. Malignant urothelial cells have invaded the muscular layer of the bladder wall.

Lupus erythematosus, kidneys. Enlarged, very pale kidneys with "flea bite" or ectasia from a patient with nephrotic syndrome or subacute glomerulonephritis as a result of lupus erythematosus.*

Normal glomerulus, microscopic, with **(A)** macula densa and **(B)** afferent and **(C)** efferent arterioles.

Thickening of basement membrane

Proliferation of mesangial cells

Systemic lupus erythematosus, kidney pathology. In the membranous glomerulonephritic pattern, "wire-loop" thickening occurs as a result of subendothelial immune complex deposition.

Polycystic kidney disease. Abdominal CT shows multiple cysts in both kidneys. PKD is an autosomal-dominant disease and is often associated with aneurysm formation in the brain. The disease occurs bilaterally and presents with flank pain and hematuria.*

Minimal change disease (lipoid nephrosis) shows normal glomeruli on light microscopy but effacement of foot processes on EM (arrowhead). The full arrow points to a normal foot process.

Kimmelstiel-Wilson nodules

Diabetic nodular glomerulosclerosis. The nodular Kimmelstiel-Wilson lesions at the periphery of the glomerulus are pathognomonic for diabetic GS.

Calcium oxalate crystals in the kidney, viewed with partially crossed polarizers. Tubular failure in oxalate nephropathy can result from vitamin C or antifreeze abuse.*

A

B

Renal cell carcinoma. (A) Gross. Notably, the tumor may extend into the renal vein and IVC and spread hematogenously. **(B)** Microscopic view, taken from the urinary tract, showing eosinophilic cell lesions. Glycogen and lipid-filled clear cells derived from tubular epithelium are common but are not shown here.*

A

B

Osteogenesis imperfecta. (A) Blue sclera caused by translucency of connective tissue over the choroid. The optic nerve is on the right side of the image. **(B)** Abnormal collagen synthesis results from a variety of gene mutations and causes brittle bones and connective tissue malformations.*

Foot gangrene. The first four toes and adjacent skin are dry, shrunken, and blackened with superficial necrosis and peeling of the skin. A well-defined line of demarcation separates the black region from the viable skin.*

Bone fracture. New bone formation with osteoblasts.*

Meningomyelocele. A neural tube defect in which the meninges and spinal cord herniate through the spinal canal; gross image of infant's lower back.*

Omphalocele in a newborn. Note that the defect is midline and is covered by peritoneum, as opposed to gastroschisis, which is not covered by peritoneum and is often not midline.*

Sarcoidosis. Necrotizing sarcoid granuloma with macrophage infiltrates and caseation.*

Amyloidosis from tongue tissue with skeletal muscle atrophy. The amyloid deposits stain red with Congo red and exhibit an apple-green birefringence with polarized light (as shown here in a section of cardiac muscle).*

Candidal vaginitis. Branched and budding *Candida albicans* is visible on KOH preparation of whitish vaginal discharge.

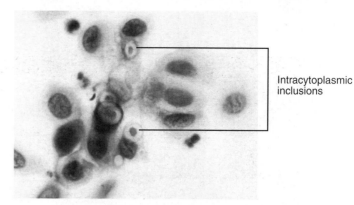

Intracytoplasmic inclusions

Trichomonas vaginalis. Trophozoites are visible on Giemsa stain.

Klinefelter's syndrome (XXY). Phenotype includes a female fat distribution with male external genitalia.

Turner's syndrome (XO). Phenotype includes short stature, webbing of the neck, and poorly developed secondary sex characteristics.

Marfan's syndrome. Patients are tall with very long extremities. The joints are hyperextensible, with slim bone structure and wiry muscles.*

Simian crease. A characteristic feature of Down syndrome (trisomy 21). The palm has a single transverse crease instead of the normal two creases.*

Duodenal ulcer. The epithelium is ulcerated, and the lamina propria is infiltrated with inflammatory cells. Necrotic debris is present in the ulcer crater.

Photomicrograph of the **small intestine.**

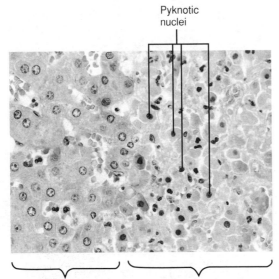

Pyknotic nuclei

Normal liver cells
Arranged in cords
Normal nuclei

Granular cytoplasm

Coagulative necrosis of liver cells
Disorganized
Pyknotic or absent nuclei
Homogeneous cytoplasm

Coagulative necrosis of hepatocytes.

Crohn's disease. Barium x-ray showing spicules, edema, and ulcers. (Reproduced, with permission, from Le T et al. *First Aid for the Wards,* 1st ed. Stamford, CT: Appleton & Lange, 1998.)

A

B

Inflammatory bowel disease (IBD). In **Crohn's disease (A),** the juxtaposition of ulcerated and normal mucosa gives a "cobblestone" appearance. In acute **ulcerative colitis (B),** the intestinal mucosa is inflamed and edematous and has a pseudopolypoid appearance. Chronically, ulcerative colitis has a more atrophic appearance.

Small bowel obstruction on supine abdominal x-ray. Note dilated loops of small bowel in a ladder-like pattern. Air-fluid levels may be seen if an upright x-ray is done. (Reproduced, with permission, from Le T et al. *First Aid for the Wards*, 1st ed. Stamford, CT: Appleton & Lange, 1998.)

Squamous cell carcinoma in the right lower lobe. (Reproduced, with permission, from Le T et al. *First Aid for the Wards*, 1st ed. Stamford, CT: Appleton & Lange, 1998.)

A

B

Compare the diffuse, patchy bilateral infiltrates of "atypical" **interstitial pneumonia (A)** with the localized, dense lesion of **lobar pneumonia (B)**.

A

B

Bronchopneumonia. (A) Gross. Note the large area of consolidation at the base plus multiple small areas of consolidation (pale) involving bronchioles and surrounding alveolar sacs throughout the lung. **(B)** Bronchopneumonia with neutrophils in alveolar spaces, microscopic.

Anterior shoulder dislocation. Note the humeral head inferior and medial to the glenoid fossa and fracture fragments from the greater tuberosity.

1—Acromion   4—Fracture fragments
2—Coracoid   5—Humeral head
3—Glenoid fossa   6—Clavicle

Multiple **leiomyomas** (fibroids) of the uterus. A common benign uterine tumor. Fibroids beneath the endometrium may present with vaginal bleeding; they also develop subserosally or within the myometrium.

Teratoma (benign) of the ovary containing teeth and hair—an incidental finding during abdominal surgery. In females, teratomas are generally benign, whereas in males they account for roughly 30% of testicular tumors.

Atherosclerosis in a coronary vessel. Calcified plaques have narrowed the lumen of the artery, increasing the risk for occlusion—i.e., myocardial infarction.

Breast mammogram diagnosis of breast cancer. The upper half of the breast shows a dense, irregularly shaped mass with long, branching tentacles extending toward the nipple. Numerous tiny calcium deposits looking like grains of sand (microcalcifications) are seen both in the mass and in the surrounding tissue.*

A

B

Subarachnoid hemorrhage. CT scan with contrast reveals blood in the subarachnoid space at the base of the brain.

Left ventricular hypertrophy (mediastinum wider than 50% of the width of the chest) from aortic valve stenosis.*

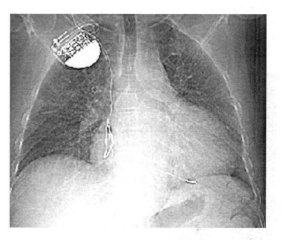

Amiodarone toxicity. Diffuse interstitial bilateral pulmonary markings in a reticular nodular pattern, most prominent in the lung bases and posteriorly, are evidence of pulmonary fibrosis.*

Pneumothorax. The right lung is collapsed; the apparent straight line off the rightmost edge of the pleural space indicated by the arrow shows the edge of the collapsed lung.*

Descending aortic dissection. Presents with severe chest pain. Type A is proximal to the subclavian artery and type B distal to the subclavian.*

CT abdomen with contrast—normal anatomy.

1—Liver	7—Splenic vein
2—IVC	8—Aorta
3—Portal vein	9—Spleen
4—Hepatic artery	10—Stomach
5—Gastroduodenal artery	11—Pancreas
6—Celiac trunk	

Left adrenal mass.

1—Large left adrenal mass	7—Spleen
2—Kidney	8—Liver
3—Vertebral body	9—Stomach with air and contrast
4—Aorta	10—Colon–splenic flexure
5—IVC	
6—Pancreas	

Pancreatic adenocarcinoma. A large, heterogeneously enhancing mass is visible at the neck of the pancreas, compressing the common bile duct, portal vein, splenic vein, superior mesenteric vein, and IVC. No liver metastases are apparent.*

Acute pancreatitis, typically from alcohol abuse or gallstone obstruction of the pancreatic duct. No evidence of necrosis or fluid collection is seen.*

Chronic pancreatitis precipitated by large duct stones. A small fatty infiltrate is visible to the left of the liver. Mild central biliary dilatation and a prominent common bile duct are also seen.*

Osteoarthritis. Increased fibrosis of the joint and a decreased amount of cartilage are apparent.*

Type 1 vs. type 2 diabetes mellitus

Variable	Type 1—juvenile onset (IDDM)	Type 2—adult onset (NIDDM)
Incidence	15%	85%
Insulin necessary in treatment	Always	Sometimes
Age (exceptions commonly occur)	< 30	> 40
Association with obesity	No	Yes
Genetic predisposition	Weak, polygenic	Strong, polygenic
Association with HLA system	Yes (HLA-DR3 and 4)	No
Glucose intolerance	Severe	Mild to moderate
Ketoacidosis	Common	Rare
β-cell numbers in the islets	↓	Variable
Serum insulin level	↓	Variable
Classic symptoms of polyuria, polydipsia, thirst, weight loss	Common	Sometimes
Theorized cause	Viral or immune destruction of β cells	↑ resistance to insulin

Diabetic ketoacidosis

One of the most important complications of type 1 diabetes. Usually due to an ↑ in insulin requirements from an ↑ in stress (e.g., infection). Excess fat breakdown and ↑ ketogenesis from the ↑ in free fatty acids, which are then made into ketone bodies.

Signs/symptoms — Kussmaul respirations (rapid/deep breathing), hyperthermia, nausea/vomiting, abdominal pain, psychosis/dementia, dehydration. Fruity breath odor.

Labs — Hyperglycemia, $\uparrow H^+$, $\downarrow HCO_3^-$ (anion gap metabolic acidosis), ↑ blood ketone levels, leukocytosis.

Complications — Life-threatening mucormycosis, *Rhizopus* infection, cerebral edema, cardiac arrhythmias, heart failure.

Treatment — Fluids, insulin, and potassium; glucose if necessary to prevent hypoglycemia.

Diabetes insipidus

Characterized by intensive thirst and polyuria together with an inability to concentrate urine with fluid restriction owing to lack of ADH (central DI) or to a lack of renal response to ADH (nephrogenic DI). Caused by lithium or demeclocycline.

Findings — Urine specific gravity < 1.006; serum osmolality > 290 mOsm/L.

Treatment — Adequate fluid intake. For central DI—intranasal desmopressin (ADH analog). For nephrogenic DI—hydrochlorothiazide, indomethacin, or amiloride.

SIADH

Syndrome of inappropriate antidiuretic hormone secretion:
1. Excessive water retention
2. Hyponatremia
3. Urine osmolarity > serum osmolarity

Very low serum sodium levels can lead to seizures (correct slowly).

Causes include:
1. Ectopic ADH (small cell lung cancer)
2. CNS disorders/head trauma
3. Pulmonary disease
4. Drugs

Hyperparathyroidism

Primary	Usually an adenoma. Hypercalcemia, hypercalciuria, hypophosphatemia, ↑ PTH, ↑ cAMP in urine. Often asymptomatic, or may present with weakness and constipation.	**Osteitis fibrosa cystica** (von Recklinghausen's syndrome)—cystic bone spaces filled with non-neoplastic fibrous tissue.
Secondary	2° hyperplasia due to ↓ serum Ca^{2+}, most often in chronic renal disease. Hypocalcemia, hyperphosphatemia, ↑ PTH.	**Renal osteodystrophy**—bone lesions due to 2° hyperparathyroidism due in turn to renal disease.

Hypoparathyroidism

Hypocalcemia, tetany. Due to accidental surgical excision (thyroid surgery) or DiGeorge syndrome.	**Pseudohypoparathyroidism**—autosomal-recessive kidney unresponsiveness to PTH. Hypocalcemia, shortened 4th/5th digits, short stature.

Carcinoid syndrome

Rare syndrome caused by carcinoid tumors (neuroendocrine cells), especially those of the small bowel; the tumors secrete high levels of serotonin (5-HT) that does not get metabolized by the liver due to liver metastases. Results in recurrent **diarrhea, cutaneous flushing, asthmatic wheezing,** and **right-sided valvular disease.** Most common tumor of appendix. ↑ 5-HIAA in urine.	**Rule of 1/3s:** 1/3 metastasize 1/3 present with 2nd malignancy 1/3 multiple Derived from neuroendocrine cells of GI tract. Treat with octreotide.

Zollinger-Ellison syndrome

Gastrin-secreting tumor that is usually located in the pancreas. Causes recurrent ulcers. May be associated with MEN type I.

Osteoporosis

	Reduction of bone mass in spite of normal bone mineralization.	Affects whites > blacks > Asians.
Type I	Postmenopausal (10–15 years after menopause); ↑ bone resorption due to ↓ estrogen levels. Treated with estrogen replacement.	Vertebral crush fractures—acute back pain, loss of height, kyphosis.
Type II	Senile osteoporosis—affects men and women > 70 years.	Distal radius (Colles') fractures, vertebral wedge fractures.

Mild compression fracture   Normal vertebra

Benign prostatic hyperplasia

Common in men > 50 years of age. May be due to an age-related increase in estradiol with possible sensitization of the prostate to the growth-promoting effects of DHT. Characterized by a nodular enlargement of the periurethral (lateral and middle) lobes of the prostate gland, compressing the urethra into a vertical slit. Often presents with ↑ frequency of urination, nocturia, difficulty starting and stopping the stream of urine, and dysuria. May lead to distention and hypertrophy of the bladder, hydronephrosis, and UTIs. Not considered a premalignant lesion.

Hydatidiform mole

A pathologic ovum ("empty egg"—ovum with no DNA) resulting in cystic swelling of chorionic villi and proliferation of chorionic epithelium (trophoblast). Most common precursor of choriocarcinoma. High β-hCG. "Honeycombed uterus," "cluster of grapes" appearance. Genotype of a **complete** mole is 46,XX and is **completely** paternal in origin (no maternal chromosomes); no associated fetus. **PART**ial mole is made up of 3 or more **PARTS** (triploid or tetraploid).

Pregnancy-induced hypertension (preeclampsia-eclampsia)

Preeclampsia is the triad of hypertension, proteinuria, and edema; eclampsia is the addition of seizures to the triad. Affects 7% of pregnant women from 20 weeks' gestation to 6 weeks postpartum. ↑ incidence in patients with preexisting hypertension, diabetes, chronic renal disease, and autoimmune disorders. Can be associated with HELLP syndrome (**H**emolysis, **E**levated **LFT**s, **L**ow **P**latelets).

Clinical features — Headache, blurred vision, abdominal pain, edema of face and extremities, altered mentation, hyperreflexia; lab findings may include thrombocytopenia, hyperuricemia.

Treatment — Delivery of fetus as soon as viable. Otherwise bed rest, salt restriction, and monitoring and treatment of hypertension. For eclampsia, a medical emergency, IV magnesium sulfate and diazepam.

Pregnancy complications

1. Abruptio placentae—premature separation of placenta. **Painful** uterine bleeding (usually during 3rd trimester). Fetal death. May be associated with DIC.
2. Placenta accreta—defective decidual layer allows placenta to attach directly to myometrium. Predisposed by prior C-section or inflammation. May have massive hemorrhage after delivery.
3. Placenta previa—attachment of placenta to lower uterine segment. May occlude cervical os. **Painless** bleeding in any trimester.
4. Ectopic pregnancy—most often in fallopian tubes, predisposed by salpingitis (PID).

Cervical pathology

Dysplasia and carcinoma in situ — Disordered epithelial growth; begins at basal layer and extends outward. Classified as CIN 1 CIN 2, or CIN 3 (carcinoma in situ), depending on extent of dysplasia. Associated with HPV. May progress to invasive carcinoma.

Invasive carcinoma — Often squamous cell carcinoma. Pap smear can catch cervical dysplasia (koilocytes) before it progresses to invasive carcinoma.

HIGH-YIELD FACTS

Pathology

Uterine pathology

Endometriosis	Non-neoplastic endometrial glands/stroma in abnormal locations outside the uterus. Characterized by cyclic bleeding (menstrual type) from ectopic endometrial tissue resulting in blood-filled, "chocolate cysts." Ovary is most common site. Manifests clinically as severe menstrual-related pain. Often results in infertility.
Adenomyosis	Endometriosis within the myometrium.
Endometrial hyperplasia	Abnormal endometrial gland proliferation usually caused by excess estrogen stimulation. ↑ risk for endometrial carcinoma. Most commonly manifests clinically as vaginal bleeding.
Endometrial carcinoma	Most common gynecologic malignancy. Peak age 55–65 years old. Clinically presents with vaginal bleeding. Typically preceded by endometrial hyperplasia. Risk factors include prolonged estrogen use (compare with carcinomas of cervix), obesity, diabetes, and hypertension.
Leiomyoma	Most common of all tumors in females. Often presents with multiple tumors. ↑ incidence in blacks. Malignant transformation is rare. Estrogen sensitive—tumor size ↑ with pregnancy and ↓ with menopause. Does not progress to leiomyosarcoma (leiomyomas are de novo).
Leiomyosarcoma	Bulky tumor with areas of necrosis and hemorrhage, typically arising de novo (not from leiomyoma). ↑ incidence in blacks. Highly aggressive tumor with tendency to recur. May protrude from cervix and bleed.

Polycystic ovarian syndrome (Stein-Leventhal syndrome)

↑ LH due to peripheral estrogen production leads to anovulation. Manifest clinically by amenorrhea, infertility, obesity, and hirsutism. Treat with weight loss, OCPs, gonadotropin analogs, or surgery.

Ovarian cysts

1. Follicular cyst—distention of unruptured graafian follicle. May be associated with hyperestrinism and endometrial hyperplasia.
2. Corpus luteum cyst—hemorrhage into persistent corpus luteum. Menstrual irregularity.
3. Theca-lutein cyst—often bilateral/multiple. Due to gonadotropin stimulation. Associated with choriocarcinoma and moles.
4. "Chocolate cyst"—blood-containing cyst from ovarian endometriosis. Varies with menstrual cycle.

Ovarian germ cell tumors

1. Dysgerminoma—analogous to male seminoma.
2. Yolk sac tumor—similar to testicular form; produces α-fetoprotein.
3. Choriocarcinoma—like testicular version. ↑ hCG.
4. Teratoma—constitutes 90% of germ cell tumors of ovary. All 3 germ layers. Mature teratoma ("dermoid cyst") is benign. Immature teratoma is an aggressive malignant tumor. Struma ovarii—monodermal, composed only of thyroid tissue.

HIGH-YIELD FACTS

Pathology

Ovarian non–germ cell tumors

1. Serous cystadenoma—20% of ovarian tumors. Frequently bilateral, lined with fallopian tube–like epithelium. Benign.
2. Serous cystadenocarcinoma—50% ovarian tumors, malignant and frequently bilateral.
3. Mucinous cystadenoma—multilocular cyst lined by mucus-secreting epithelium. Benign.
4. Mucinous cystadenocarcinoma—malignant. Pseudomyxoma peritonei—intraperitoneal accumulation of mucinous material.
5. **B**renner tumor—benign tumor that resembles **B**ladder epithelium.
6. Ovarian fibroma—bundles of spindle-shaped fibroblasts. Meigs' syndrome—triad of ovarian fibroma, ascites, and hydrothorax.
7. Granulosa cell tumor—secretes estrogen → precocious puberty (kids). Can cause endometrial hyperplasia or carcinoma in adults. Call-Exner bodies—small follicles filled with eosinophilic secretions.

Breast disease

Type	Characteristics
Fibrocystic disease	Presents with diffuse breast pain and multiple lesions, often bilateral. Biopsy shows fibrocystic elements. Usually does not indicate ↑ risk of carcinoma. Histologic types: 1. Fibrosis—hyperplasia of breast stroma. 2. Cystic—fluid filled. 3. Sclerosing—↑ acini and intralobular fibrosis. 4. Epithelial hyperplasia—↑ in number of epithelial cell layers in terminal duct lobule. ↑ risk of carcinoma with atypical cells. Occurs > 30 years.
Benign tumors	Fibroadenoma—most common tumor < 25 years. Small, mobile, firm mass with sharp edges. ↑ size and tenderness with pregnancy. Not a precursor to breast cancer. Cystosarcoma phyllodes—large, bulky mass of connective tissue and cysts. Breast surface has "leaflike" appearance. Intraductal papilloma—tumor of lactiferous ducts; presents with nipple discharge.
Malignant tumors (carcinoma)	Common postmenopause. Arise from mammary duct epithelium or lobular glands. Histologic types: 1. Comedocarcinoma—cheesy consistency of tumor tissue due to central necrosis. 2. Infiltrating ductal—most common carcinoma. Firm, fibrous mass. 3. Inflammatory—lymphatic involvement; poor prognosis. 4. Paget's disease—eczematous patches on nipple. Paget cells—large cells with clear halo; suggest underlying ductal cancer. 5. Infiltrating lobular—often multiple/bilateral. Clusters of cells fill intralobular ductules. 6. Medullary—cellular with scant stroma and lymphocytic infiltrate.
Risk factors	Gender, age, early 1st menarche (< 12 years old), delayed 1st pregnancy (> 30 years old), late menopause (> 50 years old), family history of 1st-degree relative with breast cancer at a young age. Risk is NOT increased by fibroadenoma or nonhyperplastic cysts.

Hypertension

Risk factors	↑ age, obesity, diabetes, smoking, genetics, black > white > Asian.
Features	90% of hypertension is primary (essential) and related to ↑ CO or ↑ TPR; remaining 10% mostly 2° to renal disease.
Predisposes to	CAD, cerebrovascular accidents, CHF, renal failure, and aortic dissection.
Pathology	Hyaline thickening and atherosclerosis.

Arteriosclerosis

Mönckeberg	Stiffening of the arteries. Involve the media, often at radial or ulnar arteries.
Arteriolosclerosis	Hyaline thickening of small arteries.
Atherosclerosis	Fibrous plaques and atheromas form in intima of arteries.

Atherosclerosis

Disease of elastic arteries and large and medium-sized muscular arteries.

Risk factors	Smoking, hypertension, diabetes mellitus, hyperlipidemia, family history.
Progression	Fatty streaks → proliferative plaque → complex atheromas.
Complications	Aneurysms, ischemia, infarcts, peripheral vascular disease, thrombus, emboli.
Location	Abdominal aorta > coronary artery > popliteal artery > carotid artery.
Symptoms	Angina, claudication, but can be asymptomatic.

Ischemic heart disease

Possible manifestations:

1. **Angina** (CAD narrowing > 75%):
   a. Stable—mostly 2° to atherosclerosis (retrosternal chest pain with exertion)
   b. Prinzmetal's variant—occurs at rest 2° to coronary artery spasm
   c. Unstable/crescendo—thrombosis in a branch (worsening chest pain)
2. **Myocardial infarction**—most often occurs in CAD involving the left anterior descending artery (LAD)
3. **Sudden cardiac death**—death from cardiac causes within 1 hour of onset of symptoms, most commonly due to a lethal arrhythmia
4. **Chronic ischemic heart disease**—progressive onset of CHF over many years due to chronic ischemic myocardial damage

Infarcts: red vs. pale

Red (hemorrhagic) infarcts occur in loose tissues with collaterals, such as lungs, intestine, or following reperfusion.

Pale infarcts occur in solid tissues with single blood supply, such as brain, heart, kidney, and spleen.

REd = **RE**perfusion.

HIGH-YIELD FACTS

Pathology

Evolution of MI

Coronary artery occlusion: LAD > RCA > circumflex.

Symptoms: severe retrosternal pain, pain in left arm and/or jaw, shortness of breath, fatigue, adrenergic symptoms.

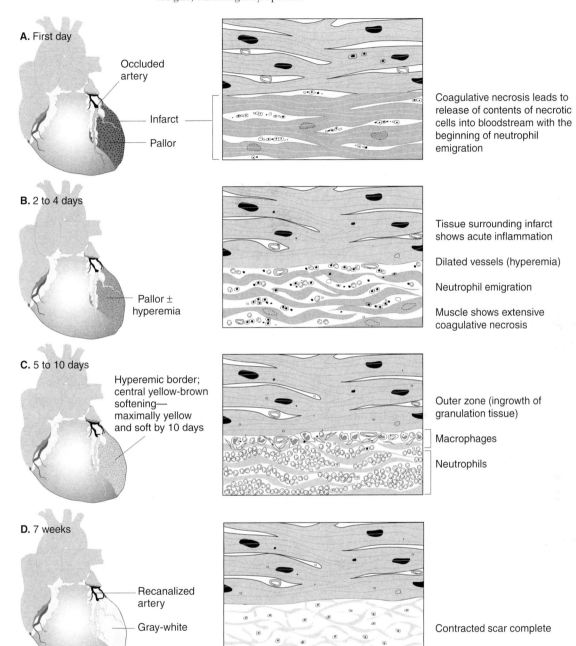

A. First day

Occluded artery

Infarct

Pallor

Coagulative necrosis leads to release of contents of necrotic cells into bloodstream with the beginning of neutrophil emigration

B. 2 to 4 days

Pallor ± hyperemia

Tissue surrounding infarct shows acute inflammation

Dilated vessels (hyperemia)

Neutrophil emigration

Muscle shows extensive coagulative necrosis

C. 5 to 10 days

Hyperemic border; central yellow-brown softening— maximally yellow and soft by 10 days

Outer zone (ingrowth of granulation tissue)

Macrophages

Neutrophils

D. 7 weeks

Recanalized artery

Gray-white

Contracted scar complete

(Adapted, with permission, from Chandrasoma P. *Pathology Notes.* Norwalk, CT: Appleton & Lange, 1991:244.)

HIGH-YIELD FACTS

Pathology

HIGH-YIELD FACTS

Pathology

Diagnosis of MI

In the 1st 6 hours, ECG is the gold standard.

Cardiac troponin I is used within the 1st 4 hours up to 7–10 days; more specific than other protein markers.

CK-MB is test of choice in the first 24 hours post-MI.

LDH_1 (former test of choice) is also elevated from 2 to 7 days post-MI.

AST is nonspecific and can be found in cardiac, liver, and skeletal muscle cells.

ECG changes can include ST elevation (transmural infarct), ST depression (subendocardial infarct), and Q waves (transmural infarct).

MI complications

1. Cardiac arrhythmia (90%); highest rise 2 days postinfarct
2. LV failure and pulmonary edema (60%)
3. Thromboembolism—mural thrombus
4. Cardiogenic shock (large infarct—high risk of mortality)
5. Rupture of ventricular free wall, interventricular septum, papillary muscle (4–10 days post-MI), cardiac tamponade
6. Fibrinous pericarditis—friction rub (3–5 days post-MI)
7. Dressler's syndrome—autoimmune phenomenon resulting in fibrinous pericarditis (several weeks post-MI)

Cardiomyopathies

Dilated (congestive) cardiomyopathy	Most common cardiomyopathy (90% of cases). Etiologies include chronic **A**lcohol abuse, **B**eriberi, postviral myocarditis by **C**oxsackievirus B, chronic **C**ocaine use, **C**hagas' disease, **D**oxorubicin toxicity, peripartum cardiomyopathy. Heart dilates and looks like a balloon on chest x-ray.	Systolic dysfunction ensues.
Hypertrophic cardiomyopathy (formerly IHSS)	Hypertrophy often asymmetric and involving the intraventricular septum. 50% of cases are familial and are inherited as an autosomal-dominant trait. Cause of sudden death in young athletes. Walls of LV are thickened and chamber becomes banana shaped on echocardiogram.	Diastolic dysfunction ensues.
Restrictive/obliterative cardiomyopathy	Major causes include sarcoidosis, amyloidosis, scleroderma, hemochromatosis, endocardial fibroelastosis, and endomyocardial fibrosis (Löffler's).	

Heart murmurs

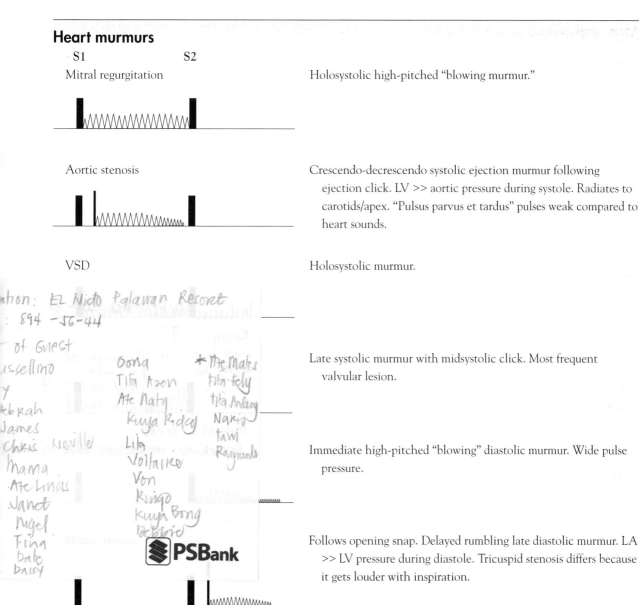

Mitral regurgitation — Holosystolic high-pitched "blowing murmur."

Aortic stenosis — Crescendo-decrescendo systolic ejection murmur following ejection click. LV >> aortic pressure during systole. Radiates to carotids/apex. "Pulsus parvus et tardus" pulses weak compared to heart sounds.

VSD — Holosystolic murmur.

Late systolic murmur with midsystolic click. Most frequent valvular lesion.

Immediate high-pitched "blowing" diastolic murmur. Wide pulse pressure.

Follows opening snap. Delayed rumbling late diastolic murmur. LA >> LV pressure during diastole. Tricuspid stenosis differs because it gets louder with inspiration.

PDA — Continuous machine-like murmur. Loudest at time of S2.

(Adapted, with permission, from Wood P. *Diseases of the Heart and Circulation*, 3rd ed. Philadelphia: Lippincott, 1968.)

Cardiac tumors

Myxomas are the most common 1° cardiac tumor in adults. 90% occur in the atria (mostly LA). Myxomas are usually described as a "ball-valve" obstruction in the LA. Rhabdomyomas are the most frequent 1° cardiac tumor in children.

Metastases most common heart tumor.

CHF

Abnormality	Cause
Ankle, sacral edema	RV failure → ↑ venous pressure → fluid transudation.
Hepatomegaly (nutmeg liver)	↑ central venous pressure → ↑ resistance to portal flow. Rarely, leads to "cardiac cirrhosis."
Pulmonary congestion	LV failure → ↑ pulmonary venous pressure → pulmonary venous distention and transudation of fluid. Presence of hemosiderin-laden macrophages ("heart failure" cells).
Dyspnea on exertion	Failure of LV output to ↑ during exercise.
Paroxysmal nocturnal dyspnea, pulmonary edema	Failure of left heart output to keep up with right heart output → acute rise in pulmonary venous and capillary pressure → transudation of fluid.
Orthopnea (shortness of breath when supine)	Pooling of blood in lungs in supine position adds volume to congested pulmonary vascular system; ↑ venous return not put out by LV.
Cardiac dilation	Greater ventricular end-diastolic volume.

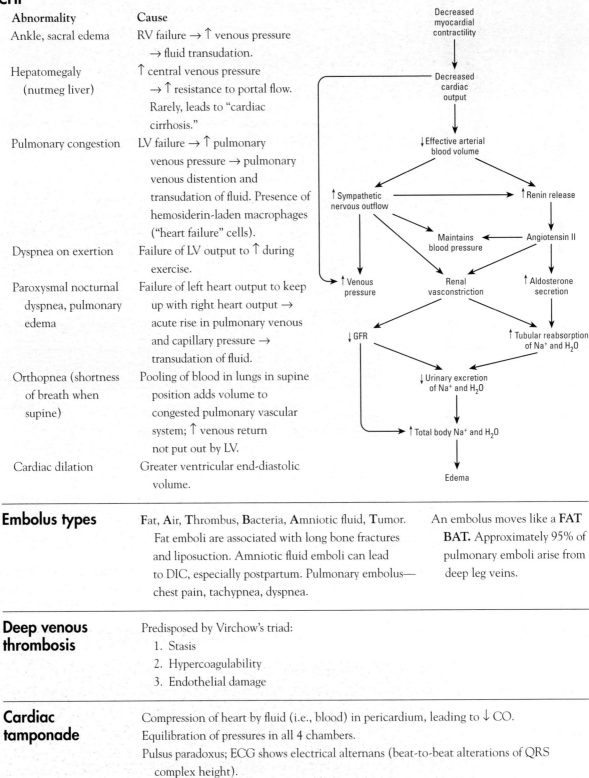

Embolus types	Fat, Air, Thrombus, Bacteria, Amniotic fluid, Tumor. Fat emboli are associated with long bone fractures and liposuction. Amniotic fluid emboli can lead to DIC, especially postpartum. Pulmonary embolus—chest pain, tachypnea, dyspnea.

An embolus moves like a **FAT BAT.** Approximately 95% of pulmonary emboli arise from deep leg veins.

Deep venous thrombosis	Predisposed by Virchow's triad: 1. Stasis 2. Hypercoagulability 3. Endothelial damage

Cardiac tamponade	Compression of heart by fluid (i.e., blood) in pericardium, leading to ↓ CO. Equilibration of pressures in all 4 chambers. Pulsus paradoxus; ECG shows electrical alternans (beat-to-beat alterations of QRS complex height).

Bacterial endocarditis	New murmur, anemia, fever, Osler nodes (tender raised lesions on finger or toe pads), Roth's spots (round white spots on retina surrounded by hemorrhage), Janeway lesions (small erythematous lesions on palm or sole), splinter hemorrhages on nail bed. Multiple blood cultures necessary for diagnosis (continuous bacteremia).
	  1. Acute—*S. aureus* (high virulence). Large vegetations on previously normal valves. Rapid onset.
	  2. Subacute—viridans streptococcus (low virulence). Smaller vegetations on congenitally abnormal or diseased valves. Sequela of dental procedures. More insidious onset.
	Endocarditis may also be nonbacterial 2° to metastasis or renal failure (marantic/thrombotic endocarditis).
		Mitral valve is most frequently involved. Tricuspid valve endocarditis is associated with IV drug abuse.
		Complications: chordae rupture, glomerulonephritis, suppurative pericarditis, emboli.
		JR = NO FAME:
		Janeway lesions
		Roth's spots
		Nail-bed hemorrhage
		Osler nodes
		Fever
		Anemia
		Murmur
		Emboli

Rheumatic fever/ rheumatic heart disease	Rheumatic fever is a consequence of pharyngeal infection with group A β-hemolytic streptococci. Late sequelae include rheumatic heart disease, which affects heart valves— mitral > aortic >> tricuspid (high-pressure valves affected most). Associated with Aschoff bodies, migratory polyarthritis, erythema marginatum, elevated ASO titers. Due to cross-reactivity, not direct effect of bacteria.	**FEVERSS:** **F**ever **E**rythema marginatum **V**alvular damage **E**SR ↑ **R**ed-hot joints (polyarthritis) **S**ubcutaneous nodules **St**. Vitus' dance (chorea)

Pericarditis
  Serous
  Fibrinous
  Hemorrhagic
	Caused by SLE, rheumatoid arthritis, infection, uremia.
	Uremia, MI, rheumatic fever.
	TB, malignancy (e.g., melanoma).
	Findings: pericardial pain, friction rub, ECG changes (diffuse ST elevations in all leads), pulsus paradoxus, distant heart sounds.
	Can resolve without scarring or lead to chronic adhesive or chronic constrictive pericarditis.	

Syphilitic heart disease	3° syphilis disrupts the vasa vasorum of the aorta with consequent dilation of the aorta and valve ring. Often affects the aortic root and ascending aorta. Associated with a tree-bark appearance of the aorta.	Can result in aneurysm of the ascending aorta or aortic arch and aortic valve incompetence.

Buerger's disease

Known as smoker's disease and thromboangiitis obliterans; idiopathic, segmental, thrombosing vasculitis of intermediate and small peripheral arteries and veins.

Findings

Intermittent claudication, superficial nodular phlebitis, cold sensitivity (Raynaud's phenomenon), severe pain in affected part; may lead to gangrene.

Treatment

Quit smoking.

Takayasu's arteritis

Known as "pulseless disease"—thickening of aortic arch and/or proximal great vessels. Associated with an elevated ESR. Primarily affects young Asian females. **F**ever, **A**rthritis, **N**ight sweats, **MY**algia, **SKIN** nodules, **O**cular disturbances, **W**eak pulses in upper extremities.

Affects medium and large arteries.

FAN MY SKIN On Wednesday.

Temporal arteritis (giant cell arteritis)

Most common vasculitis that affects medium and small arteries, usually branches of carotid artery. Findings include unilateral headache, jaw claudication, impaired vision (occlusion of ophthalmic artery, which can lead to blindness). Half of patients have systemic involvement and syndrome of polymyalgia rheumatica (proximal muscle pain, periarticular pain). Associated with elevated ESR. Responds well to steroids.

TEMporal = signs near **TEM**ples. ESR is markedly elevated. Affects elderly females.

Polyarteritis nodosa

Characterized by necrotizing immune complex inflammation of small or medium-sized muscular arteries, typically involving renal and visceral vessels.

PAN = P-ANCA.
Lesions are of different ages.
Churg-Strauss—variant associated with eosinophilia and asthma.

Symptoms

Fever, weight loss, malaise, abdominal pain, headache, myalgia, hypertension.

Findings

Cotton-wool spots, microaneurysms, pericarditis, myocarditis, palpable purpura. ↑ ESR.
Associated with hepatitis B infection in 30% of patients.
P-ANCA (perinuclear pattern of antineutrophil cytoplasmic antibodies) is often present in the serum and correlates with disease activity, primarily in small vessel disease. Typically affects young males.

Treatment

Corticosteroids, azathioprine, and/or cyclophosphamide.

Wegener's granulomatosis

Characterized by focal necrotizing vasculitis and necrotizing granulomas in the lung and upper airway and by necrotizing glomerulonephritis.

Symptoms

Perforation of nasal septum, chronic sinusitis, otitis media, mastoiditis, cough, dyspnea, hemoptysis.

Findings

C-ANCA is a strong marker of disease; chest x-ray may reveal large nodular densities; hematuria and red cell casts.

Treatment

Cyclophosphamide, corticosteroids, and/or methotrexate.

Kawasaki disease

Acute, self-limiting disease of infants/kids. Acute necrotizing vasculitis of small/medium-sized vessels. Fever, congested conjunctiva, changes in lips/oral mucosa, lymphadenitis. May develop coronary aneurysms.

Glomerular pathology

NephrItic syndrome—hematuria, hypertension, oliguria, azotemia.

1. **Acute poststreptococcal glomerulonephritis**— LM: glomeruli enlarged and hypercellular, neutrophils, "lumpy-bumpy." EM: subepithelial humps. IF: granular pattern.
2. **Rapidly progressive (crescentic) glomerulonephritis**—LM and IF: crescent-moon shape.
3. **Goodpasture's syndrome (type II hypersensitivity)**—IF: linear pattern, anti-GBM antibodies.
4. **Membranoproliferative glomerulonephritis**— EM: subendothelial humps, "tram track."
5. **IgA nephropathy (Berger's disease)**— IF and EM: mesangial deposits of IgA.
6. **Alport's syndrome**—split basement membrane.

NephrOtic syndrome—massive proteinuria, hypoalbuminemia, generalized edema, hyperlipidemia.

1. **Membranous glomerulonephritis**—LM: diffuse capillary and basement membrane thickening. IF: granular pattern. EM: "spike and dome."
2. **Minimal change disease (lipoid nephrosis)**— LM: normal glomeruli. EM: foot process effacement.
3. **Focal segmental glomerular sclerosis**— LM: segmental sclerosis and hyalinosis.
4. **Diabetic nephropathy**—LM: Kimmelstiel-Wilson lesions, basement membrane thickening.
5. **SLE** (5 patterns of renal involvement)— LM: wire-loop appearance with extensive granular subendothelial basement membrane deposits in membranous glomerulonephritis pattern.

(LM = light microscopy; EM = electron microscopy; IF = immunofluorescence)

I = **i**nflammation.

Most frequently seen in children. Peripheral, periorbital edema. Resolves spontaneously.

Rapid course to renal failure from one of many causes.

Hemoptysis, hematuria.

Slowly progresses to renal failure.

Mild disease. Often postinfectious.

Collagen IV mutation. Nerve deafness and ocular disorders.

O = pr**O**teinuria.

A common cause of adult nephrotic syndrome.

Most common cause of childhood nephrotic syndrome. Responds well to steroids.

More severe disease in HIV patients.

EP = epithelium with foot processes
US = urinary space
GBM = glomerular basement membrane
EN = fenestrated endothelium
MC = mesangial cells
EM = extracellular matrix

1 = subepithelium deposits (membranous nephropathy)
2 = large irregular subepithelium deposits or "humps" (acute glomerulonephritis)
3 = subendothelial deposits in lupus glomerulonephritis
4 = mesangial deposits (IgA nephropathy)
5 = antibody binding to GBM—smooth linear pattern on immunofluorescence (Goodpasture's)
6 = effacement of epithelial foot processes (common in all forms of glomerular injury with proteinuria)

(Adapted, with permission, from Luke RG et al. "Nephrology and hypertension." In *Medical Knowledge Self-Assessment Program IX.* Philadelphia: American College of Physicians, 1992.)

HIGH-YIELD FACTS

Pathology

Kidney stones

Can lead to severe complications such as hydronephrosis and pyelonephritis. 4 major types:

1. Calcium—constitute the majority of kidney stones (80–85%). Calcium oxalate or calcium phosphate or both. Stones are radiopaque. Disorders or conditions that cause hypercalcemia (e.g., cancer, increased PTH, increased vitamin D, milk-alkali syndrome) can all lead to hypercalciuria and stones. Tend to recur.
2. Ammonium magnesium phosphate (struvite)—2nd most common kidney stone. Radiopaque and urease-positive bugs such as *Proteus vulgaris* or *Staphylococcus*. Can form large struvite calculi that can be a nidus for UTIs.
3. Uric acid—strong association with hyperuricemia (e.g., gout). Often seen as a result of diseases with ↑ cell proliferation and turnover, such as leukemia and myeloproliferative disorders. Radiolucent.
4. Cystine—most often 2° to cystinuria. Radiolucent.

Renal cell carcinoma

Most common renal malignancy. Most common in men ages 50–70. ↑ incidence in smokers. Associated with von Hippel–Lindau and gene deletion in chromosome 3. Originates in renal tubule cells → polygonal clear cells. Manifests clinically with hematuria, palpable mass, 2° polycythemia, flank pain, and fever. Invades IVC and spreads hematogenously. Associated with paraneoplastic syndromes (ectopic EPO, ACTH, PTHrP, and prolactin).

Wilms' tumor

Most common renal malignancy of early childhood (ages 2–4). Presents with huge, palpable flank mass, hemihypertrophy. Deletion of tumor suppression gene *WT1* on chromosome 11. Can be part of **WAGR** complex: **W**ilms' tumor, **A**niridia, **G**enitourinary malformation, and mental-motor **R**etardation.

Transitional cell carcinoma

Most common tumor of urinary tract system (can occur in renal calyces, renal pelvis, ureters, and bladder). Often recurs after removal. Presents with hematuria and may spread to adjacent tissue. Associated with problems in your **P**ee **SAC**: **P**henacetin, **S**moking, **A**niline dyes, and **C**yclophosphamide.

Acid-base physiology

	pH	P_{CO_2}	$[HCO_3^-]$	Cause	Compensatory response
Metabolic acidosis	↓	↓	↓	Diabetic ketoacidosis, diarrhea, lactic acidosis, salicylate OD, acetazolamide OD	Hyperventilation
Respiratory acidosis	↓	↑	↑	COPD, airway obstruction	Renal $[HCO_3^-]$ reabsorption
Respiratory alkalosis	↑	↓	↓	High altitude, hyperventilation	Renal $[HCO_3^-]$ secretion
Metabolic alkalosis	↑	↑	↑	Vomiting	Hypoventilation

Henderson-Hasselbalch equation: $pH = pKa + \log \dfrac{[HCO_3^-]}{0.03\, P_{CO_2}}$

Key: ↑ ↓ = primary disturbance; ↓ ↑ = compensatory response.

Acid-base nomogram

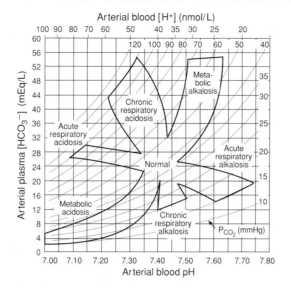

(Adapted, with permission, from Ganong WF. *Review of Medical Physiology,* 20th ed. New York: McGraw-Hill, 2003:709.)

Acidosis/alkalosis

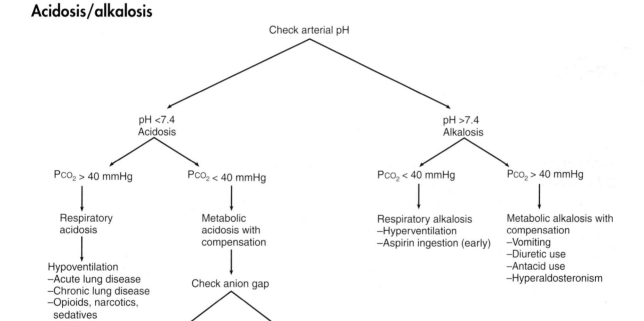

Check arterial pH

pH <7.4
Acidosis

pH >7.4
Alkalosis

P_{CO_2} > 40 mmHg

P_{CO_2} < 40 mmHg

P_{CO_2} < 40 mmHg

P_{CO_2} > 40 mmHg

Respiratory
acidosis

Metabolic
acidosis with
compensation

Respiratory alkalosis
–Hyperventilation
–Aspirin ingestion (early)

Metabolic alkalosis with
compensation
–Vomiting
–Diuretic use
–Antacid use
–Hyperaldosteronism

Hypoventilation
–Acute lung disease
–Chronic lung disease
–Opioids, narcotics,
sedatives
–Weakening of
respiratory
muscles

Check anion gap

↑Anion gap
–Renal failure
–Lactic acidosis
–Ketoacidosis (DM)
–Aspirin ingestion

Normal anion gap (8–12 mEq/L)
–Diarrhea
–Glue sniffing
–Renal tubular acidosis
–Hyperchloremia

Anion gap acidosis	Gap is $Na^+ - (Cl^- + HCO_3^-) = 8–12$ mEq/L.
	If elevated, may be due to:
	  Methanol
	  Uremia (chronic renal failure)
	  Diabetic ketoacidosis
	  Paraldehyde or **P**henformin
	  Iron tablets or **I**NH
	  Lactic acidosis (CN^-, CO, shock)
	  Ethanol or **E**thylene glycol
	  Salicylates
		MUD PILES.

Acid-base compensations	The following formulas give appropriate compensations for a single disorder. If the formula does not match the actual values, suspect a mixed disorder.
Metabolic acidosis	Winter's formula: $P_{CO_2} = 1.5 (HCO_3^-) + 8 \pm 2$.
Metabolic alkalosis	$P_{CO_2} \uparrow 0.7$ mmHg for every $\uparrow 1$ mEq/L HCO_3^-.
Respiratory acidosis	Acute— $\uparrow 1$ mEq/L HCO_3^- for every $\uparrow 10$ mmHg P_{CO_2}. Chronic— $\uparrow 3.5$ mEq/L HCO_3^- for every $\uparrow 10$ mmHg P_{CO_2}.
Respiratory alkalosis	Acute— $\downarrow 2$ mEq/L HCO_3^- for every $\downarrow 10$ mmHg P_{CO_2}. Chronic— $\downarrow 5$ mEq/L HCO_3^- for every $\downarrow 10$ mmHg P_{CO_2}.

Pyelonephritis	
Acute	Affects cortex with relative sparing of glomeruli/vessels. White cell casts in urine are pathognomonic.
Chronic	Coarse, asymmetric corticomedullary scarring. Tubules can contain eosinophilic casts (thyroidization of kidney).

Diffuse cortical necrosis	Acute generalized infarction of cortices of both kidneys. Likely due to a combination of vasospasm and DIC. Associated with obstetric catastrophes (e.g., abruptio placentae) and septic shock.

Acute tubular necrosis	Most common cause of acute renal failure. Reversible, but fatal if left untreated. Associated with renal ischemia (e.g., shock), crush injury (myoglobulinuria), toxins. Death most often occurs during initial oliguric phase. Recovery in 2–3 weeks.

Renal papillary necrosis	Associated with: 1. Diabetes mellitus 2. Acute pyelonephritis 3. Chronic phenacetin use

Acute renal failure

Abrupt decline in renal function with ↑ creatinine and ↑ BUN over a period of several days.

1. Prerenal azotemia—decreased RBF (e.g., hypotension) → ↓ GFR. Na+/H_2O retained by kidney.
2. Intrinsic renal—generally due to acute tubular necrosis or ischemia/toxins. Patchy necrosis leads to debris obstructing tubule and fluid backflow across necrotic tubule → ↓ GFR. Urine has epithelial/granular casts.
3. Postrenal—outflow obstruction (stones, BPH, neoplasia). Develops only with bilateral obstruction.

Variable	Prerenal	Renal	Postrenal
Urine osmolality	> 500	< 350	< 350
Urine Na	< 10	> 20	> 40
Fe_{Na}	< 1%	> 2%	> 4%
BUN/Cr ratio	> 20	< 15	> 15

Consequences of renal failure

Failure to make urine and excrete nitrogenous wastes. Consequences:

1. Anemia (failure of erythropoietin production)
2. Renal osteodystrophy (failure of active vitamin D production)
3. Hyperkalemia, which can lead to cardiac arrhythmias
4. Metabolic acidosis due to ↓ acid secretion and ↓ generation of HCO_3^-
5. Uremia (↑ BUN, creatinine)
6. Sodium and H_2O excess → CHF and pulmonary edema
7. Chronic pyelonephritis
8. Hypertension

2 forms of renal failure—acute renal failure (often due to hypoxia) and chronic renal failure (e.g., due to hypertension and diabetes).

Alcoholism   Physiologic tolerance and dependence with symptoms of withdrawal (tremor, tachycardia, hypertension, malaise, nausea, delirium tremens) when intake is interrupted.
Continued drinking despite medical and social contraindications and life disruptions.
Treatment: disulfiram to condition the patient negatively against alcohol use. Supportive treatment of other systemic manifestations. Alcoholics Anonymous and other peer support groups are most successful in sustaining abstinence.

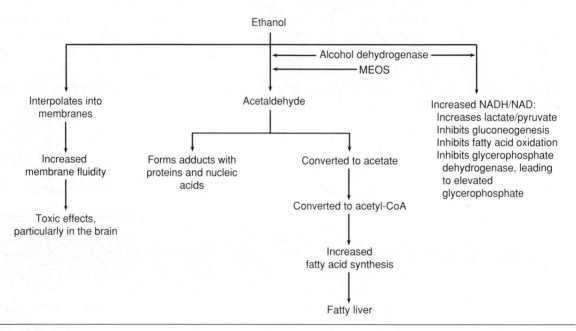

Complications of alcoholism

Alcoholic hepatitis and cirrhosis, pancreatitis, dilated cardiomyopathy, peripheral neuropathy, cerebellar degeneration, Wernicke-Korsakoff syndrome, testicular atrophy and hyperestrinism, and Mallory-Weiss syndrome.

Alcoholic cirrhosis   Long-term alcohol use leads to micronodular cirrhosis with accompanying symptoms of jaundice, hypoalbuminemia, coagulation factor deficiencies, and portal hypertension, leading to peripheral edema and ascites, encephalopathy, and neurologic manifestations (e.g., asterixis, flapping tremor of the hands).

Wernicke-Korsakoff syndrome   Caused by vitamin B_1 (thiamine) deficiency in alcoholics. Classically may present with triad of psychosis, ophthalmoplegia, and ataxia (Wernicke's encephalopathy). May progress to memory loss, confabulation, confusion (Korsakoff's syndrome; irreversible). Associated with periventricular hemorrhage/necrosis, especially in mammillary bodies. Treatment: IV vitamin B_1 (thiamine).

Mallory-Weiss syndrome   Longitudinal lacerations at the gastroesophageal junction caused by excessive vomiting with failure of LES relaxation that could lead to fatal hematemesis.

HIGH-YIELD FACTS

Pathology

Argyll Robertson pupil	Argyll Robertson pupil constricts with accommodation but is not reactive to light. Pathognomonic for 3° syphilis.	"Prostitute's pupil—" accommodates but does not react.
Amyloidosis	1° (light chain deposition) seen with multiple myeloma (most common cause) or Waldenström's macroglobulinemia; 2° (amyloid associated) can cause nephrotic syndrome in kidney. Apple-green birefringence on Congo red stain.	Alzheimer's disease associated with β-amyloid deposition in the cerebral cortex; islet cell amyloid deposition characteristic of diabetes mellitus type 2.
Aschoff body	Aschoff bodies (granuloma with giant cells) and Anitschkow's cells (activated histiocytes) are found in rheumatic heart disease.	Think of two **RH**ussians with **RH**eumatic heart disease (Aschoff and Anitschkow).
Auer bodies (rods)	Auer rods are peroxidase-positive cytoplasmic inclusions in granulocytes and myeloblasts. Primarily seen in acute promyelocytic leukemia (M3). Treatment of AML M3 can release Auer rods → DIC.	
Casts	Casts in urine: RBC casts—glomerular inflammation (nephritic syndromes), ischemia, or malignant hypertension. WBC casts—inflammation in renal interstitium, tubules, and glomeruli. Hyaline casts often seen in normal urine. Waxy casts seen in chronic renal failure.	Presence of casts indicates that hematuria/pyuria is of renal origin. Bladder cancer → RBCs. Acute cystitis → WBCs.

Red blood cell casts   White blood cell casts   Hyaline casts   Granular casts

Erythrocyte sedimentation rate	Nonspecific test that measures acute-phase reactants. Dramatically ↑ with infection, malignancy, connective tissue disease. Also ↑ with pregnancy, inflammatory disease, and anemia. ↓ with sickle cell anemia, CHF, and polycythemia.	Simple and cheap but nonspecific. Should not be used for asymptomatic screening; can be used to diagnose and monitor temporal arteritis and polymyalgia rheumatica.
Ghon complex	TB granulomas with lobar or perihilar lymph node involvement (Ghon focus and lymph node involvement). Reflects 1° infection or exposure.	

HIGH-YIELD FACTS

Pathology

HIGH-YIELD FACTS

Pathology

Hyperlipidemia signs

Atheromata	Plaques in blood vessel walls.
Xanthoma	Plaques or nodules composed of lipid-laden histiocytes in the skin, especially the eyelids.
Tendinous xanthoma	Lipid deposit in tendon, especially Achilles.
Corneal arcus	Lipid deposit in cornea, nonspecific (arcus senilis).

Psammoma bodies

Laminated, concentric, calcific spherules seen in:

1. Papillary adenocarcinoma of thyroid
2. Serous papillary cystadenocarcinoma of ovary
3. Meningioma
4. Malignant mesothelioma

PSaMMoma:

Papillary (thyroid)
Serous (ovary)
Meningioma
Mesothelioma

RBC forms

Biconcave	Normal.
Spherocytes	Hereditary spherocytosis, autoimmune hemolysis.
Elliptocyte	Hereditary elliptocytosis.
Macro-ovalocyte	Megaloblastic anemia, marrow failure.
Helmet cell, schistocyte	DIC, traumatic hemolysis.
Sickle cell	Sickle cell anemia.
Teardrop cell	Myeloid metaplasia with myelofibrosis.
Acanthocyte	Spiny appearance in abetalipoproteinemia.
Target cell	Thalassemia, liver disease, HbC.
Poikilocytes	Nonuniform shapes in TTP/HUS, microvascular damage, DIC.
Burr cell	TTP/HUS.

HLA subtypes

B27	**P**soriasis, **A**nkylosing spondylitis, **I**nflammatory bowel disease, **R**eiter's syndrome.	**PAIR.**
13, 17	Psoriasis.	
DR2	Multiple sclerosis, hay fever.	
DR3, DR4	Diabetes mellitus type 1.	
DR4	Rheumatoid arthritis.	
DR5	Pernicious anemia $\rightarrow$ B_{12} deficiency.	
DR7	Steroid-responsive nephrotic syndrome.	

Reed-Sternberg cells

Distinctive tumor giant cell seen in Hodgkin's disease; binucleate or bilobed with the 2 halves as mirror images ("owl's eyes"). Necessary but not sufficient for a diagnosis of Hodgkin's disease. Variants include lacunar cells in nodular sclerosis variant.

There are 4 types of Hodgkin's disease; nodular sclerosis variant is the only one seen in women > men (excellent prognosis).

Virchow's (sentinel) node

A firm supraclavicular lymph node, often on left side, easily palpable (can be detected by medical students), also known as "jugular gland." Presumptive evidence of malignant visceral neoplasm (classically stomach).

Peripheral blood smears

Normal

Microcytic hypochromic anemia

—normally 2° to **iron deficiency**

—low serum ferritin

—elevated serum iron-binding capacity

—lead poisoning

Megaloblastic anemia

—2° to **folate or B$_{12}$ deficiency**

—hypersegmented (5–7 lobes) PMNs

—large red blood cells (MCV > 100)

—**never** give folate to a patient who is deficient in B$_{12}$

—**pernicious anemia**—autoimmune disease that causes B$_{12}$ deficiency by depleting **intrinsic factor,** which is needed to absorb B$_{12}$ in **terminal ileum**

—anisocytosis, poikilocytosis

Target cells

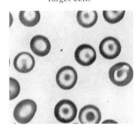

—**HALT:**

—**H**emoglobin **C** disease

—**A**splenia

—**L**iver disease

—**T**halassemia

Hemoglobin SS with sickle cells

—**HbS**—β-globin GLU → VAL at #6; 8% of U.S. blacks are HbS carriers

—cells will sickle 2° to hypoxia, dehydration, and ↑ blood viscosity

—anemia

—vaso-occlusive crises +/– chest pain

—aplastic crises (B19 virus)

—splenic sequestration crises

—CVA

(Adapted, with permission, from Stobo J et al. *The Principles and Practice of Medicine,* 23rd ed. Stamford, CT: Appleton & Lange, 1996:704.)

Enzyme markers

Serum enzyme	Major diagnostic use
Aminotransferases (AST and ALT)	Myocardial infarction (AST only)
	Viral hepatitis (ALT > AST)
	Alcoholic hepatitis (AST > ALT)
Amylase	Acute pancreatitis, mumps
Ceruloplasmin ($\downarrow$)	Wilson's disease
CPK (creatine phosphokinase)	Muscle disorders (e.g., Duchenne's muscular dystrophy) and MI (CPK-MB)
GGT (γ-glutamyl transpeptidase)	Various liver diseases
LDH-1 (lactate dehydrogenase fraction 1)	MI (LDH-1 > LDH-2)
Lipase	Acute pancreatitis
Alkaline phosphatase	Bone disease (Paget's disease of bone), obstructive liver disease (hepatocellular carcinoma)

Immunohistochemical stains

Stain	Cell type
Vimentin	Connective tissue
Desmin	Muscle
Cytokeratin	Epithelial cells
Glial fibrillary acid proteins (GFAP)	Neuroglia
Neurofilaments	Neurons

Pharmacology

"Take me, I am the drug; take me, I am hallucinogenic."
—Salvador Dali

"I was under medication when I made the decision not to burn the tapes."
—Richard Nixon

Preparation for questions on pharmacology is straightforward. Memorizing all the key drugs and their characteristics (e.g., mechanisms, clinical use, and important side effects) is high yield. Focus on understanding the prototype drugs in each class. Avoid memorizing obscure derivatives. Learn the "classic" and distinguishing toxicities of the major drugs. Do not bother with drug dosages or trade names. Reviewing associated biochemistry, physiology, and microbiology can be useful while studying pharmacology. There is a strong emphasis on ANS, CNS, antimicrobial, and cardiovascular agents as well as on NSAIDs. Much of the material is clinically relevant. Newer drugs on the market are also fair game.

High-Yield Clinical Vignettes
Pharmacokinetics
Antimicrobials
CNS/Neurologic Drugs
Psychiatric Drugs
Analgesics/Anesthetics
Cardiovascular Drugs
Respiratory Drugs
Gastrointestinal Drugs
Hematologic Drugs
Endocrine Drugs
Reproductive Drugs
Rheumatologic Drugs
Oncologic Drugs
Immunosuppressant and Cytokine Therapy
Toxicology
Miscellaneous

These abstracted case vignettes are designed to demonstrate the thought processes necessary to answer multistep clinical reasoning questions.

Vignette	Question	Answer
28-year-old chemist presents with MPTP exposure.	What neurotransmitter is depleted?	Dopamine.
Woman taking tetracycline exhibits photosensitivity.	What are the clinical manifestations?	Rash on sun-exposed regions of the body.
Nondiabetic patient presents with hypoglycemia but low levels of C peptide.	What is the diagnosis?	Surreptitious insulin injection.
African-American man who goes to Africa develops a hemolytic anemia after taking malarial prophylaxis.	What is the enzyme deficiency?	Glucose-6-phosphate dehydrogenase.
27-year-old female with a history of psychiatric illness now has urinary retention due to a neuroleptic.	What do you treat it with?	Bethanechol.
Farmer presents with dyspnea, salivation, miosis, diarrhea, cramping, and blurry vision.	What caused this, and what is the mechanism of action?	Insecticide poisoning; inhibition of acetylcholinesterase.
Patient with recent kidney transplant is on cyclosporine for immunosuppression. Requires antifungal agent for candidiasis.	What antifungal drug would result in cyclosporine toxicity?	Ketoconazole.
Man on several medications, including antidepressants and antihypertensives, has mydriasis and becomes constipated.	What is the cause of his symptoms?	TCA.
55-year-old postmenopausal woman is on tamoxifen therapy.	What is she at ↑ risk of acquiring?	Endometrial carcinoma.
Woman on MAO inhibitor has hypertensive crisis after a meal.	What did she ingest?	Tyramine (wine or cheese).
After taking clindamycin, patient develops toxic megacolon and diarrhea.	What is the mechanism of diarrhea?	*Clostridium difficile* overgrowth.

Vignette	Question	Answer
■ Man starts a medication for hyperlipidemia. He then develops a rash, pruritus, and GI upset.	What drug was it?	Niacin.
■ Patient is on carbamazepine.	What routine workup should always be done?	LFTs.
■ 23-year-old female who is on rifampin for TB prophylaxis and on birth control (estrogen) gets pregnant.	Why?	Rifampin augments estrogen metabolism in the liver, rendering it less effective.
■ Patient develops cough and must discontinue captopril.	What is a good replacement drug, and why doesn't it have the same side effects?	Losartan, an angiotensin II receptor antagonist, does not ↑ bradykinin as captopril does.

Pharmacokinetics

Volume of distribution (V_d)	Relates the amount of drug in the body to the plasma concentration. V_d of plasma protein–bound drugs can be altered by liver and kidney disease.

$$V_d = \frac{\text{amount of drug in the body}}{\text{plasma drug concentration}}$$

Clearance (CL)	Relates the rate of elimination to the plasma concentration.

$$CL = \frac{\text{rate of elimination of drug}}{\text{plasma drug concentration}}$$

Half-life ($t_{1/2}$)	The time required to change the amount of drug in the body by ½ during elimination (or during a constant infusion). A drug infused at a constant rate reaches about 94% of steady state after 4 $t_{1/2}$.

$$t_{1/2} = \frac{0.7 \times V_d}{CL}$$

# of half-lives	1	2	3	3.3
Concentration	50%	75%	87.5%	90%

Dosage calculations

Loading dose = $C_p \times V_d/F$.
Maintenance dose = $C_p \times CL/F$
  where C_p = target plasma concentration
  and F = bioavailability.

In patients with impaired renal or hepatic function, the loading dose remains unchanged, although the maintenance dose is ↓.

Elimination of drugs

Zero-order elimination	Rate of elimination is constant regardless of C (i.e., constant **amount** of drug eliminated per unit time). C_p ↓ linearly with time. Examples of drugs—ethanol, phenytoin, and aspirin (at high or toxic concentrations).
First-order elimination	Rate of elimination is proportional to the drug concentration (i.e., constant **fraction** of drug eliminated per unit time). C_p ↓ exponentially with time.

In drugs with first-order kinetics (see left panel above), rate of elimination is proportional to plasma concentration (C_p); in the case of zero-order elimination (right panel), the rate is constant and independent of concentration.

(Adapted, with permission, from Katzung BG, Trevor AJ. *Examination & Board Review: Pharmacology*, 5th ed. Stamford, CT: Appleton & Lange, 1998:5.)

Phase I vs. phase II metabolism	Phase I (reduction, oxidation, hydrolysis) yields slightly polar, water-soluble metabolites (often still active). Phase II (acetylation, glucuronidation, sulfation) yields very polar, inactive metabolites (renally excreted).	Phase I—cytochrome P-450. Phase II—conjugation. Geriatric patients lose phase I first.

Drug development

(Adapted, with permission, from Katzung BG, Trevor AJ. *Examination & Board Review: Pharmacology*, 5th ed. Stamford, CT: Appleton & Lange, 1998:365.)

Pharmacodynamics

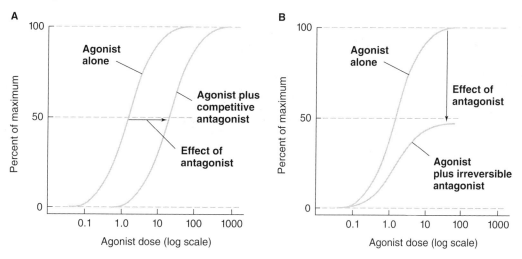

(Adapted, with permission, from Katzung BG, Trevor AJ. *Examination & Board Review: Pharmacology*, 5th ed. Stamford, CT: Appleton & Lange, 1998:13–14.)

Shown above are agonist dose-response curves in the presence of competitive and irreversible antagonists. Note the use of a logarithmic scale for drug concentration. **A.** A competitive antagonist has an effect illustrated by the shift of the agonist curve to the right. **B.** A noncompetitive antagonist shifts the agonist curve downward.

Pharmacodynamics
(*continued*)

(Adapted, with permission, from Katzung BG. *Basic and Clinical Pharmacology*, 7th ed. Stamford, CT: Appleton & Lange, 1997:13.)

C. In a system with spare receptors, the EC_{50} is lower than the K_d, indicating that to achieve 50% of maximum effect, < 50% of the receptors must be activated.

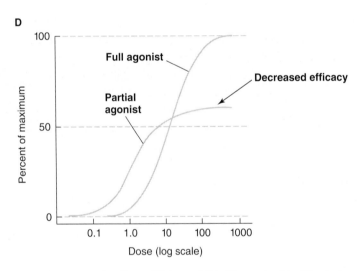

(Adapted, with permission, from Katzung BG. *Basic and Clinical Pharmacology*, 7th ed. Stamford, CT: Appleton & Lange, 1997:13.)

D. Comparison of dose-response curves for a full agonist and a partial agonist. The partial agonist acts on the same receptor system as the full agonist but cannot produce an equivalently large effect (it has lower maximal efficacy) no matter how much the dose is increased. A partial agonist may be more potent (as in the figure), less potent, or equally potent; potency is an independent factor.

Antimicrobial therapy

Mechanism of action	Drugs
Block cell wall synthesis by inhibition of peptidoglycan cross-linking	Penicillin, ampicillin, ticarcillin, piperacillin, imipenem, aztreonam, cephalosporins
Block peptidoglycan synthesis	Bacitracin, vancomycin, cycloserine
Block protein synthesis at 50S ribosomal subunit	Chloramphenicol, erythromycin/macrolides, lincomycin, clindamycin, streptogramins (quinupristin, dalfopristin), linezolid
Block protein synthesis at 30S ribosomal subunit	Aminoglycosides, tetracyclines
Block nucleotide synthesis	Sulfonamides, trimethoprim
Block DNA topoisomerases	Quinolones
Block mRNA synthesis	Rifampin
Bactericidal antibiotics	Penicillin, cephalosporins, vancomycin, aminoglycosides, fluoroquinolones, metronidazole
Disrupt bacterial/fungal cell membranes	Polymyxins
Disrupt fungal cell membranes	Amphotericin B, nystatin, fluconazole/azoles
Unknown	Pentamidine

Penicillin

Penicillin G (IV form), penicillin V (oral).

Mechanism	1. Binds penicillin-binding proteins
	2. Blocks transpeptidase cross-linking of cell wall
	3. Activates autolytic enzymes
Clinical use	Bactericidal for gram-positive cocci, gram-positive rods, gram-negative cocci, and spirochetes. Not penicillinase resistant.
Toxicity	Hypersensitivity reactions, hemolytic anemia.

Methicillin, nafcillin, dicloxacillin

Mechanism	Same as penicillin. Narrow spectrum; penicillinase resistant because of bulkier R group.
Clinical use	*S. aureus.*
Toxicity	Hypersensitivity reactions; methicillin—interstitial nephritis.

Ampicillin, amoxicillin

Mechanism	Same as penicillin. Wider spectrum; penicillinase sensitive. Also combine with clavulanic acid (penicillinase inhibitor) to enhance spectrum. AmOxicillin has greater Oral bioavailability than ampicillin.
Clinical use	Extended-spectrum penicillin—certain gram-positive bacteria and gram-negative rods (*Haemophilus influenzae*, *E. coli*, *Listeria monocytogenes*, *Proteus mirabilis*, *Salmonella*, enterococci).
Toxicity	Hypersensitivity reactions; ampicillin rash; pseudomembranous colitis.

Coverage: ampicillin/amoxicillin **HELPS** kill enterococci.

Carbenicillin, piperacillin, ticarcillin

Mechanism	Same as penicillin. Extended spectrum.
Clinical use	*Pseudomonas* spp. and gram-negative rods; susceptible to penicillinase; use with clavulanic acid.
Toxicity	Hypersensitivity reactions.

Cephalosporins

Mechanism	β-lactam drugs that inhibit cell wall synthesis but are less susceptible to penicillinases. Bactericidal.
Clinical use	1st generation—gram-positive cocci, *Proteus mirabilis*, *E. coli*, *Klebsiella pneumoniae*.

1st generation—**PEcK.**

2nd generation—gram-positive cocci, *Haemophilus influenzae*, *Enterobacter aerogenes*, *Neisseria* spp., *Proteus mirabilis*, *E. coli*, *Klebsiella pneumoniae*, *Serratia marcescens*.

2nd generation—**HEN PEcKS.**

3rd generation—serious gram-negative infections resistant to other β-lactams; meningitis (most penetrate the blood-brain barrier). Examples: ceftazidime for *Pseudomonas*; ceftriaxone for gonorrhea.

4th generation—increased activity against *Pseudomonas* and gram-positive organisms.

Toxicity	Hypersensitivity reactions, ↑ nephrotoxicity of aminoglycosides, disulfiram-like reaction with ethanol (in cephalosporins with a methylthiotetrazole group, e.g., cefamandole).

Aztreonam

Mechanism	A monobactam resistant to β-lactamases. Inhibits cell wall synthesis (binds to PBP3). Synergistic with aminoglycosides. No cross-allergenicity with penicillins.
Clinical use	Gram-negative rods—*Klebsiella* spp., *Pseudomonas* spp., *Serratia* spp. No activity against gram-positives or anaerobes. For penicillin-allergic patients and those with renal insufficiency who cannot tolerate aminoglycosides.
Toxicity	Usually nontoxic; occasional GI upset.

Imipenem/cilastatin

Mechanism	Imipenem is a broad-spectrum, β-lactamase-resistant carbapenem. Always administered with cilastatin (inhibitor of renal dihydropeptidase I) to ↓ inactivation in renal tubules.	With imipenem, "the kill is **LASTIN'** with ci**LASTATIN**."
Clinical use	Gram-positive cocci, gram-negative rods, and anaerobes. Drug of choice for *Enterobacter*.	
Toxicity	GI distress, skin rash, and CNS toxicity (seizures) at high plasma levels.	

Vancomycin

Mechanism	Inhibits cell wall mucopeptide formation by binding D-ala D-ala portion of cell wall precursors. Bactericidal. Resistance occurs with amino acid change of D-ala D-ala to D-ala D-lac.
Clinical use	Used for serious, gram-positive multidrug-resistant organisms, including *S. aureus* and *Clostridium difficile* (pseudomembranous colitis).
Toxicity	**N**ephrotoxicity, **O**totoxicity, **T**hrombophlebitis, diffuse flushing—"red man syndrome" (can largely prevent by pretreatment with antihistamines and slow infusion rate). Well tolerated in general—does **NOT** have many problems.

Protein synthesis inhibitors

30S inhibitors:

A = **A**minoglycosides (streptomycin, gentamicin, tobramycin, amikacin) [bactericidal]

T = **T**etracyclines [bacteriostatic]

50S inhibitors:

C = **C**hloramphenicol [bacteriostatic]

E = **E**rythromycin [bacteriostatic]

L = **L**incomycin [bacteriostatic]

L = c**L**indamycin [bacteriostatic]

"Buy **AT 30, CELL** at 50."

Ribosomal subunits

P = growing peptide chain
A = amino acid

Aminoglycosides

Gentamicin, neomycin, amikacin, tobramycin, streptomycin.

Mechanism	Bactericidal; inhibit formation of initiation complex and cause misreading of mRNA. Require O_2 for uptake; therefore ineffective against anaerobes.	
Clinical use	Severe gram-negative rod infections. Synergistic with β-lactam antibiotics. Neomycin for bowel surgery.	
Toxicity	**N**ephrotoxicity (especially when used with cephalosporins), **O**totoxicity (especially when used with loop diuretics).	Ami**NO**glycosides. Teratogen.

Tetracyclines

Tetracycline, doxycycline, demeclocycline, minocycline.

Mechanism	Bacteriostatic; bind to 30S and prevent attachment of aminoacyl-tRNA; limited CNS penetration. Doxycycline is fecally eliminated and can be used in patients with renal failure. Must NOT take with milk, antacids, or iron-containing preparations because divalent cations inhibit its absorption in the gut.	
Clinical use	*Vibrio cholerae*, **A**cne, *Chlamydia*, *Ureaplasma Urealyticum*, **M**ycoplasma *pneumoniae*, **B**orrelia *burgdorferi* (Lyme disease), **R**ickettsia, tularemia.	**VACUUM** your **B**ed**R**oom.
Toxicity	GI distress, discoloration of teeth and inhibition of bone growth in children, Fanconi's syndrome, photosensitivity.	

Macrolides

Erythromycin, azithromycin, clarithromycin.

Mechanism	Inhibit protein synthesis by blocking translocation; bind to the 23S rRNA of the 50S ribosomal subunit. Bacteriostatic.
Clinical use	URIs, pneumonias, STDs—gram-positive cocci (streptococcal infections in patients allergic to penicillin), *Mycoplasma*, *Legionella*, *Chlamydia*, *Neisseria*.
Toxicity	GI discomfort (most common cause of noncompliance), acute cholestatic hepatitis, eosinophilia, skin rashes.

Chloramphenicol

Mechanism	Inhibits 50S peptidyltransferase. Bacteriostatic.
Clinical use	Meningitis (*Haemophilus influenzae*, *Neisseria meningitidis*, *Streptococcus pneumoniae*). Conservative use owing to toxicities.
Toxicity	Anemia (dose dependent), aplastic anemia (dose independent), gray baby syndrome (in premature infants because they lack liver UDP-glucuronyl transferase).

Clindamycin

Mechanism	Blocks peptide bond formation at 50S ribosomal subunit. Bacteriostatic.	Treats anaerobes above the diaphragm.
Clinical use	Treat anaerobic infections (e.g., *Bacteroides fragilis*, *Clostridium perfringens*).	
Toxicity	Pseudomembranous colitis (*C. difficile* overgrowth), fever, diarrhea.	

Sulfonamides

Sulfamethoxazole (SMX), sulfisoxazole, triple sulfas, sulfadiazine.

Mechanism PABA antimetabolites inhibit dihydropteroate synthase. Bacteriostatic.

Clinical use Gram-positive, gram-negative, *Nocardia*, *Chlamydia*. Triple sulfas or SMX for simple UTI.

Toxicity Hypersensitivity reactions, hemolysis if G6PD deficient, nephrotoxicity (tubulointerstitial nephritis), kernicterus in infants, displace other drugs from albumin (e.g., warfarin).

(Adapted, with permission, from Katzung BG. *Basic and Clinical Pharmacology,* 7th ed. Stamford, CT: Appleton & Lange, 1997:762.)

Trimethoprim

Mechanism Inhibits bacterial dihydrofolate reductase. Bacteriostatic. Trimethoprim = **TMP:**

Clinical use Used in combination with sulfonamides (trimethoprim-sulfamethoxazole [TMP-SMX]), causing sequential block of folate synthesis. Combination used for recurrent UTIs, *Shigella, Salmonella, Pneumocystis carinii* pneumonia. "**T**reats **M**arrow **P**oorly."

Toxicity Megaloblastic anemia, leukopenia, granulocytopenia. (May alleviate with supplemental folinic acid.)

Fluoroquinolones

Ciprofloxacin, norfloxacin, ofloxacin, sparfloxacin, moxifloxacin, gatifloxacin, enoxacin (fluoroquinolones), nalidixic acid (a quinolone).

Mechanism Inhibit DNA gyrase (topoisomerase II). Bactericidal. Fluoroquino**LONES** hurt

Clinical use Gram-negative rods of urinary and GI tracts (including *Pseudomonas*), *Neisseria*, some gram-positive organisms. attachments to your **BONES.**

Toxicity GI upset, superinfections, skin rashes, headache, dizziness. Contraindicated in pregnant women and in children because animal studies show damage to cartilage. Tendonitis and tendon rupture in adults.

HIGH-YIELD FACTS

Pharmacology

Metronidazole

Mechanism	Forms toxic metabolites in the bacterial cell. Bactericidal.	
Clinical use	Antiprotozoal. *Giardia*, *Entamoeba*, *Trichomonas*, *Gardnerella vaginalis*, anaerobes (*Bacteroides*, *Clostridium*). Used with bismuth and amoxicillin (or tetracycline) for "triple therapy" against *H. pylori*.	**GET** on the **Metro!** Anaerobic infection below the diaphragm.
Toxicity	Disulfiram-like reaction with alcohol, headache.	

Polymyxins

Polymyxin B, polymyxin E.

Mechanism	Bind to cell membranes of bacteria and disrupt their osmotic properties. Polymyxins are cationic, basic proteins that act like detergents.
Clinical use	Resistant gram-negative infections.
Toxicity	Neurotoxicity, acute renal tubular necrosis.

Isoniazid (INH)

Mechanism	Decreases synthesis of mycolic acids.	**INH** **I**njures **N**eurons and **H**epatocytes.
Clinical use	*Mycobacterium tuberculosis*. The only agent used as solo prophylaxis against TB.	Different INH half-lives in fast vs. slow acetylators.
Toxicity	Hemolysis if G6PD deficient, neurotoxicity, hepatotoxicity, SLE-like syndrome. Pyridoxine (vitamin B_6) can prevent neurotoxicity.	

Rifampin

Mechanism	Inhibits DNA-dependent RNA polymerase.	**R**ifampin's **4 R's:**
Clinical use	*Mycobacterium tuberculosis*; delays resistance to dapsone when used for leprosy. Used for meningococcal prophylaxis and chemoprophylaxis in contacts of children with *Haemophilus influenzae* type B.	**R**NA polymerase inhibitor **R**evs up microsomal P-450 **R**ed/orange body fluids **R**apid resistance if used alone
Toxicity	Minor hepatotoxicity and drug interactions (increased P-450).	

Anti-TB drugs

Rifampin, **E**thambutol, **S**treptomycin, **P**yrazinamide, **I**soniazid (INH). Cycloserine (2nd-line therapy)	**RESPI**re. INH is used alone for TB prophylaxis. All are hepatotoxic.

Resistance mechanisms for various antibiotics

Drug	Most common mechanism
Penicillins/ cephalosporins	β-lactamase cleavage of β-lactam ring
Aminoglycosides	Modification via acetylation, adenylation, or phosphorylation
Vancomycin	Terminal D-ala of cell wall component replaced with D-lac; ↓ affinity.
Chloramphenicol	Modification via acetylation
Macrolides	Methylation of rRNA near erythromycin's ribosome-binding site
Tetracycline	↓ uptake or ↑ transport out of cell
Sulfonamides	Altered enzyme (bacterial dihydropteroate synthetase), ↓ uptake, or ↑ PABA synthesis

Nonsurgical antimicrobial prophylaxis

Meningococcal infection	Rifampin (drug of choice), minocycline.
Gonorrhea	Ceftriaxone.
Syphilis	Benzathine penicillin G.
History of recurrent UTIs	TMP-SMX.
Pneumocystis carinii pneumonia	TMP-SMX (drug of choice), aerosolized pentamidine.

Antifungal therapy

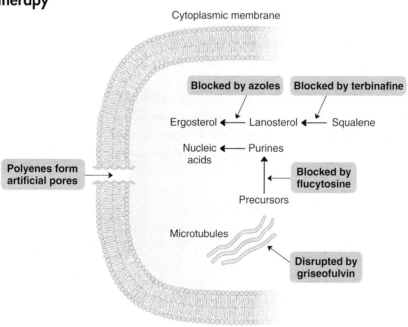

(Adapted, with permission, from Katzung BG, Trevor AJ. *USMLE Road Map: Pharmacology*, 1st ed. New York: McGraw-Hill, 2003:120.)

Amphotericin B

Mechanism	Binds ergosterol (unique to fungi); forms membrane pores that allow leakage of electrolytes and disrupt homeostasis.
Clinical use	Used for wide spectrum of systemic mycoses. *Cryptococcus, Blastomyces, Coccidioides, Aspergillus, Histoplasma, Candida, Mucor* (systemic mycoses). Intrathecally for fungal meningitis; does not cross blood-brain barrier.
Toxicity	Fever/chills ("shake and bake"), hypotension, nephrotoxicity, arrhythmias ("amphoterrible").

Amphotericin "tears" holes in the fungal membrane by forming pores.

Nystatin

Mechanism	Binds to ergosterol, disrupting fungal membranes.
Clinical use	"Swish and swallow" for oral candidiasis (thrush).

Fluconazole, ketoconazole, clotrimazole, miconazole, itraconazole, voriconazole

Mechanism	Inhibit fungal steroid (ergosterol) synthesis.
Clinical use	Systemic mycoses. Fluconazole for cryptococcal meningitis in AIDS patients and candidal infections of all types (i.e., yeast infections). Ketoconazole for *Blastomyces, Coccidioides, Histoplasma, Candida albicans*; hypercortisolism.
Toxicity	Hormone synthesis inhibition (gynecomastia), liver dysfunction (inhibits cytochrome P-450), fever, chills.

Flucytosine

Mechanism	Inhibits DNA synthesis by conversion to fluorouracil, which competes with uracil.
Clinical use	Used in systemic fungal infections (e.g., *Candida, Cryptococcus*).
Toxicity	Nausea, vomiting, diarrhea, bone marrow suppression.

Caspofungin

Mechanism	Inhibits cell wall synthesis.
Clinical use	Invasive aspergillosis.
Toxicity	GI upset, flushing.

Terbinafine

Mechanism	Inhibits the fungal enzyme squalene epoxidase.
Clinical use	Used to treat dermatophytoses (especially onychomycosis).

Griseofulvin

Mechanism	Interferes with microtubule function; disrupts mitosis. Deposits in keratin-containing tissues (e.g., nails).
Clinical use	Oral treatment of superficial infections; inhibits growth of dermatophytes (tinea, ringworm).
Toxicity	Teratogenic, carcinogenic, confusion, headaches, ↑ warfarin metabolism.

HIGH-YIELD FACTS

Pharmacology

Antiviral chemotherapy

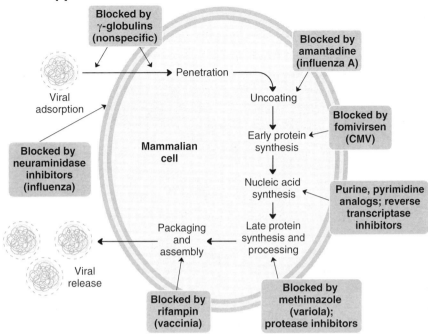

(Adapted, with permission, from Katzung BG, Trevor AJ. *USMLE Road Map: Pharmacology*, 1st ed. New York: McGraw-Hill, 2003:120.)

Amantadine

Mechanism	Blocks viral penetration/uncoating; may buffer pH of endosome. Also causes the release of dopamine from intact nerve terminals.
Clinical use	Prophylaxis for influenza A; Parkinson's disease.
Toxicity	Ataxia, dizziness, slurred speech.

Amantadine blocks influenza **A** and rubell**A** and causes problems with the cerebell**A**.

Rimantidine is a derivative with fewer CNS side effects.

Zanamivir

Mechanism	Inhibits influenza neuraminidase.
Clinical use	Both influenza A and B.

Ribavirin

Mechanism	Inhibits synthesis of guanine nucleotides by competitively inhibiting IMP dehydrogenase.
Clinical use	RSV.
Toxicity	Hemolytic anemia. Severe teratogen.

Acyclovir

Mechanism	Preferentially inhibits viral DNA polymerase when phosphorylated by viral thymidine kinase.
Clinical use	HSV, VZV, EBV. Mucocutaneous and genital herpes lesions. Prophylaxis in immunocompromised patients.
Toxicity	Delirium, tremor, nephrotoxicity.

Ganciclovir   DHPG (dihydroxy-2-propoxymethyl guanine)

    Mechanism   Phosphorylation by viral kinase; preferentially inhibits CMV DNA polymerase.

    Clinical use   CMV, especially in immunocompromised patients.

    Toxicity   Leukopenia, neutropenia, thrombocytopenia, renal toxicity. More toxic to host enzymes than acyclovir.

Foscarnet

    Mechanism   Viral DNA polymerase inhibitor that binds to the pyrophosphate binding site of the enzyme. Does not require activation by viral kinase.   **FOS**carnet = pyro**FOS**phate analog.

    Clinical use   CMV retinitis in immunocompromised patients when ganciclovir fails.

    Toxicity   Nephrotoxicity.

HIV therapy

    Protease inhibitors   Saquinavir, ritonavir, indinavir, nelfinavir, amprenavir.

        Mechanism   Inhibit assembly of new virus by blocking protease enzyme.

        Toxicity   GI intolerance (nausea, diarrhea), hyperglycemia, lipid abnormalities, thrombocytopenia (indinavir).

    Reverse transcriptase inhibitors

        Nucleosides   Zidovudine (AZT), didanosine (ddI), zalcitabine (ddC), stavudine (d4T), lamivudine (3TC), abacavir.

        Non-nucleosides   Nevirapine, delavirdine, efavirenz.

        Mechanism   Preferentially inhibit reverse transcriptase of HIV; prevent incorporation of viral genome into host DNA.

        Toxicity   Bone marrow suppression (neutropenia, anemia), peripheral neuropathy, lactic acidosis (nucleosides), rash (non-nucleosides), megaloblastic anemia (AZT).

    Clinical use   Highly active antiretroviral therapy (HAART) generally entails combination therapy with protease inhibitors and reverse transcriptase inhibitors. Initiated when patients have low CD4 counts (< 500 cells/mm^3) or high viral load. AZT is used during pregnancy to reduce risk of fetal transmission.

Interferons

    Mechanism   Glycoproteins from human leukocytes that block various stages of viral RNA and DNA synthesis.

    Clinical use   Chronic hepatitis B and C, Kaposi's sarcoma.

    Toxicity   Neutropenia.

Antiparasitic drugs

Ivermectin	Onchocerciasis (r**IVER** blindness treated with **IVER**mectin).
Mebendazole/ thiabendazole	Nematode/roundworm (e.g., pinworm, whipworm) infections.
Pyrantel pamoate	Giant roundworm (*Ascaris*), hookworm (*Necator/Ancylostoma*), pinworm (*Enterobius*).
Praziquantel	Trematode/fluke (e.g., schistosomes, *Paragonimus*, *Clonorchis*) and cysticercosis.
Niclosamide	Cestode/tapeworm (e.g., *Diphyllobothrium latum*, *Taenia* species) infections except cysticercosis.
Pentavalent antimony	Leishmaniasis.
Chloroquine, quinine, mefloquine, atovaquone, proguanil	Malaria.
Primaquine	Latent hypnozoite (liver) forms of malaria (*Plasmodium vivax*, *P. ovale*).
Metronidazole	Giardiasis, amebic dysentery (*Entamoeba histolytica*), bacterial vaginitis (*Gardnerella vaginalis*), *Trichomonas*.
Pentamidine	*Pneumocystis carinii* pneumonia prophylaxis.
Nifurtimox	Chagas' disease, American trypanosomiasis (*Trypanosoma cruzi*).
Suramin	African trypanosomiasis (sleeping sickness).

PHARMACOLOGY—CNS/NEUROLOGIC DRUGS

Central and peripheral nervous system

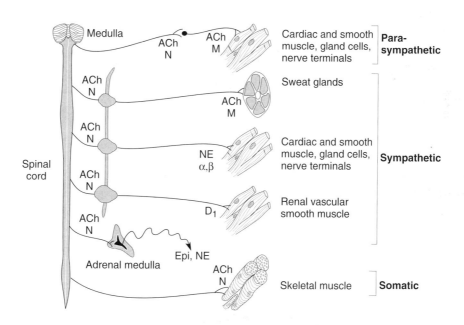

(Adapted, with permission, from Katzung BG. *Basic and Clinical Pharmacology*, 7th ed. Stamford, CT: Appleton & Lange, 1997:74.)

Autonomic drugs

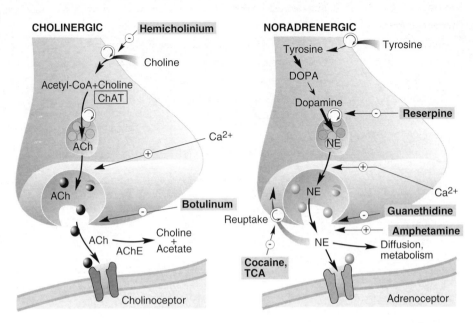

(Adapted, with permission, from Katzung BG, Trevor AJ. *Examination & Board Review: Pharmacology*, 5th ed. Stamford, CT: Appleton & Lange, 1998:42.)

Circles with rotating arrows represent transporters; ChAT, choline acetyltransferase; ACh, acetylcholine; AChE, acetylcholinesterase; NE, norepinephrine.

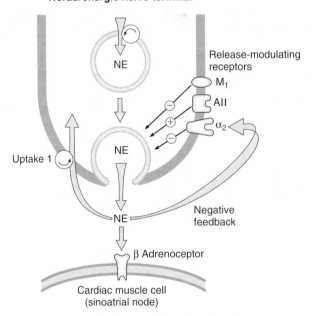

(Adapted, with permission, from Katzung BG, Trevor AJ. *Examination & Board Review: Pharmacology*, 5th ed. Stamford, CT: Appleton & Lange, 1998:42.)

Release of NE from a sympathetic nerve ending is modulated by NE itself, acting on presynaptic α_2 autoreceptors, and by ACh, angiotensin II, and other substances.

Cholinomimetics

Drug	Clinical applications	Action
Direct agonists		
Bethanechol	Postoperative and neurogenic ileus and urinary retention	Activates bowel and bladder smooth muscle
Carbachol, pilocarpine	Glaucoma	Activates ciliary muscle of eye (open angle), pupillary sphincter (narrow angle)
Indirect agonists (anticholinesterases)		
Neostigmine	Postoperative and neurogenic ileus and urinary retention, myasthenia gravis, reversal of neuromuscular junction blockade (postoperative)	$\uparrow$ endogenous ACh
Pyridostigmine	Myasthenia gravis	$\uparrow$ endogenous ACh; $\uparrow$ strength
Edrophonium	Diagnosis of myasthenia gravis (extremely short acting)	$\uparrow$ endogenous ACh
Physostigmine	Glaucoma (crosses blood-brain barrier $\rightarrow$ CNS) and atropine overdose	$\uparrow$ endogenous ACh
Echothiophate	Glaucoma	$\uparrow$ endogenous ACh

Cholinesterase inhibitor poisoning

Symptoms include **D**iarrhea, **U**rination, **M**iosis, **B**ronchospasm, **B**radycardia, **E**xcitation of skeletal muscle and CNS, **L**acrimation, **S**weating, **S**alivation (also abdominal cramping).

Cholinesterase regenerator (antidote)—pralidoxime regenerates active cholinesterase, chemical antagonist, used to treat organophosphate exposure.

DUMBBELSS.

Parathion and other organophosphates.

Cholinoreceptor blockers

Muscarinic antagonists	Atropine is used to dilate pupil, $\downarrow$ acid secretion in acid-peptic disease, $\downarrow$ urgency in mild cystitis, $\downarrow$ GI motility, reduce airway secretions, and treat organophosphate poisoning. Causes $\uparrow$ body temperature, rapid pulse, dry mouth, dry/flushed skin, disorientation, mydriasis with cycloplegia, and constipation.	Blocks **SLUD**: Salivation Lacrimation Urination Defecation Atropine parasympathetic block side effects: Blind as a bat Red as a beet Mad as a hatter Hot as a hare Dry as a bone
Nicotinic antagonists	Hexamethonium—ganglionic blocker.	

Antimuscarinic drugs

Organ system	Drugs	Application
CNS	Benztropine	Parkinson's disease
	Scopolamine	Motion sickness
Eye	Atropine, homatropine, tropicamide	Produce mydriasis and cycloplegia
Respiratory	Ipratropium	Asthma, COPD

Neuromuscular blocking drugs

Used for muscle paralysis in surgery or mechanical ventilation.

Depolarizing — Succinylcholine.

Reversal of blockade:

Phase I (prolonged depolarization)—no antidote. Block potentiated by cholinesterase inhibitors.

Phase II (repolarized but blocked)—antidote consists of cholinesterase inhibitors (e.g., neostigmine).

Nondepolarizing — Tubocurarine, atracurium, mivacurium, pancuronium, vecuronium, rapacuronium.

Reversal of blockade—neostigmine, edrophonium, and other cholinesterase inhibitors.

Dantrolene

Used in the treatment of malignant hyperthermia, which is caused by the concomitant use of inhation anesthetics (except N_2O) and succinylcholine. Also used to treat neuroleptic malignant syndrome (a toxicity of antipsychotic drugs).

Mechanism: prevents the release of Ca^{2+} from the sarcoplasmic reticulum of skeletal muscle.

Sympathomimetics

Drug	Mechanism/selectivity	Applications
Catecholamines		
Epinephrine	Direct general agonist (α_1, α_2, β_1, β_2)	Anaphylaxis, glaucoma (open angle), asthma, hypotension
NE	α_1, α_2, β_1	Hypotension (but $\downarrow$ renal perfusion)
Isoproterenol	$\beta_1 = \beta_2$	AV block (rare)
Dopamine	$D_1 = D_2 > \beta > \alpha$	Shock ($\uparrow$ renal perfusion), heart failure
Dobutamine	$\beta_1 > \beta_2$	Shock, heart failure
Other		
Amphetamine	Indirect general agonist, releases stored catecholamines	Narcolepsy, obesity, attention deficit disorder
Ephedrine	Indirect general agonist, releases stored catecholamines	Nasal decongestion, urinary incontinence, hypotension
Phenylephrine	$\alpha_1 > \alpha_2$	Pupil dilator, vasoconstriction, nasal decongestion
Albuterol, terbutaline	$\beta_2 > \beta_1$	Asthma
Cocaine	Indirect general agonist, uptake inhibitor	Causes vasoconstriction and local anesthesia
Clonidine, α-methyldopa	Centrally acting α-agonist, $\downarrow$ central adrenergic outflow	Hypertension, especially with renal disease (no $\downarrow$ in blood flow to kidney)

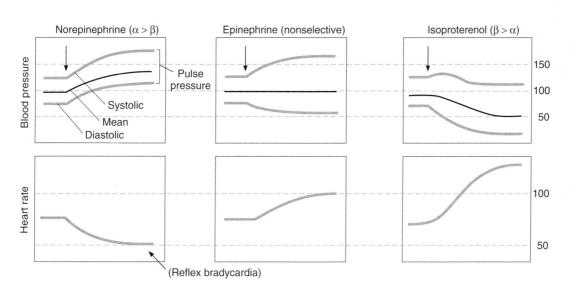

(Adapted, with permission, from Katzung BG, Trevor AJ. *Examination & Board Review: Pharmacology*, 5th ed. Stamford, CT: Appleton & Lange, 1998:72.)

α-blockers

Drugs	Application	Toxicity
Nonselective		
Phenoxybenzamine (irreversible) and phentolamine (reversible)	Pheochromocytoma	Orthostatic hypotension, reflex tachycardia
α_1 selective		
Prazosin, terazosin, doxazosin	Hypertension, urinary retention in BPH	1st-dose orthostatic hypotension, dizziness, headache
α_2 selective		
Yohimbine	Impotence (effectiveness is controversial)	

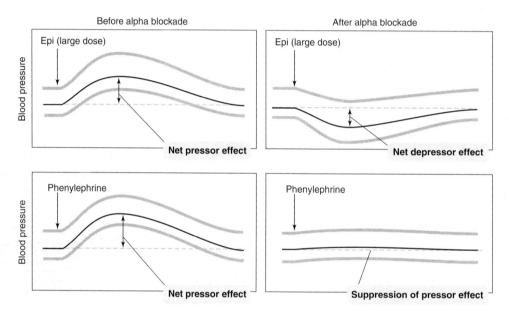

(Adapted, with permission, from Katzung BG, Trevor AJ. *Examination & Board Review: Pharmacology*, 5th ed. Stamford, CT: Appleton & Lange, 1998:80.)

Shown above are the effects of an α-blocker (e.g., phentolamine) on blood pressure responses to epinephrine and phenylephrine. The epinephrine response exhibits reversal of the mean blood pressure change, from a net increase (the α response) to a net decrease (the β_2 response). The response to phenylephrine is suppressed but not reversed because phenylephrine is a "pure" α-agonist without β action.

β-blockers

Propranolol, metoprolol, atenolol, nadolol, timolol, pindolol, esmolol, labetalol.

Application	Effect	
Hypertension	↓ cardiac output, ↓ renin secretion	
Angina pectoris	↓ heart rate and contractility, resulting in ↓ O_2 consumption	
MI	β-blockers ↓ mortality	
SVT (propranolol, esmolol)	↓ AV conduction velocity	
CHF	Slows progression of chronic failure	
Glaucoma (timolol)	↓ secretion of aqueous humor	

Toxicity — Impotence, exacerbation of asthma, cardiovascular adverse effects (bradycardia, AV block, CHF), CNS adverse effects (sedation, sleep alterations); use with caution in diabetics

Selectivity — Nonselective ($β_1 = β_2$)—propranolol, timolol, pindolol, nadolol, and labetalol (also blocks $α_1$ receptors)

$β_1$ selective ($β_1 > β_2$)—**A**cebutolol, **B**etaxolol, **E**smolol (short acting), **A**tenolol, **M**etoprolol — **A BEAM** of $β_1$ blockers.

Glaucoma drugs

Drug	Mechanism	Side effects
α-agonists		
Epinephrine	↑ outflow of aqueous humor	Mydriasis, stinging; do not use in closed-angle glaucoma
Brimonidine	↓ aqueous humor synthesis	No pupillary or vision changes
β-blockers		
Timolol, betaxolol, carteolol	↓ aqueous humor secretion	No pupillary or vision changes
Cholinomimetics		
Pilocarpine, carbachol, physostigmine, echothiophate	Ciliary muscle contraction, opening of trabecular meshwork; ↑ outflow of aqueous humor	Miosis, cyclospasm
Diuretics		
Acetazolamide, dorzolamide, brinzolamide	↓ aqueous humor secretion due to decreased HCO_3^- (via inhibition of carbonic anhydrase)	No pupillary or vision changes
Prostaglandin		
Latanoprost	↑ outflow of aqueous humor	Darkens color of iris (browning)

L-dopa (levodopa)/carbidopa

Mechanism	↑ level of dopamine in brain. Parkinsonism thought to be due to loss of dopaminergic neurons and excess cholinergic function. Unlike dopamine, L-dopa can cross blood-brain barrier and is converted by dopa decarboxylase in the CNS to dopamine.
Clinical use	Parkinsonism.
Toxicity	Arrhythmias from peripheral conversion to dopamine. Carbidopa, a peripheral decarboxylase inhibitor, is given with L-dopa in order to ↑ the bioavailability of L-dopa in the brain and to limit peripheral side effects. Dyskinesias also occur.

Parkinson's disease drugs

Dopamine agonists	L-dopa/carbidopa, bromocriptine (an ergot alkaloid and partial dopamine agonist), pramipexole, ropinirole, amantadine (enhances dopamine release).	**BALSA:** **B**romocriptine **A**mantadine
MAO inhibitors	Selegiline (selective MAO type B inhibitor).	**L**evodopa
Antimuscarinics	Benztropine (improves tremor and rigidity but has little effect on bradykinesia).	**S**elegiline **A**ntimuscarinics

Sumatriptan

Mechanism	5-HT$_{1D}$ agonist. Half-life < 2 hours.
Clinical use	Acute migraine, cluster headache attacks.
Toxicity	Chest discomfort, mild tingling (contraindicated in patients with CAD or Prinzmetal's angina).

Epilepsy drugs

	PARTIAL		GENERALIZED			
	Simple	Complex	Tonic-Clonic	Absence	Status	Notes
Phenytoin	✓	✓	✓		✓	Also a class IB antiarrhythmic
Carbamazepine	✓	✓	✓			Monitor LFTs weekly
Lamotrigine	✓	✓	✓			
Gabapentin	✓	✓	✓			Adjunct in refractory seizures, renal excretion
Topiramate	✓	✓				Adjunct use
Phenobarbital	✓	✓	✓			Safer in pregnant women Crigler-Najjar II
Valproate			✓	✓		
Ethosuximide				✓		
Benzodiazepines (diazepam or lorazepam)					✓	

Epilepsy drug toxicities

Benzodiazepines	Sedation, tolerance, dependence.
Carbamazepine	Diplopia, ataxia, induction of cytochrome P-450, blood dyscrasias (agranulocytosis, aplastic anemia), liver toxicity (always check LFTs).
Ethosuximide	GI distress, lethargy, headache, urticaria, Stevens-Johnson syndrome.
Phenobarbital	Sedation, induction of cytochrome P-450, tolerance, dependence.
Phenytoin	Nystagmus, diplopia, ataxia, sedation, gingival hyperplasia, hirsutism, anemias, birth defects (teratogenic).
Valproic acid	GI distress, rare but fatal hepatotoxicity (measure LFTs), neural tube defects in fetus (spina bifida).
Lamotrigine	Life-threatening rash, Stevens-Johnson syndrome.
Gabapentin	Sedation, movement disorders.
Topiramate	Sedation, mental dulling, kidney stones, weight loss.

Phenytoin

Mechanism	Use-dependent blockade of Na^+ channels.
Clinical use	Grand mal seizures.
Toxicity	Nystagmus, ataxia, diplopia, lethargy. Chronic use produces gingival hyperplasia in children, peripheral neuropathy, hirsutism, megaloblastic anemia ($\downarrow$ vitamin B_{12}), and malignant hyperthermia (rare); teratogenic (fetal hydantoin syndrome).

PHARMACOLOGY—PSYCHIATRIC DRUGS

Barbiturates
Phenobarbital, pentobarbital, thiopental, secobarbital.

Mechanism	Facilitate $GABA_A$ action by $\uparrow$ **duration** of Cl⁻ channel opening, thus $\downarrow$ neuron firing.	Barbi**DURAT**e (increased **DURAT**ion).
Clinical use	Sedative for anxiety, seizures, insomnia, induction of anesthesia (thiopental).	Contraindicated in porphyria.
Toxicity	Dependence, additive CNS depression effects with alcohol, respiratory or cardiovascular depression (can lead to death), drug interactions owing to induction of liver microsomal enzymes (cytochrome P-450).	

Benzodiazepines
Diazepam, lorazepam, triazolam, temazepam, oxazepam, midazolam, chlordiazepoxide.

Mechanism	Facilitate $GABA_A$ action by $\uparrow$ **frequency** of Cl⁻ channel opening. Most have long half-lives and active metabolites.	**FRE**nzodiazepines (increased **FRE**quency).
Clinical use	Anxiety, spasticity, status epilepticus (diazepam), detoxification (especially alcohol withdrawal–DTs).	Short acting = **TOM** Thumb = **T**riazolam, **O**xazepam, **M**idazolam.
Toxicity	Dependence, additive CNS depression effects with alcohol. Less risk of respiratory depression and coma than with barbiturates.	
	Treat overdose with flumazenil (competitive antagonist at GABA receptor).	

Antipsychotics (neuroleptics)

Thioridazine, haloperidol, fluphenazine, chlorpromazine.

Mechanism	Most antipsychotics block dopamine D_2 receptors (excess dopamine effects connected with schizophrenia).	Evolution of EPS side effects:
		4 h acute dystonia
		4 d akinesia
Clinical use	Schizophrenia, psychosis.	4 wk akathisia
Toxicity	Extrapyramidal system (EPS) side effects, sedation, endocrine side effects, and side effects arising from blocking muscarinic, α, and histamine receptors.	4 mo tardive dyskinesia (often irreversible)

Neuroleptic malignant syndrome—rigidity, autonomic instability, hyperpyrexia (treat with dantrolene and dopamine agonists).

Tardive dyskinesia—stereotypic oral-facial movements probably due to dopamine receptor sensitization; results of long-term antipsychotic use.

Atypical antipsychotics

Clozapine, olanzapine, risperidone.

Mechanism	Block 5-HT_2 and dopamine receptors.
Clinical use	Treatment of schizophrenia; useful for positive and negative symptoms. **Olanzapine** is also used for OCD, anxiety disorder, and depression.
Toxicity	Fewer extrapyramidal and anticholinergic side effects than other antipsychotics. **Clozapine** may cause agranulocytosis (requires weekly WBC monitoring).

Lithium

Mechanism	Not established; possibly related to inhibition of phosphoinositol cascade.
Clinical use	Mood stabilizer for bipolar affective disorder; blocks relapse and acute manic events.
Toxicity	Tremor, hypothyroidism, polyuria (ADH antagonist causing nephrogenic diabetes insipidus), teratogenesis. Narrow therapeutic window requiring close monitoring of serum levels.

Antidepressants

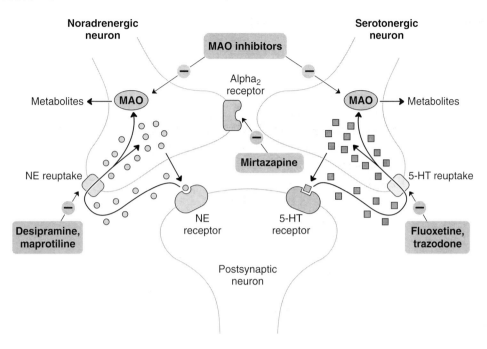

(Adapted, with permission, from Katzung BG, Trevor AJ. *USMLE Road Map: Pharmacology*, 1st ed. New York: McGraw-Hill, 2003:80.)

Tricyclic antidepressants	Imipramine, amitriptyline, desipramine, nortriptyline, clomipramine, doxepin.	
Mechanism	Block reuptake of NE and serotonin.	
Clinical use	Endogenous depression, bedwetting (imipramine), OCD (clomipramine).	
Side effects	Sedation, α-blocking effects, atropine-like (anticholinergic) side effects (tachycardia, urinary retention). 3° TCAs (amitriptyline) have more anticholinergic effects than do 2° TCAs (nortriptyline). Desipramine is the least sedating.	
Toxicity	**Tri-C**s: **C**onvulsions, **C**oma, **C**ardiotoxicity (arrhythmias); also respiratory depression, hyperpyrexia. Confusion and hallucinations in elderly due to anticholinergic side effects.	
SSRIs	Fluoxetine, sertraline, paroxetine, citalopram.	
Mechanism	Serotonin-specific reuptake inhibitors.	It normally takes 2–3 weeks
Clinical use	Endogenous depression.	for antidepressants to have
Toxicity	Fewer than TCAs. CNS stimulation—anxiety, insomnia, tremor, anorexia, nausea, and vomiting. "Serotonin syndrome" with MAO inhibitors—hyperthermia, muscle rigidity, cardiovascular collapse.	an effect.

Heterocyclics

2nd- and 3rd-generation antidepressants with varied and mixed mechanisms of action. Used in major depressive disorders.

Trazodone	Primarily inhibit serotonin reuptake. Toxicity: sedation, nausea, priapism, postural hypotension.
Buproprion	Also used for smoking cessation. Mechanism not well known. Toxicity: stimulant effects (tachycardia, agitation), dry mouth, aggravation of psychosis.
Venlafaxine	Also used in generalized anxiety disorder. Inhibits serotonin and dopamine reuptake. Toxicity: stimulant effects (anxiety, agitation, headache, insomnia).
Mirtazapine	α_2 antagonist ($\uparrow$ release of NE and serotonin) and potent 5-HT$_2$ receptor antagonist. Toxicity: sedation, $\uparrow$ serum cholesterol, $\uparrow$ appetite.
Maprotiline	Blocks NE reuptake.

Monoamine oxidase (MAO) inhibitors

Phenelzine, tranylcypromine.

Mechanism	Nonselective MAO inhibition.
Clinical use	Atypical depressions (i.e., with psychotic or phobic features), anxiety, hypochondriasis.
Toxicity	Hypertensive crisis with tyramine ingestion (in many foods) and meperidine; CNS stimulation. Contraindication with SSRIs or β-agonists.

Selegiline (deprenyl)

Mechanism	Selectively inhibits MAO-B, thereby increasing the availability of dopamine.
Clinical use	Adjunctive agent to L-dopa in treatment of Parkinson's disease.
Toxicity	May enhance adverse effects of L-dopa.

Anesthetics— general principles

Drugs with $\downarrow$ solubility in blood = rapid induction and recovery times.

Drugs with $\uparrow$ solubility in lipids = $\uparrow$ potency = $\dfrac{1}{MAC}$.

Examples: N$_2$O has low blood and lipid solubility, and thus fast induction and low potency. Halothane, in contrast, has $\uparrow$ lipid and blood solubility, and thus high potency and slow induction.

Inhaled anesthetics

Halothane, enflurane, isoflurane, sevoflurane, methoxyflurane, nitrous oxide.

Mechanism	The lower the solubility in blood, the quicker the anesthetic induction and the quicker the recovery.
Effects	Myocardial depression, respiratory depression, nausea/emesis, $\uparrow$ cerebral blood flow.
Toxicity	Hepatotoxicity (halothane), nephrotoxicity (methoxyflurane), proconvulsant (enflurane), malignant hyperthermia (rare).

Intravenous anesthetics

Barbiturates	Thiopental—high lipid solubility, rapid entry into brain. Used for induction of anesthesia and short surgical procedures. Effect terminated by redistribution from brain. ↓ cerebral blood flow.
Benzodiazepines	Midazolam most common drug used for endoscopy; used adjunctively with gaseous anesthetics and narcotics. May cause severe postoperative respiratory depression and amnesia.
Arylcyclohexylamines	Ketamine (PCP analog) acts as dissociative anesthetic. Cardiovascular stimulant. Causes disorientation, hallucination, and bad dreams. Increases cerebral blood flow.
Narcotic analgesics	Morphine, fentanyl used with other CNS depressants during general anesthesia.
Other	Propofol used for rapid anesthesia induction and short procedures. Less postoperative nausea than thiopental.

Local anesthetics

	Esters—procaine, cocaine, tetracaine; amides—lIdocaine, bupIvacaine (amIdes have 2 **I**'s in name).
Mechanism	Block Na$^+$ channels by binding to specific receptors on inner portion of channel. 3° amine local anesthetics penetrate membrane in uncharged form, then bind in charged form.
Principle	1. In infected (acidic) tissue, anesthetics are charged and cannot penetrate membrane effectively. Therefore, more anesthetic is needed in these cases.
	2. Order of nerve blockade—small-diameter fibers > large diameter. Myelinated fibers > unmyelinated fibers. Overall, size factor predominates over myelination such that small unmyelinated pain fibers > small myelinated autonomic fibers > large myelinated autonomic fibers. Order of loss—pain (lose first) > temperature > touch > pressure (lose last).
	3. Given with vasoconstrictors (usually epinephrine) to enhance local action.
Clinical use	Minor surgical procedures, spinal anesthesia. If allergic to esters, give amides.
Toxicity	CNS excitation, severe cardiovascular toxicity (bupivacaine), hypertension, and arrhythmias (cocaine).

Opioid analgesics

	Morphine, fentanyl, codeine, heroin, methadone, meperidine, dextromethorphan.
Mechanism	Act as agonists at opioid receptors (mu = morphine, delta = enkephalin, kappa = dynorphin) to modulate synaptic transmission.
Clinical use	Pain, cough suppression (dextromethorphan), diarrhea (loperamide and diphenoxylate), acute pulmonary edema, maintenance programs for addicts (methadone).
Toxicity	Addiction, **respiratory depression,** constipation, miosis (**pinpoint pupils**), additive **CNS depression** with other drugs. Tolerance does not develop to miosis and constipation. Toxicity treated with naloxone or naltrexone (opioid receptor antagonist).

Other NSAIDs

	Ibuprofen, naproxen, indomethacin.
Mechanism	Reversibly inhibit cyclooxygenase (both COX-1 and COX-2). Block prostaglandin synthesis.
Clinical use	Antipyretic, analgesic, anti-inflammatory. Indomethacin is used to close a PDA.
Toxicity	Renal damage, aplastic anemia, GI distress, ulcers.

COX-2 inhibitors (celecoxib, rofecoxib)

Mechanism	Selectively inhibit cyclooxygenase (COX) isoform 2, which is found in inflammatory cells and mediates inflammation and pain; spares COX-1, which helps maintain the gastric mucosa. Thus, should not have the corrosive effects of other NSAIDs on the GI lining.
Clinical use	Rheumatoid and osteoarthritis.
Toxicity	Similar to other NSAIDs; may have less toxicity to GI mucosa (i.e., lower incidence of ulcers, bleeding).

Acetaminophen

Mechanism	Reversibly inhibits cyclooxygenase, mostly in CNS. Inactivated peripherally.
Clinical use	Antipyretic, analgesic, but lacking anti-inflammatory properties.
Toxicity	Overdose produces hepatic necrosis; acetaminophen metabolite depletes glutathione and forms toxic tissue adducts in liver.

Cardiovascular therapy

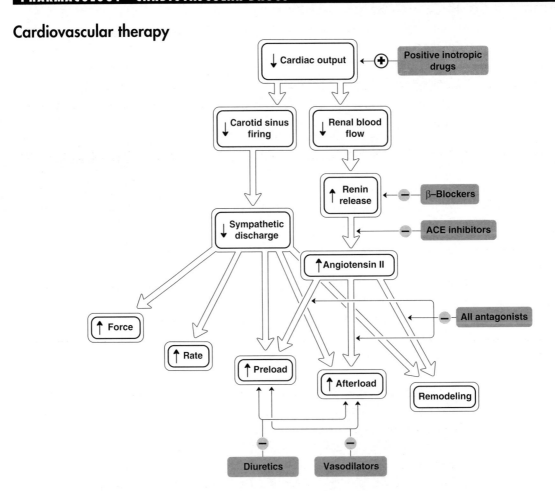

(Adapted, with permission, from Katzung BG, Trevor AJ. *USMLE Road Map: Pharmacology*, 1st ed. New York: McGraw-Hill, 2003:39.)

Antihypertensive drugs

Drug	Adverse effects
Diuretics	
Hydrochlorothiazide	Hypokalemia, slight hyperlipidemia, hyperuricemia, lassitude, hypercalcemia, hyperglycemia
Loop diuretics	Potassium wasting, metabolic alkalosis, hypotension, ototoxicity
Sympathoplegics	
Clonidine	Dry mouth, sedation, severe rebound hypertension
Methyldopa	Sedation, positive Coombs' test
Ganglionic blockers	Severe orthostatic hypotension, blurred vision, constipation, sexual dysfunction
Reserpine	Sedation, depression, nasal stuffiness, diarrhea
Guanethidine	Orthostatic and exercise hypotension, sexual dysfunction, diarrhea
Prazosin	1st-dose orthostatic hypotension, dizziness, headache
β-blockers	Impotence, asthma, cardiovascular effects (bradycardia, CHF, AV block), CNS effects (sedation, sleep alterations)
Vasodilators	
Hydralazine[a]	Nausea, headache, lupus-like syndrome, reflex tachycardia, angina, salt retention
Minoxidil[a]	Hypertrichosis, pericardial effusion, reflex tachycardia, angina, salt retention
Nifedipine, verapamil	Dizziness, flushing, constipation (verapamil), nausea
Nitroprusside	Cyanide toxicity (releases CN)
ACE inhibitors	
Captopril	Fetal renal toxicity, hyperkalemia, **C**ough, **A**ngioedema, **P**roteinuria, **T**aste changes, hyp**O**tension, **P**regnancy problems (fetal renal damage), **R**ash, **I**ncreased renin, **L**ower angiotensin II.
Angiotensin II receptor inhibitors	
Losartan	Fetal renal toxicity, hyperkalemia

[a]Use with β-blockers to prevent reflex tachycardia, diuretic to block salt retention.

Hydralazine

Mechanism	↑ cGMP → smooth muscle relaxation. Vasodilates arterioles > veins; afterload reduction.
Clinical use	Severe hypertension, CHF.
Toxicity	Compensatory tachycardia, fluid retention. Lupus-like syndrome.

Calcium channel blockers

Nifedipine, verapamil, diltiazem.

Mechanism	Block voltage-dependent L-type calcium channels of cardiac and smooth muscle and thereby reduce muscle contractility. Vascular smooth muscle—nifedipine > diltiazem > verapamil. Heart—verapamil > diltiazem > nifedipine.
Clinical use	Hypertension, angina, arrhythmias (not nifedipine).
Toxicity	Cardiac depression, peripheral edema, flushing, dizziness, and constipation.

ACE inhibitors

Captopril, enalapril, lisinopril.

Mechanism
: Inhibit angiotensin-converting enzyme, reducing levels of angiotensin II and preventing inactivation of bradykinin, a potent vasodilator. Renin release is ↑ due to loss of feedback inhibition.

Clinical use
: Hypertension, CHF, diabetic renal disease.

Toxicity
: **C**ough, **A**ngioedema, **P**roteinuria, **T**aste changes, hyp**O**tension, **P**regnancy problems (fetal renal damage), **R**ash, **I**ncreased renin, **L**ower angiotensin II, hyperkalemia.

Losartan is an angiotensin II receptor antagonist. It is **not** an ACE inhibitor and does not cause cough.

CAPTOPRIL.

Diuretics: site of action

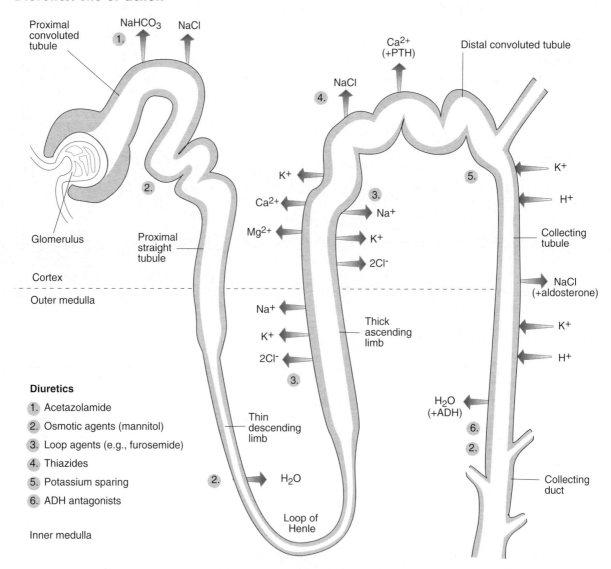

Diuretics

1. Acetazolamide
2. Osmotic agents (mannitol)
3. Loop agents (e.g., furosemide)
4. Thiazides
5. Potassium sparing
6. ADH antagonists

(Adapted, with permission, from Katzung BG. *Basic and Clinical Pharmacology*, 7th ed. Stamford, CT: Appleton & Lange, 1997:243.)

Mannitol

Mechanism   Osmotic diuretic, $\uparrow$ tubular fluid osmolarity, producing $\uparrow$ urine flow.

Clinical use   Shock, drug overdose, $\downarrow$ intracranial/intraocular pressure.

Toxicity   Pulmonary edema, dehydration. Contraindicated in anuria, CHF.

Acetazolamide

Mechanism   Carbonic anhydrase inhibitor. Causes self-limited $NaHCO_3$ diuresis and reduction in total-body HCO_3^- stores. Acts at the proximal convoluted tubule.

Clinical use   Glaucoma, urinary alkalinization, metabolic alkalosis, altitude sickness.

Toxicity   Hyperchloremic metabolic acidosis, neuropathy, NH_3 toxicity, sulfa allergy.

ACIDazolamide causes **ACID**osis.

Furosemide

Mechanism   Sulfonamide loop diuretic. Inhibits cotransport system (Na^+, K^+, 2 Cl^-) of thick ascending limb of loop of Henle. Abolishes hypertonicity of medulla, preventing concentration of urine. $\uparrow$ Ca^{2+} excretion. **L**oops **L**ose calcium.

Clinical use   Edematous states (CHF, cirrhosis, nephrotic syndrome, pulmonary edema), hypertension, hypercalcemia.

Toxicity   **O**totoxicity, **H**ypokalemia, **D**ehydration, **A**llergy (sulfa), **N**ephritis (interstitial), **G**out.

OH DANG!

Ethacrynic acid

Mechanism   Phenoxyacetic acid derivative (NOT a sulfonamide). Essentially same action as furosemide.

Clinical use   Diuresis in patients allergic to sulfa drugs.

Toxicity   Similar to furosemide; can be used in hyperuricemia, acute gout (never used to treat gout).

Hydrochlorothiazide

Mechanism	Thiazide diuretic. Inhibits NaCl reabsorption in early distal tubule, reducing diluting capacity of the nephron. Decreases Ca^{2+} excretion.
Clinical use	Hypertension, CHF, idiopathic hypercalciuria, nephrogenic diabetes insipidus.
Toxicity	Hypokalemic metabolic alkalosis, hyponatremia, hyperGlycemia, hyperLipidemia, hyperUricemia, and hyperCalcemia. Sulfa allergy.

Hyper**GLUC.**

K⁺-sparing diuretics   Spironolactone, Triamterene, Amiloride.

The K⁺ **STA**ys.

Mechanism	Spironolactone is a competitive aldosterone receptor antagonist in the cortical collecting tubule. Triamterene and amiloride act at the same part of the tubule by blocking Na^+ channels in the CCT.
Clinical use	Hyperaldosteronism, K⁺ depletion, CHF.
Toxicity	Hyperkalemia, endocrine effects (e.g., spironolactone causes gynecomastia, antiandrogen effects).

Diuretics: electrolyte changes

Urine NaCl	↑ (all diuretics—carbonic anhydrase inhibitors, loop diuretics, thiazides, K⁺-sparing diuretics).
Urine K⁺	↑ (all except K⁺-sparing diuretics).
Blood pH	↓ (acidosis)—carbonic anhydrase inhibitors, K⁺-sparing diuretics; ↑ (alkalosis)—loop diuretics, thiazides.
Urine Ca⁺	↑ loop diuretics, ↓ thiazides.

Antianginal therapy

Goal—reduction of myocardial O_2 consumption (MVO_2) by decreasing 1 or more of the determinants of MVO_2: end diastolic volume, blood pressure, heart rate, contractility, ejection time.

Component	Nitrates (affect preload)	β-blockers (affect afterload)	Nitrates + β-blockers
End diastolic volume	↓	↑	No effect or ↓
Blood pressure	↓	↓	↓
Contractility	↑ (reflex response)	↓	Little/no effect
Heart rate	↑ (reflex response)	↓	↓
Ejection time	↓	↑	Little/no effect
MVO_2	↓	↓	↓↓

Calcium channel blockers—**N**ifedipine is similar to **N**itrates in effect; verapamil is similar to β-blockers in effect.

Nitroglycerin, isosorbide dinitrate

Mechanism	Vasodilate by releasing nitric oxide in smooth muscle, causing ↑ in cGMP and smooth muscle relaxation. Dilate veins >> arteries.
Clinical use	Angina, pulmonary edema. Also used as an aphrodisiac and erection enhancer.
Toxicity	Tachycardia, hypotension, headache, "Monday disease" in industrial exposure, development of tolerance for the vasodilating action during the work week and loss of tolerance over the weekend, resulting in tachycardia, dizziness, and headache.

Cardiac drugs: sites of action

(Adapted, with permission, from Katzung BG. *Basic and Clinical Pharmacology*, 7th ed. Stamford, CT: Appleton & Lange, 1998:198.)

Cardiac sarcomere is shown above with the cellular components involved in excitation-contraction coupling. Factors involved in excitation-contraction coupling are numbered. (1) Na^+/K^+ ATPase; (2) Na^+-Ca^{2+} exchanger; (3) voltage-gated calcium channel; (4) calcium pump in the wall of the sarcoplasmic reticulum (SR); (5) calcium release channel in the SR; (6) site of calcium interaction with troponin-tropomyosin system.

Cardiac glycosides	Digoxin—75% bioavailability, 20–40% protein bound, $t_{1/2}$ = 40 hours, urinary excretion.
Mechanism	Inhibit the Na^+/K^+ ATPase of cell membrane, causing ↑ intracellular Na^+. Na^+-Ca^{2+} antiport does not function as efficiently, causing ↑ intracellular Ca^{2+}; leads to positive inotropy. May cause ↑ PR, ↓ QT, scooping of ST segment, T-wave inversion on ECG.
Clinical use	CHF (↑ contractility); atrial fibrillation (↓ conduction at AV node).
Toxicity	Nausea, vomiting, diarrhea. Blurry yellow vision (think Van Gogh). Arrhythmia. Toxicities of digoxin are ↑ by renal failure (↓ excretion), hypokalemia (potentiates drug's effects), and quinidine (↓ digoxin clearance; displaces digoxin from tissue binding sites).
Antidote	Slowly normalize K^+, lidocaine, cardiac pacer, anti-dig Fab fragments.

Antiarrhythmics— Na⁺ channel blockers (class I)

Local anesthetics. Slow or block (↓) conduction (especially in depolarized cells). ↓ slope of phase 4 depolarization and ↑ threshold for firing in abnormal pacemaker cells. Are state dependent (selectively depress tissue that is frequently depolarized, e.g., fast tachycardia).

Class IA

Quinidine, Amiodarone, Procainamide, Disopyramide. ↑ AP duration, ↑ effective refractory period (ERP), ↑ QT interval. Affect both atrial and ventricular arrhythmias.

Toxicity: quinidine (cinchonism—headache, tinnitus; thrombocytopenia; torsades de pointes due to increased QT interval); procainamide (reversible SLE-like syndrome).

"Queen Amy Proclaims Diso's **pyramid**."

Class IB

Lidocaine, mexiletine, tocainide. ↓ AP duration. Affect ischemic or depolarized Purkinje and ventricular tissue. Useful in acute ventricular arrhythmias (especially post-MI) and in digitalis-induced arrhythmias.

Toxicity: Local anesthetic. CNS stimulation/depression, cardiovascular depression.

Class IC

Flecainide, encainide, propafenone. No effect on AP duration. Useful in V-tachs that progress to VF and in intractable SVT. Usually used only as last resort in refractory tachyarrhythmias because of toxicities.

Toxicity: proarrhythmic.

(Adapted, with permission, from Katzung BG, Trevor AJ. *Examination & Board Review: Pharmacology*, 5th ed. Stamford, CT: Appleton & Lange, 1998:118.)

Antiarrhythmics— β-blockers (class II)

Propranolol, esmolol, metoprolol, atenolol, timolol.

Mechanism
$\downarrow$ cAMP, $\downarrow$ Ca^{2+} currents. Suppress abnormal pacemakers by $\downarrow$ slope of phase 4. AV node particularly sensitive—$\uparrow$ PR interval. Esmolol very short acting.

Toxicity
Impotence, exacerbation of asthma, cardiovascular effects (bradycardia, AV block, CHF), CNS effects (sedation, sleep alterations). May mask the signs of hypoglycemia.

Antiarrhythmics— K⁺ channel blockers (class III)

Sotalol, ibutilide, bretylium, amiodarone.

Mechanism
$\uparrow$ AP duration, $\uparrow$ ERP. Used when other antiarrhythmics fail. $\uparrow$ QT interval.

Remember to check **PFT**s, **LFT**s, and **TFT**s when using amiodarone.

Toxicity
Sotalol—torsades de pointes, excessive β block; ibutilide—torsades; bretylium—new arrhythmias, hypotension; amiodarone—**pulmonary fibrosis,** corneal deposits, **hepatotoxicity,** skin deposits resulting in photodermatitis, neurologic effects, constipation, cardiovascular effects (bradycardia, heart block, CHF), **hypothyroidism/hyperthyroidism.**

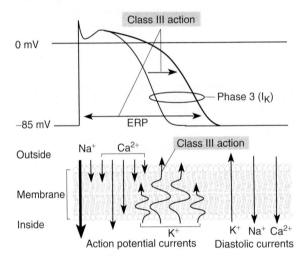

(Adapted, with permission, from Katzung BG, Trevor AJ. *Examination & Board Review: Pharmacology,* 5th ed. Stamford, CT: Appleton & Lange, 1998:120.)

Antiarrhythmics— Ca²⁺ channel blockers (class IV)

Verapamil, diltiazem.

Mechanism	Primarily affect AV nodal cells. $\downarrow$ conduction velocity, $\uparrow$ ERP, $\uparrow$ PR interval. Used in prevention of nodal arrhythmias (e.g., SVT).
Toxicity	Constipation, flushing, edema, CV effects (CHF, AV block, sinus node depression); torsades de pointes (bepridil).

(Adapted, with permission, from Katzung BG, Trevor AJ. *Examination & Board Review: Pharmacology,* 5th ed. Stamford, CT: Appleton & Lange, 1998:121.)

Other antiarrhythmics

Adenosine	Drug of choice in diagnosing/abolishing AV nodal arrhythmias.
K⁺	Depresses ectopic pacemakers, especially in digoxin toxicity.
Mg⁺	Effective in torsades de pointes and digoxin toxicity.

Lipid-lowering agents

Drug	Effect on LDL "bad cholesterol"	Effect on HDL "good cholesterol"	Effect on triglycerides	Side effects/problems
Bile acid resins (cholestyramine, colestipol)	↓↓	—	Slightly ↑	Patients hate it—tastes bad and causes GI discomfort
HMG-CoA reductase inhibitors (lovastatin, pravastatin, simvastatin, atorvastatin)	↓↓↓	↑	↓	Expensive, reversible ↑ LFTs, myositis
Niacin	↓↓	↑↑	↓	Red, flushed face, which is ↓ by aspirin or long-term use
"Fibrates" (gemfibrozil, clofibrate, bezafibrate, fenofibrate)	↓	↑	↓↓↓	Myositis, ↑ LFTs
Cholestrol absorption blocker (ezetimibe	↓↓	—	—	Rare ↑ LFTs

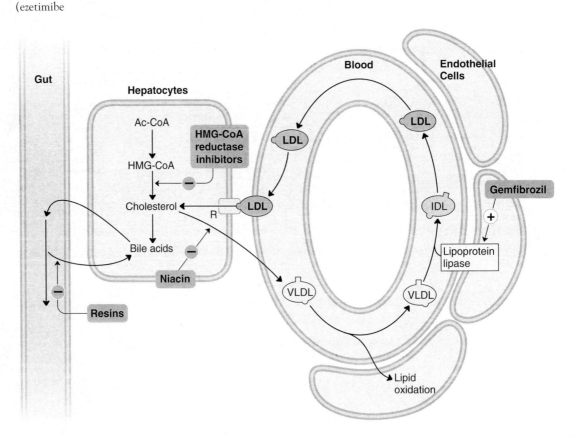

(Adapted, with permission, from Katzung BG, Trevor AJ. *USMLE Road Map: Pharmacology*, 1st ed. New York: McGraw-Hill, 2003:56.)

Arachidonic acid products

Membrane lipid (e.g., phosphatidylinositol)

Phospholipase A$_2$ ← ⊖ **Corticosteroids**

Arachidonic acid

Lipoxygenase

Cyclooxygenase (COX-1, COX-2)

⊖ Protein synthesis

Zileuton — ⊖

⊖ — **NSAIDs, acetaminophen, COX-2 inhibitors**

Hydroperoxides (HPETEs)

Endoperoxides (PGG, PGH)

Leukotrienes (LTB, LTC, LTD)

Prostacyclin (PGI)

Thromboxane (TXA)

Prostaglandins (PGE, PGF)

Zafirlukast — ⊖ →

↑ Bronchial tone

↓ Platelet aggregation
↓ Vascular tone
↓ Bronchial tone
↓ Uterine tone

↑ Uterine tone
↓ Vascular tone
↓ Bronchial tone

↑ Platelet aggregation
↑ Vascular tone
↑ Bronchial tone

(Adapted, with permission, from Katzung BG, Trevor AJ. *Examination & Board Review: Pharmacology,* 5th ed. Stamford, CT: Appleton & Lange, 1998:150.)

HIGH-YIELD FACTS

Pharmacology

Asthma drugs

Nonspecific β-agonists	**Isoproterenol**—relaxes bronchial smooth muscle (β_2). Adverse effect is tachycardia (β_1).
β_2 agonists	**Albuterol**—relaxes bronchial smooth muscle (β_2). Use during acute exacerbation.
	Salmeterol—long-acting agent for prophylaxis. Adverse effects are tremor and arrhythmia.
Methylxanthines	**Theophylline**—likely causes bronchodilation by inhibiting phosphodiesterase, thereby ↓ cAMP hydrolysis. The usage is limited because of narrow therapeutic index (cardiotoxicity, neurotoxicity).
Muscarinic antagonists	**Ipratropium**—competitive block of muscarinic receptors, preventing bronchoconstriction.
Cromolyn	Prevents release of mediators from mast cells. Effective only for the prophylaxis of asthma. Not effective during an acute asthmatic attack. Toxicity is rare.
Corticosteroids	**Beclomethasone, prednisone**—inhibits the synthesis of virtually all cytokines. Inactivates NF-κB, the transcription factor that induces the production of TNF-α, among other inflammatory agents. 1st-line therapy for chronic asthma.
Antileukotrienes	**Zileuton**—A 5-lipoxygenase pathway inhibitor. Blocks conversion of arachidonic acid to leukotrienes.
	Zafirlukast—blocks leukotriene receptors.

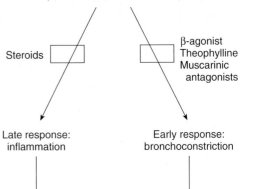

Treatment strategies in asthma

(Adapted, with permission, from Katzung BG, Trevor AJ. *Examination & Board Review: Pharmacology,* 5th ed. Stamford, CT: Appleton & Lange, 1998:159 and 161.)

GI therapy

(Adapted, with permission, from Katzung BG, Trevor AJ. *USMLE Road Map: Pharmacology*, 1st ed. New York: McGraw-Hill, 2003:159.)

H$_2$ blockers

Cimetidine, ranitidine, famotidine, nizatidine.

Mechanism	Reversible block of histamine H$_2$ receptors.
Clinical use	Peptic ulcer, gastritis, esophageal reflux, Zollinger-Ellison syndrome.
Toxicity	Cimetidine is a potent inhibitor of P-450; it also has an antiandrogenic effect and ↓ renal excretion of creatinine. Other H$_2$ blockers are relatively free of these effects.

Omeprazole, lansoprazole

Mechanism	Irreversibly inhibits H$^+$/K$^+$ ATPase in stomach parietal cells.
Clinical use	Peptic ulcer, gastritis, esophageal reflux, Zollinger-Ellison syndrome.

Bismuth, sucralfate

Mechanism	Bind to ulcer base, providing physical protection, and allow HCO$_3^-$ secretion to reestablish pH gradient in the mucus layer.
Clinical use	↑ ulcer healing.

Misoprostol

Mechanism	A PGE$_1$ analog. ↑ production and secretion of gastric mucous barrier.
Clinical use	Prevention of NSAID-induced peptic ulcers, maintains a PDA. Also used to induce labor.
Toxicity	Diarrhea. Contraindicated in women of childbearing potential (abortifacient).

Infliximab

Mechanism	A monoclonal antibody to TNF-α, proinflammatory cytokine.
Clinical use	Acute refractory Crohn's, along with fistula healing.
Toxicity	Respiratory infection, fever, hypotension.

Sulfasalazine

Mechanism	A combination of sulfapyridine and mesalamine, offering antibacterial action and anti-inflammatory effects, respectively.
Clinical use	Ulcerative colitis, remission of Crohn's disease.
Toxicity	Malaise, nausea, sulfonamide toxicity.

Ondansetron

Mechanism	5-HT_3 antagonist. Powerful central-acting antiemetic.	You will not vomit with
Clinical use	Control vomiting postoperatively and in patients undergoing cancer chemotherapy.	**ONDANS**etron, so you can go **ON DANC**ing.
Toxicity	Headache, constipation.	

Antacid overuse

Can affect absorption, bioavailability, or urinary excretion of other drugs by altering gastric and urinary pH or by delaying gastric emptying.

Overuse can also cause the following problems:

1. Aluminum hydroxide—constipation and hypophosphatemia

   Alu**minimum** amount of feces.
2. Magnesium hydroxide—diarrhea

   Mg = Must **g**o to the bathroom.
3. Calcium carbonate—hypercalcemia, rebound acid ↑

All can cause hypokalemia.

Heparin

Mechanism	Catalyzes the activation of antithrombin III, ↓ thrombin and Xa. Short half-life. Check PTT.
Clinical use	Immediate anticoagulation for pulmonary embolism, stroke, angina, MI, DVT. Used during pregnancy (does not cross placenta). Follow PTT.
Toxicity	Bleeding, thrombocytopenia, drug-drug interactions. Use **protamine sulfate** for rapid reversal of heparinization (positively charged molecule that acts by binding negatively charged heparin).
Note	Newer **low-molecular-weight heparins** (enoxaparin) act more on Xa, have better bioavailability and 2–4 times longer half-life. Can be administered subcutaneously and without laboratory monitoring.

Warfarin (Coumadin)

Mechanism	Interferes with normal synthesis and γ-carboxylation of vitamin K–dependent clotting factors II, VII, IX, and X, protein C and S via vitamin K antagonism. Long half-life.	**WEPT**—**W**arfarin affects the **E**xtrinsic **p**athway and prolongs **PT**.
Clinical use	Chronic anticoagulation. Not used in pregnant women (because warfarin, unlike heparin, can cross the placenta). Follow PT values.	
Toxicity	Bleeding, teratogenic, drug-drug interactions.	

Heparin vs. warfarin

	Heparin	Warfarin
Structure	Large anionic polymer, acidic	Small lipid-soluble molecule
Route of administration	Parenteral (IV, SC)	Oral
Site of action	Blood	Liver
Onset of action	Rapid (seconds)	Slow, limited by half-lives of normal clotting factors
Mechanism of action	Activates antithrombin III, IIa (thrombin) and Xa	Impairs the synthesis of vitamin K–dependent clotting factors II, VII, IX, and X (vitamin K antagonist)
Duration of action	Acute (hours)	Chronic (weeks or months)
Inhibits coagulation in vitro	Yes	No
Treatment of acute overdose	Protamine sulfate	IV vitamin K and fresh frozen plasma
Monitoring	PTT (intrinsic pathway)	PT (extrinsic pathway)

Thrombolytics

Streptokinase, urokinase, tPA (alteplase), APSAC (anistreplase).

Mechanism Directly or indirectly aid conversion of plasminogen to plasmin, which cleaves thrombin and fibrin clots. It is claimed that tPA specifically converts fibrin-bound plasminogen to plasmin.

Clinical use Early MI.

Toxicity Bleeding.

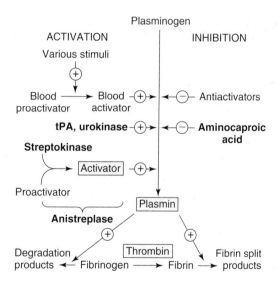

(Adapted, with permission, from Katzung BG. *Basic and Clinical Examination & Board Review: Pharmacology*, 7th ed. Stamford, CT: Appleton & Lange, 1997:550.)

Thrombolytic drugs are shown on the left in bold type. These drugs ↑ the formation of plasmin, the major fibrinolytic enzyme. Aminocaproic acid, a useful inhibitor of fibrinolysis, is shown on the right.

Mechanism of antiplatelet interaction

Clopidogrel, ticlopidine

Mechanism	Inhibit platelet aggregation by irreversibly inhibiting the ADP pathway involved in the binding of fibrinogen.
Clinical use	Acute coronary syndrome; coronary stenting. ↓ incidence or recurrence of thrombotic stroke.
Toxicity	Neutropenia (ticlopidine); reserved for those who cannot tolerate aspirin.

Abciximab

Mechanism	Binds to the glycoprotein receptor IIb/IIa on activated platelets.
Clinical use	Acute coronary syndromes, percutaneous transluminal coronary angioplasty.
Toxicity	Bleeding, thrombocytopenia.

Aspirin

Mechanism	Acetylates and irreversibly inhibits cyclooxygenase (both COX-1 and COX-2) to prevent conversion of arachidonic acid to prostaglandins. No effect on PT, PTT.
Clinical use	Antipyretic, analgesic, anti-inflammatory, antiplatelet drug.
Toxicity	Gastric ulceration, bleeding, hyperventilation, Reye's syndrome, tinnitus (CN VIII).

Diabetes drugs

Insulin	Binds insulin receptor, which has tyrosine kinase activity. In liver, ↑ storage of glucose as glycogen. In muscle, stimulates glycogen and protein synthesis, and K^+ uptake. In adipose tissue, facilitates triglyceride storage.
	Clinical use (in addition to diabetes) includes life-threatening hyperkalemia and stress-induced hyperglycemia.
	Toxicities are hypoglycemia and (rarely) hypersensitivity reaction.
Sulfonylureas	Tolbutamide, chlorpropamide, glyburide, glipizide.
	Oral hypoglycemic agents used to stimulate release of endogenous insulin in NIDDM (type 2).
	Close K^+ channels in β-cell membrane → cell depolarizes → insulin release triggered owing to ↑ Ca^{2+} influx.
	Inactive in IDDM (type 1) because requires some residual islet function.
	Toxicities includes hypoglycemia (more common with 2nd-generation drugs—glyburide, glipizide) and disulfiram-like effects (not seen with 2nd-generation drugs—glyburide, glipizide).
Metformin	Mechanism unknown; possibly inhibits gluconeogenesis and increases glycolysis; ↓ serum glucose levels.
	Used as an oral hypoglycemic. Can be used in patients without islet function.
	Most grave adverse effect is lactic acidosis.
Glitazones	Pioglitazone, rosiglitazone, troglitazone.
	↑ target cell response to insulin. Used as monotherapy in type 2 diabetes or in combination with above agents.
	Toxicity: weight gain, hepatotoxic (troglitazone).
α-glucosidase inhibitors	Acarbose, miglitol.
	Inhibit intestinal brush border α-glucosidases; delayed hydrolysis of sugars and absorption of glucose lead to ↓ postprandial hyperglycemia.
	Used as monotherapy in type 2 diabetes or in combination with above agents.
	Toxicity: GI disturbances.

Leuprolide

Mechanism	GnRH analog with agonist properties when used in pulsatile fashion; antagonist properties when used in continuous fashion.	When used in continuous fashion, it causes a transient initial burst of LH and FSH.
Clinical use	Infertility (pulsatile), prostate cancer (continuous—use with flutamide), uterine fibroids.	
Toxicity	Antiandrogen, nausea, vomiting.	

Propylthiouracil

Mechanism	Inhibits organification and coupling of thyroid hormone synthesis. Also ↓ peripheral conversion of T_4 to T_3.
Clinical use	Hyperthyroidism.
Toxicity	Skin rash, agranulocytosis (rare), aplastic anemia.

Antiandrogens

Finasteride	A 5α-reductase inhibitor (↓ conversion of testosterone to dihydrotestosterone). Useful in BPH. Also promote hair growth—used to treat male-pattern baldness.
Flutamide	A nonsteroidal competitive inhibitor of androgens at the testosterone receptor. Used in prostate carcinoma.
Ketoconazole, spironolactone	Inhibit steroid synthesis; used in the treatment of polycystic ovarian syndrome to prevent hirsutism.

HIGH-YIELD FACTS

Pharmacology

331

Glucocorticoids
Hydrocortisone, prednisone, triamcinolone, dexamethasone, beclomethasone.

Mechanism
$\downarrow$ the production of leukotrienes and prostaglandins by inhibiting phospholipase A_2 and expression of COX-2.

Clinical use
Addison's disease, inflammation, immune suppression, asthma.

Toxicity
Iatrogenic Cushing's syndrome—buffalo hump, moon facies, truncal obesity, muscle wasting, thin skin, easy bruisability, osteoporosis, adrenocortical atrophy, peptic ulcers.

PHARMACOLOGY—REPRODUCTIVE DRUGS

cGMP inhibitors, sildenafil, vardenafil

Mechanism
Inhibits cGMP phosphodiesterase, causing $\uparrow$ cGMP, smooth muscle relaxation in the corpus cavernosum, $\uparrow$ blood flow, and penile erection.

Sildena**fil** and vardena**fil** **fill** the penis.

Clinical use
Treatment of erectile dysfunction.

Toxicity
Headache, flushing, dyspepsia, blue-green color vision. Risk of life-threatening hypotension in patients taking nitrates.

Clomiphene

Mechanism
A partial agonist at estrogen receptors in the pituitary gland. Prevents normal feedback inhibition and $\uparrow$ release of LH and FSH from the pituitary, which stimulates ovulation.

Clinical use
Treatment of infertility.

Toxicity
Hot flashes, ovarian enlargement, multiple simultaneous pregnancies, visual disturbances.

Mifepristone (RU-486)

Mechanism
Competitive inhibitor of progestins at progesterone receptors.

Clinical use
Abortifacient.

Toxicity
Heavy bleeding, GI effects (nausea, vomiting, anorexia), abdominal pain.

Oral contraception (synthetic progestins, estrogen)

Advantages	Disadvantages
Reliable (<1% failure)	Taken daily
$\downarrow$ risk of endometrial and ovarian cancer	No protection against STDs
$\downarrow$ incidence of ectopic pregnancy	$\uparrow$ triglycerides
$\downarrow$ pelvic infections	Depression, weight gain, nausea, hypertension
Regulation of menses	Hypercoagulable state

HIGH-YIELD FACTS

Pharmacology

Gout drugs

Colchicine	Acute gout. Depolymerizes microtubules, impairing leukocyte chemotaxis and degranulation. GI side effects, especially if given orally. (Note: indomethacin is less toxic, more commonly used.)
Probenecid	Chronic gout. Inhibits reabsorption of uric acid (also inhibits secretion of penicillin).
Allopurinol	Chronic gout. Inhibits xanthine oxidase, ↓ conversion of xanthine to uric acid.

Cancer drugs—site of action

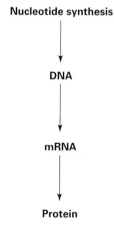

1. Methotrexate— ↓ thymidine + purine synthesis
2. 5-FU— ↓ thymidine + purine synthesis
3. 6-MP

4. Alkylating agents + cisplatin—DNA cross-linkage
5. Dactinomycin + doxorubicin—intercalate DNA strands
6. Bleomycin
7. Etoposide—strand breakage
8. Steroids
9. Tamoxifen

10. Vinca alkaloids—inhibit microtubule formation
11. Paclitaxel

Cell cycle specific—antimetabolites, plant alkaloids, steroid hormones, bleomycin, paclitaxel, etoposide.
Cell cycle nonspecific—alkylating agents, antibiotics.

HIGH-YIELD FACTS

Pharmacology

333

Cancer drugs—cell cycle

(Adapted, with permission, from Katzung BG, Trevor AJ. *USMLE Road Map: Pharmacology*, 1st ed. New York: McGraw-Hill, 2003:133.)

Methotrexate

Mechanism	S-phase-specific antimetabolite. Folic acid analog that inhibits dihydrofolate reductase, resulting in decreased dTMP and therefore ↓ DNA and protein synthesis.
Clinical use	Leukemias, lymphomas, choriocarcinoma, sarcomas. Abortion, ectopic pregnancy, rheumatoid arthritis, psoriasis.
Toxicity	Myelosuppression, which is reversible with leucovorin (folinic acid) "rescue." Macrovesicular fatty change in liver.

5-fluorouracil (5-FU)

Mechanism	S-phase-specific antimetabolite. Pyrimidine analog bioactivated to 5F-dUMP, which covalently complexes folic acid. This complex inhibits thymidylate synthase, resulting in ↓ dTMP and same effects as methotrexate.
Clinical use	Colon cancer and other solid tumors, basal cell carcinoma (topical). Synergy with methotrexate.
Toxicity	Myelosuppression, which is NOT reversible with leucovorin; photosensitivity.

6-mercaptopurine (6-MP)

Mechanism	Blocks purine synthesis.
Clinical use	Leukemias, lymphomas (not CLL or Hodgkin's).
Toxicity	Bone marrow, GI, liver. Metabolized by xanthine oxidase; thus ↑ toxicity with allopurinol.

Busulfan

Mechanism	Alkylates DNA.
Clinical use	CML.
Toxicity	Pulmonary fibrosis, hyperpigmentation.

Cytarabine

Mechanism	Inhibits DNA polymerase.
Clinical use	AML.
Toxicity	Leukopenia, thrombocytopenia, megaloblastic anemia.

Cyclophosphamide

Mechanism	Alkylating agent; covalently x-links (interstrand) DNA at guanine N-7. Requires bioactivation by liver.
Clinical use	Non-Hodgkin's lymphoma, breast and ovarian carcinomas. Also an immunosuppressant.
Toxicity	Myelosuppression, hemorrhagic cystitis.

Nitrosoureas

	Carmustine, lomustine, semustine, streptozocin.
Mechanism	Alkylate DNA. Require bioactivation. Cross blood-brain barrier → CNS.
Clinical use	Brain tumors (including glioblastoma multiforme).
Toxicity	CNS toxicity (dizziness, ataxia).

Cisplatin

Mechanism	Acts like an alkylating agent. X-links via hydrolysis of Cl^- groups and reaction with platinum.
Clinical use	Testicular, bladder, ovary, and lung carcinomas.
Toxicity	Nephrotoxicity and acoustic nerve damage.

Doxorubicin (Adriamycin)

Mechanism	Noncovalently intercalates in DNA, creating breaks to ↓ replication and transcription and generate free radicals.
Clinical use	Part of the **A**BVD combination regimen for Hodgkin's and for myelomas, sarcomas, and solid tumors (breast, ovary, lung).
Toxicity	Cardiotoxicity; also myelosuppression and marked alopecia. Toxic extravasation.

Bleomycin, dactinomycin

Mechanism	Intercalates DNA strands and induces free radical formation, causing strand breaks.
Clinical use	Testicular cancer, lymphomas.
Toxicity	Pulmonary fibrosis, skin changes, minimal myelosuppression (bleomycin).

Etoposide

Mechanism	G_2-phase-specific inhibits topoisomerase II so that double-strand breaks remain in DNA following replication with subsequent DNA degradation.
Clinical use	Oat cell carcinoma of the lung and prostate, testicular carcinoma.
Toxicity	Myelosuppression, GI irritation, alopecia.

Prednisone

Mechanism	May trigger apoptosis. May even work on nondividing cells.
Clinical use	Most commonly used glucocorticoid in cancer chemotherapy. Used in CLL, Hodgkin's lymphomas (part of the MOP**P** regimen). Also an immunosuppressant used in autoimmune diseases.
Toxicity	Cushing-like symptoms; immunosuppression, cataracts, acne, osteoporosis, hypertension, peptic ulcers, hyperglycemia, psychosis.

Tamoxifen/raloxifene

Mechanism	Estrogen receptor mixed agonist/antagonists ("SERMs") that block the binding of estrogen to ER+ cells.
Clinical use	Breast cancer.
Toxicity	Tamoxifen may increase the risk of endometrial carcinoma via partial agonist effects; "hot flashes."

Vincristine and vinblastine

Mechanism	M-phase-specific alkaloids that bind to tubulin and block polymerization of microtubules so that mitotic spindle cannot form.
Clinical use	Part of the MOPP (Oncovin [vincristine]) regimen for lymphoma, Wilms' tumor, choriocarcinoma.
Toxicity	Vincristine—neurotoxicity (areflexia, peripheral neuritis), paralytic ileus. VinBLASTine BLASTs Bone marrow (suppression).

Paclitaxel

Mechanism	M-phase-specific agent obtained from yew tree that binds to tubulin and hyperstabilizes polymerized microtubules so that mitotic spindle cannot break down (anaphase cannot occur).
Clinical use	Ovarian and breast carcinomas.
Toxicity	Myelosuppression and hypersensitivity.

Immunosuppressive agents: sites of action

Agent	Site
Prednisone	2, 5
Cyclosporine	2, 3
Azathioprine	2
Methotrexate	2
Dactinomycin	2, 3
Cyclophosphamide	2
Antilymphocytic globulin and monoclonal anti-T-cell antibodies	1, 2, 3
Rh₃(D) immune globulin	1
Tacrolimus	4

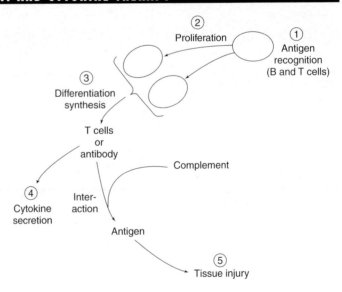

(Adapted, with permission, from Katzung BG. *Basic and Clinical Pharmacology,* 7th ed. Stamford, CT: Appleton & Lange, 1997:924.)

HIGH-YIELD FACTS

Pharmacology

Cyclosporine

Mechanism	Binds to cyclophilins (peptidyl proline *cis-trans* isomerase), blocking the differentiation and activation of T cells mainly by inhibiting the production of IL-2 and its receptor.
Clinical use	Suppresses organ rejection after transplantation; selected autoimmune disorders.
Toxicity	Predisposes patients to viral infections and lymphoma; nephrotoxic (preventable with mannitol diuresis).

Azathioprine

Mechanism	Antimetabolite derivative of 6-mercaptopurine that interferes with the metabolism and synthesis of nucleic acid. Toxic to proliferating lymphocytes after antigenic stimulus.
Clinical use	Kidney transplantation, autoimmune disorders (including glomerulonephritis and hemolytic anemia).

Tacrolimus (FK506)

Mechanism	Similar to cyclosporine; binds to FK-binding protein, inhibiting secretion of IL-2 and other cytokines.
Clinical use	Potent immunosuppressive used in organ transplant recipients.
Toxicity	Significant—nephrotoxicity, peripheral neuropathy, hypertension, pleural effusion, hyperglycemia.

Recombinant cytokines and clinical uses

Agent	Clinical uses
Aldesleukin (interleukin-2)	Renal cell carcinoma, metastatic melanoma
Erythropoietin (epoetin)	Anemias (especially in renal failure)
Filgrastim (granulocyte colony-stimulating factor)	Recovery of bone marrow
α-interferon	Hepatitis B and C, Kaposi's sarcoma, leukemias, malignant melanoma
β-interferon	Multiple sclerosis
γ-interferon	Chronic granulomatous disease
Oprelvekin (interleukin-2)	Thrombocytopenia
Sargramostim (granulocyte-macrophage colony-stimulating factor)	Recovery of bone marrow
Thrombopoietin	Thrombocytopenia

(Adapted, with permission, from Katzung BG, Trevor AJ. *USMLE Road Map: Pharmacology*, 1st ed. New York: McGraw-Hill, 2003.)

Specific antidotes

Toxin	Antidote/treatment
1. Acetaminophen	1. N-acetylcysteine
2. Salicylates	2. Alkalinize urine, dialysis
3. Anticholinesterases, organophosphates	3. Atropine, pralidoxime
4. Antimuscarinic, anticholinergic agents	4. Physostigmine salicylate
5. β-blockers	5. Glucagon
6. Digitalis	6. Stop dig, normalize K+, lidocaine, anti-dig Fab fragments, Mg^{2+}
7. Iron	7. Deferoxamine
8. Lead	8. CaEDTA, dimercaprol, succimer, penicillamine
9. Arsenic, mercury, gold	9. Dimercaprol (BAL), succimer
10. Copper, arsenic, gold	10. Penicillamine
11. Cyanide	11. Nitrite, hydroxocobalamin, thiosulfate
12. Methemoglobin	12. Methylene blue
13. Carbon monoxide	13. 100% O_2, hyperbaric O_2
14. Methanol, ethylene glycol (antifreeze)	14. Ethanol, dialysis, fomepizole
15. Opioids	15. Naloxone/naltrexone
16. Benzodiazepines	16. Flumazenil
17. TCAs	17. $NaHCO_3$ (nonspecific)
18. Heparin	18. Protamine
19. Warfarin	19. Vitamin K, fresh frozen plasma
20. tPA, streptokinase	20. Aminocaproic acid

Lead poisoning

Lead Lines on gingivae and on epiphyses of long bones on x-ray.

Encephalopathy and **E**rythrocyte basophilic stippling.

Abdominal colic and sideroblastic **A**nemia.

Drops—wrist and foot drop. **D**imercaprol and EDTA 1st line of treatment.

LEAD.

High risk in houses with chipped paint.

Urine pH and drug elimination

Weak acids (phenobarbital, methotrexate, aspirin) alkalinize urine with bicarbonate to ↑ clearance.

Weak bases (amphetamines) acidify urine to ↑ clearance (give NH_4Cl).

Drug reactions

Drug reaction	Causal agent
1. Pulmonary fibrosis	1. Bleomycin, amiodarone, busulfan
2. Hepatitis	2. Isoniazid (INH), halothane
3. Focal to massive hepatic necrosis	3. Halothane, valproic acid, acetaminophen, *Amanita phalloides*
4. Anaphylaxis	4. Penicillin
5. SLE-like syndrome	5. **H**ydralazine, **I**NH, **P**rocainamide, **P**henytoin (it's not **HIPP** to have lupus)
6. Hemolysis in G6PD-deficient patients	6. Sulfonamides, INH, aspirin, ibuprofen, primaquine, nitrofurantoin, pyrimethamine, chloramphenicol
7. Thrombotic complications	7. OCPs (e.g., estrogens and progestins)
8. Adrenocortical insufficiency	8. Withdrawal of glucocorticoids (HPA suppression)
9. Photosensitivity reactions	9. **S**ulfonamides, **A**miodarone, **T**etracycline (**SAT** for a photo)
10. Induce ($\uparrow$) P-450 system	10. Barbiturates, phenytoin, carbamazepine, rifampin, griseofulvin, quinidine
11. Inhibit ($\downarrow$) P-450 system	11. Cimetidine, ketoconazole, grapefruit, erythromycin, INH, sulfonamides
12. Tubulointerstitial nephritis	12. Sulfonamides, furosemide, methicillin, rifampin, NSAIDs (except aspirin)
13. Hot flashes	13. Tamoxifen
14. Cutaneous flushing	14. Niacin, Ca^{2+} channel blockers, adenosine, vancomycin
15. Cardiac toxicity	15. Doxorubicin (Adriamycin), daunorubicin
16. Agranulocytosis	16. Clozapine, carbamazepine, colchicine
17. Stevens-Johnson syndrome	17. Ethosuximide, sulfonamides, lamotrigine
18. Cinchonism	18. Quinidine, quinine
19. Tendonitis, tendon rupture and cartilage damage (kids)	19. Fluoroquinolones
20. Disulfiram-like reaction	20. Metronidazole, certain cephalosporins, procarbazine, sulfonylureas
21. Ototoxicity and nephrotoxicity	21. Aminoglycosides, loop diuretics, cisplatin
22. Drug-induced Parkinson's	22. Haloperidol, chlorpromazine, reserpine, MPTP
23. Torsades de pointes	23. Class III (sotalol), class IA (quinidine) antiarrhythmics
24. Aplastic anemia	24. Chloramphenicol, benzene, NSAIDs
25. Neuro/nephrotoxicity	25. Polymyxins
26. Pseudomembranous colitis	26. Clindamycin, ampicillin
27. Gynecomastia	27. **S**pironolactone, **D**igitalis, **C**imetidine, chronic **A**lcohol use, estrogens, **K**etoconazole (**S**ome **D**rugs **C**reate **A**wesome **K**nockers)

Drug reactions (*continued*)

28. Atropine-like side effects	28. Tricyclics
29. Cough	29. ACE inhibitors (losartan → no cough)
30. Gingival hyperplasia	30. Phenytoin
31. Diabetes insipidus	31. Lithium
32. Tardive dyskinesia	32. Antipsychotics
33. Fanconi's syndrome	33. Tetracycline
34. Gray baby syndrome	34. Chloramphenicol
35. Extrapyramidal side effects	35. Chlorpromazine, thioridazine, haloperidol
36. Osteoporosis	36. Corticosteroids, heparin

Alcohol toxicity

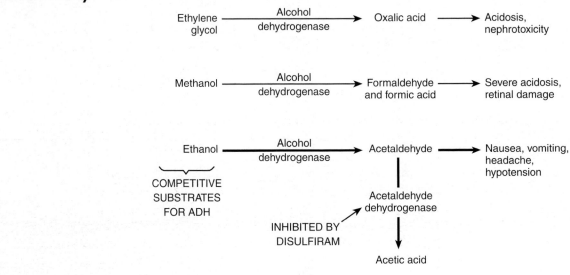

340

Herbal agents

Agent	Clinical uses	Toxicities
Echinacea	Common cold	GI distress, dizziness, and headache
Ephedra	As for ephedrine	CNS and cardiovascular stimulation; arrhythmias, stroke, and seizures at high doses
Feverfew	Migraine	GI distress, mouth ulcers, antiplatelet actions
Ginkgo	Intermittent claudication	GI distress, anxiety, insomnia, headache, antiplatelet actions
Kava	Chronic anxiety	GI distress, sedation, ataxia, hepatotoxicity, phototoxicity, dermatotoxicity
Milk thistle	Viral hepatitis	Loose stools
Saw palmetto	Benign prostatic hyperplasia	GI distress, decreased libido, hypertension
St. John's wort	Mild to moderate depression	GI distress and phototoxicity; serotonin syndrome with SSRIs
Dehydroepi-androsterone	Symptomatic improvement in females with SLE or AIDS	Androgenization (premenopausal women), estrogenic effects (postmenopausal), feminization (young men)
Melatonin	Jet lag, insomnia	Sedation, suppresses midcycle LH, hypoprolactinemia

(Adapted, with permission, from Katzung BG, Trevor AJ. *USMLE Road Map: Pharmacology*, 1st ed. New York: McGraw-Hill, 2003.)

Drug name

Ending	Category	Example
-ane	Inhalational general anesthetic	Halothane
-azepam	Benzodiazepine	Diazepam
-azine	Phenothiazine (neuroleptic, antiemetic)	Chlorpromazine
-azole	Antifungal	Ketoconazole
-barbital	Barbiturate	Phenobarbital
-caine	Local anesthetic	Lidocaine
-cillin	Penicillin	Methicillin
-cycline	Antibiotic, protein synthesis inhibitor	Tetracycline
-ipramine	TCA	Imipramine
-navir	Protease inhibitor	Saquinavir
-olol	β-antagonist	Propranolol
-operidol	Butyrophenone (neuroleptic)	Haloperidol
-oxin	Cardiac glycoside (inotropic agent)	Digoxin
-phylline	Methylxanthine	Theophylline
-pril	ACE inhibitor	Captopril
-terol	β_2 agonist	Albuterol
-tidine	H_2 antagonist	Cimetidine
-triptyline	TCA	Amitriptyline
-tropin	Pituitary hormone	Somatotropin
-zosin	α_1 antagonist	Prazosin

Physiology

"When I investigate and when I discover that the forces of the heavens and the planets are within ourselves, then truly I seem to be living among the gods."
—Leon Battista Alberti

The portion of the examination dealing with physiology is broad and concept oriented and thus does not lend itself as well to fact-based review. Diagrams are often the best study aids, especially given the increasing number of questions requiring the interpretation of diagrams. Learn to apply basic physiologic relationships in a variety of ways (e.g., Fick equation, clearance equations). You are seldom asked to perform complex calculations. Hormones are the focus of many questions. Learn their sites of production and action as well as their regulatory mechanisms.

A large portion of the physiology tested on the USMLE Step 1 is now clinically relevant and involves understanding physiologic changes associated with pathologic processes (e.g., changes in pulmonary function with COPD). Thus, it is worthwhile to review the physiologic changes that are found with common pathologies of the major organ systems (e.g., heart, lungs, kidneys, GI tract) and endocrine glands.

Cardiovascular
Renal
Endocrine/Reproductive
Respiratory
Gastrointestinal

Myocardial action potential

Occurs in atrial and ventricular myocytes and Purkinje fibers.

Phase 0 = rapid upstroke—voltage-gated Na⁺ channels open.

Phase 1 = initial repolarization—inactivation of voltage-gated Na⁺ channels. Voltage-gated K⁺ channels begin to open.

Phase 2 = plateau—Ca^{2+} influx through voltage-gated Ca^{2+} channels balances K⁺ efflux. Ca^{2+} influx triggers another Ca^{2+} release from sarcoplasmic reticulum and myocyte contraction.

Phase 3 = rapid repolarization—massive K⁺ efflux due to opening of voltage-gated slow K⁺ channels and closure of voltage-gated Ca^{2+} channels.

Phase 4 = resting potential—high K⁺ permeability through K⁺ channels.

Pacemaker action potential

Occurs in the SA and AV nodes. Key differences from the ventricular action potential include:

Phase 0 = upstroke—opening of voltage-gated Ca^{2+} channels. These cells lack fast voltage-gated Na⁺ channels. Results in a slow conduction velocity that is used by the AV node to prolong transmission from the atria to ventricles.

Phase 2 = plateau is absent.

Phase 4 = slow diastolic depolarization—membrane potential spontaneously depolarizes as Na⁺ conductance ↑ (I_f different from I_{Na} above). Accounts for automaticity of SA and AV nodes. The slope of phase 4 in the SA node determines heart rate. ACh ↓ and catecholamines ↑ the rate of diastolic depolarization, decreasing or increasing heart rate, respectively.

(Adapted, with permission, from Ganong WF et al. *Review of Medical Physiology*, 20th ed. New York: McGraw-Hill, 2001.)

Cardiac output (CO)

Cardiac output = (stroke volume) × (heart rate).

Fick principle:

$$CO = \frac{\text{rate of } O_2 \text{ consumption}}{\text{arterial } O_2 \text{ content} - \text{venous } O_2 \text{ content}}$$

$$\text{Mean arterial pressure} = \left(\begin{array}{c}\text{cardiac}\\\text{output}\end{array}\right) \times \left(\begin{array}{c}\text{total peripheral}\\\text{resistance}\end{array}\right)$$

Similar to Ohm's law:

Voltage = (current) × (resistance)

MAP = ⅓ systolic + ⅔ diastolic.

Pulse pressure = systolic − diastolic.

Pulse pressure ≈ stroke volume.

$$SV = \frac{CO}{HR} = EDV - ESV$$

$$EF = \frac{SV}{EDV} \times 100\% \ (\text{normal} \geq 55\%)$$

During exercise, CO ↑ initially as a result of an ↑ in SV. After prolonged exercise, CO ↑ as a result of an ↑ in HR.

If HR is too high, diastolic filling is incomplete and CO ↓ (e.g., ventricular tachycardia).

Cardiac output variables

Stroke Volume affected by Contractility, Afterload, and Preload. ↑ SV when ↑ preload, ↓ afterload, or ↑ contractility.

Contractility (and SV) ↑ with:
1. Catecholamines (↑ activity of Ca^{2+} pump in sarcoplasmic reticulum)
2. ↑ intracellular calcium
3. ↓ extracellular sodium
4. Digitalis (↑ intracellular Na^+, resulting in ↑ Ca^{2+})

Contractility (and SV) ↓ with:
1. β_1 blockade
2. Heart failure
3. Acidosis
4. Hypoxia/hypercapnea

SV CAP.

SV ↑ in anxiety, exercise, and pregnancy.

A failing heart has ↓ SV.

Myocardial O_2 demand is ↑ by:
1. ↑ afterload (∝ diastolic BP)
2. ↑ contractility
3. ↑ heart rate
4. ↑ heart size (↑ wall tension)

Preload and afterload

Preload = ventricular EDV.

Afterload = diastolic arterial pressure (proportional to peripheral resistance).

Venous dilators (e.g., nitroglycerin) ↓ preload.

Vasodilators (e.g., hydralazine) ↓ afterload.

Preload ↑ with exercise (slightly), ↑ blood volume (overtransfusion), and excitement (sympathetics).

Preload pumps up the heart.

345

Starling curve

Force of contraction is proportional to initial length of cardiac muscle fiber (preload).

CONTRACTILE STATE OF MYOCARDIUM

$\oplus$	$\ominus$
Circulating catecholamines	Pharmacologic depressants
Digitalis	Loss of myocardium (MI)
Sympathetic stimulation	

Ejection fraction

$$EF = \frac{EDV - ESV}{EDV} = \frac{SV}{EDV}$$

EF is an index of ventricular contractility.
EF is normally ≥ 55%.

Resistance, pressure, flow

$$Resistance = \frac{driving\ pressure\ (\Delta P)}{flow\ (Q)} = \frac{8\eta\ (viscosity) \times length}{\pi\ r^4}$$

Viscosity depends mostly on hematocrit.

Viscosity increases in:

1. Polycythemia
2. Hyperproteinemic states (e.g., multiple myeloma)
3. Hereditary spherocytosis

Resistance is directly proportional to viscosity and inversely proportional to the radius to the 4th power.

Cardiac and vascular function curves

Cardiac cycle

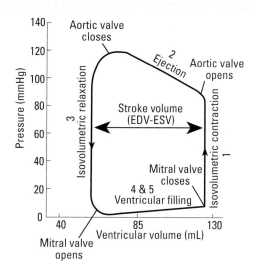

Phases:

1. Isovolumetric contraction—period between mitral valve closure and aortic valve opening; period of highest O_2 consumption
2. Systolic ejection—period between aortic valve opening and closing
3. Isovolumetric relaxation—period between aortic valve closing and mitral valve opening
4. Rapid filling—period just after mitral valve opening
5. Slow filling—period just before mitral valve closure

Sounds:

S1—mitral and tricuspid valve closure.
S2—aortic and pulmonary valve closure.
S3—at end of rapid ventricular filling.
S4—high atrial pressure/stiff ventricle.

S3 is associated with dilated CHF.
S4 ("atrial kick") is associated with a hypertrophic ventricle.

a wave—atrial contraction.
c wave—RV contraction (tricuspid valve bulging into atrium).
v wave— ↑ atrial pressure due to filling against closed tricuspid valve.

Jugular venous distention is seen in right heart failure.

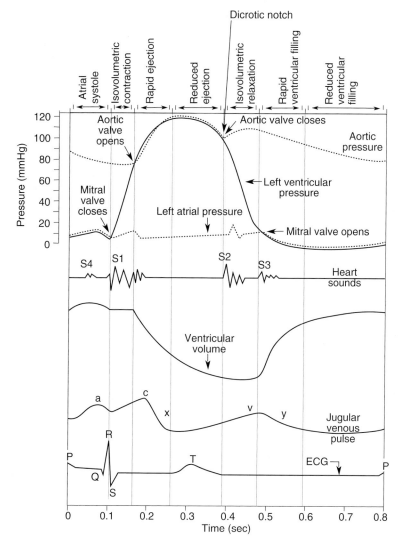

(Adapted, with permission, from Ganong WF. *Review of Medical Physiology*, 19th ed. Stamford, CT: Appleton & Lange, 1999:541.)

HIGH-YIELD FACTS

Physiology

347

Conduction to contraction

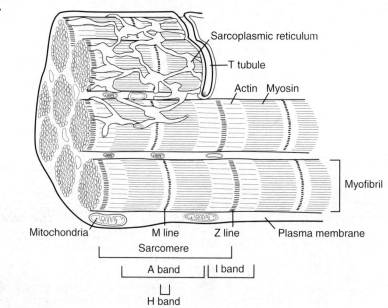

Action potential reaches axon terminal → depolarization opens voltage-gated Ca^{2+} channels and causes neurotransmitter vesicle fusion and exocytosis. Postsynaptic ligand binding leads to depolarization of the postsynaptic (muscle) cell **(A).** Depolarization travels down T tubule. A dihydropyridine receptor (voltage-sensing Ca^{2+} channel protein) lies in the T-tubule membrane next to a ryanodine receptor (voltage-sensing Ca^{2+} channel protein), which lies in the sarcoplasmic reticulum **(B).** Released calcium binds to troponin C, which causes a conformational change and moves tropomyosin out of myosin-binding groove on actin filament. Myosin hydrolyzes its bound ATP and is displaced on the actin filament (power stroke). Contraction results in **HIZ** shrinkage—H, I, and Z bands contract **(B).** A band length stays constant throughout the cycle.

Cardiac myocyte physiology

Cardiac muscle contraction is dependent on extracellular calcium, which enters the cells during plateau of action potential and stimulates calcium release from the cardiac muscle sarcoplasmic reticulum (calcium-induced calcium release).

In contrast to skeletal muscle:

1. Cardiac muscle action potential has a plateau, which is due to Ca^{2+} influx
2. Cardiac nodal cells spontaneously depolarize, resulting in automaticity
3. Cardiac myocytes are electrically coupled to each other by gap junctions

---

Smooth muscle contraction

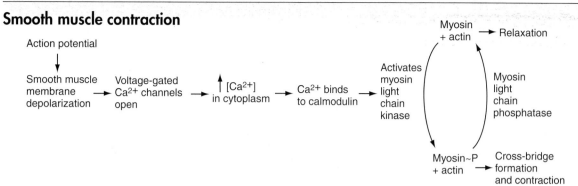

Action potential

Smooth muscle membrane depolarization → Voltage-gated Ca^{2+} channels open → ↑ $[Ca^{2+}]$ in cytoplasm → Ca^{2+} binds to calmodulin → Activates myosin light chain kinase

Myosin + actin → Relaxation

Myosin light chain phosphatase

Myosin~P + actin → Cross-bridge formation and contraction

Skeletal muscle contraction

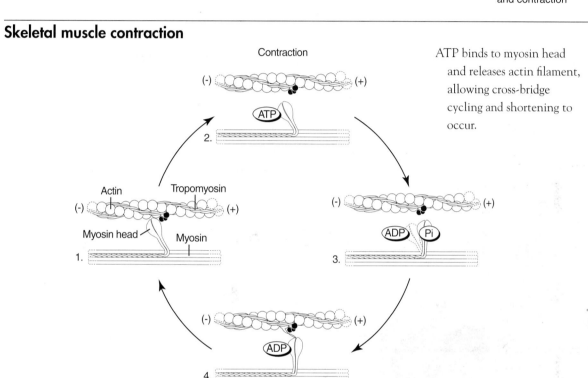

Contraction

(-) (+)

ATP

2.

Actin Tropomyosin

(-) (+)

Myosin head Myosin

1.

(-) (+)

ADP Pi

3.

(-) (+)

ADP

4.

ATP binds to myosin head and releases actin filament, allowing cross-bridge cycling and shortening to occur.

Electrocardiogram

P wave—atrial depolarization.

PR segment—conduction delay through AV node (normally < 200 msec).

QRS complex—ventricular depolarization (normally < 120 msec).

QT interval—mechanical contraction of the ventricles.

T wave—ventricular repolarization.

Atrial repolarization is masked by QRS complex.

ST segment—isoelectric, ventricles depolarized.

U wave—caused by hypokalemia.

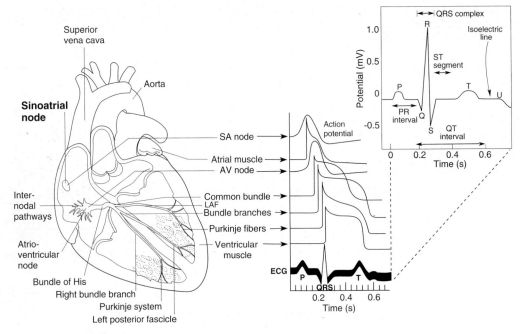

SA node "pacemaker" inherent dominance with slow phase of upstroke
AV node - 100-msec delay - atrioventricular delay

(Adapted, with permission, from Ganong WF. *Review of Medical Physiology*, 20th ed. New York: McGraw-Hill, 2001.)

ECG tracings

Atrial fibrillation   Chaotic and erratic baseline with no discrete P waves in between irregularly spaced QRS complexes.

Atrial flutter   A rapid succession of identical, back-to-back atrial depolarization waves. The identical appearance accounts for the "sawtooth" appearance of the flutter waves.

AV block

1st degree   The PR interval is prolonged (> 200 msec). Asymptomatic.

Prolonged PR interval

2nd degree

Mobitz type I   Progressive lengthening of the PR interval until a beat is "dropped" (a P wave not
(Wenckebach)   followed by a QRS complex). Usually asymptomatic.

Note progressive increase in PR length before dropped beat

ECG tracings (*continued*)

Mobitz type II
Dropped beats that are not preceded by a change in the length of the PR interval (as in type I). These abrupt, nonconducted P waves result in a pathologic condition. It is often found as 2:1 block, where there are 2 P waves to 1 QRS response. May progress to 3rd-degree block.

No QRS following P wave, normal PR intervals

3rd degree (complete)
The atria and ventricles beat independently of each other. Both P waves and QRS complexes are present, although the P waves bear no relation to the QRS complexes. The atrial rate is faster than the ventricular rate. Usually treat with pacemaker.

P on T wave   P wave on ST-T complex

Ventricular fibrillation
A completely erratic rhythm with no identifiable waves. Fatal arrhythmia without immediate defibrillation.

(Adapted, with permission, from Hurst JW. *Introduction to Electrocardiography.* New York: McGraw-Hill, 2001.)

HIGH-YIELD FACTS

Physiology

Control of mean arterial pressure

Arterial baroreceptors

Receptors:
1. Aortic arch transmits via vagus nerve to medulla (responds only to ↑ blood pressure)
2. Carotid sinus transmits via glossopharyngeal nerve to medulla

Hypotension— ↓ arterial pressure → ↓ stretch → ↓ afferent baroreceptor firing → ↑ efferent sympathetic firing and ↓ efferent parasympathetic stimulation → vasoconstriction, ↑ HR, ↑ contractility, ↑ BP. Important in the response to severe hemorrhage.

Carotid massage— ↑ pressure on carotid artery → ↑ stretch → ↓ HR.

Chemoreceptors

Peripheral   Carotid and aortic bodies respond to ↓ P_{O_2} (< 60 mmHg), ↑ P_{CO_2}, and ↓ pH of blood.

Central   Respond to changes in pH and P_{CO_2} of brain interstitial fluid, which in turn are influenced by arterial CO_2. Do not directly respond to P_{O_2}. Responsible for Cushing reaction, response to cerebral ischemia, response to ↑ intracranial pressure → hypertension (sympathetic response) and bradycardia (parasympathetic response).

Circulation through organs

Liver   Largest share of systemic cardiac output.

Kidney   Highest blood flow per gram of tissue.

Heart   Large arteriovenous O_2 difference. ↑ O_2 demand is met by ↑ coronary blood flow, not by ↑ extraction of O_2.

Normal pressures

PCWP—pulmonary capillary wedge pressure (in mmHg) is a good approximation of left atrial pressure. Measured with Swan-Ganz catheter.

Autoregulation

Mechanism—blood flow is altered to meet demands of tissue.

Organ	Factors determining autoregulation
Heart	Local metabolites: O_2, adenosine, NO
Brain	Local metabolites: CO_2 (pH)
Kidneys	Myogenic and tubuloglomerular feedback
Lungs	Hypoxia causes vasoconstriction
Skeletal muscle	Local metabolites: lactate, adenosine, K+
Skin	Sympathetic stimulation most important mechanism—temperature control

Note: the pulmonary vasculature is unique in that hypoxia causes vasoconstriction (in other organs hypoxia causes vasodilation).

Blood

Normal adult blood composition. Note that serum = plasma – clotting factors (e.g., fibrinogen).

Coagulation cascade

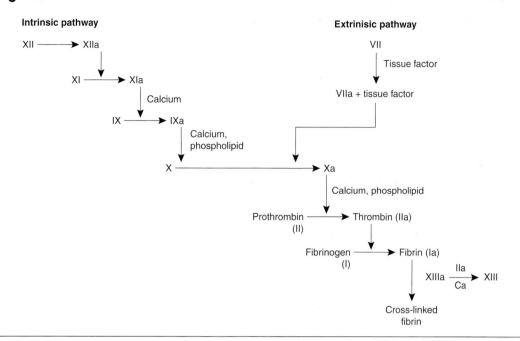

Intrinsic pathway

XII ⟶ XIIa

XI ⟶ XIa

Calcium

IX ⟶ IXa

Calcium, phospholipid

X ⟶ Xa

Extrinsic pathway

VII

Tissue factor

VIIa + tissue factor

Calcium, phospholipid

Prothrombin (II) ⟶ Thrombin (IIa)

Fibrinogen (I) ⟶ Fibrin (Ia)

XIIIa $\xrightarrow{\text{IIa}/\text{Ca}}$ XIII

Cross-linked fibrin

Convergence of coagulation, complement, and kinin pathways

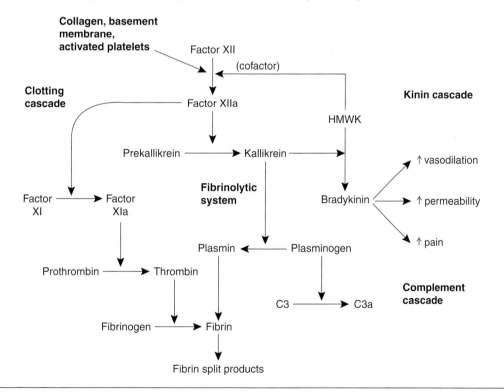

Collagen, basement membrane, activated platelets

Factor XII

(cofactor)

Clotting cascade

Factor XIIa

Prekallikrein ⟶ Kallikrein

Kinin cascade

HMWK

Fibrinolytic system

Factor XI ⟶ Factor XIa

Bradykinin ⟶ ↑vasodilation

⟶ ↑permeability

⟶ ↑pain

Prothrombin ⟶ Thrombin

Plasmin ⟵ Plasminogen

Fibrinogen ⟶ Fibrin

C3 ⟶ C3a

Complement cascade

Fibrin split products

Capillary fluid exchange

Starling forces determine fluid movement by osmosis through capillary membranes:

1. P_c = capillary pressure—tends to move fluid out of capillary
2. P_i = interstitial fluid pressure—tends to move fluid into capillary
3. π_c = plasma colloid osmotic pressure—tends to move fluid into capillary
4. π_i = interstitial fluid colloid osmotic pressure—tends to move fluid out of capillary

Thus, net filtration pressure = P_{net} = $[(P_c - P_i) - (\pi_c - \pi_i)]$.

K_f = filtration constant (capillary permeability).

Net fluid flow = $(P_{net})(K_f)$.

Edema—excess fluid outflow into interstitium that is commonly caused by:

1. ↑ capillary pressure (↑ P_c; heart failure)
2. ↓ plasma proteins (↓ π_c; nephrotic syndrome, liver failure)
3. ↑ capillary permeability (↑ K_f; toxins, infections, burns)
4. ↑ interstitial fluid colloid osmotic pressure (↑ π_i; lymphatic blockage)

Fluid compartments

Total body weight (kg)
- 40% nonwater mass
- 60% total body water (L)
  - 1/3 extracellular fluid
    - 1/4 plasma vol.
    - 3/4 interstitial vol.
  - 2/3 intracellular fluid

TBW – ECF = ICF.

ECF – PV = interstitial volume.

60–40–20 rule (% of body weight):
- 60% total body water
- 40% ICF
- 20% ECF

Renal clearance

$C_x = U_xV/P_x$ = volume of plasma from which the substance is cleared completely per unit time.

If $C_x < GFR$, then there is net tubular reabsorption of X.

If $C_x > GFR$, then there is net tubular secretion of X.

If $C_x = GFR$, then there is no net secretion or reabsorption.

Be familiar with calculations.

C_x = clearance of X.

U_x = urine concentration of X.

P_x = plasma concentration of X.

V = urine flow rate.

Glomerular filtration barrier

Composed of:

1. Fenestrated capillary endothelium (size barrier)
2. Fused basement membrane with heparan sulfate (negative charge barrier)
3. Epithelial layer consisting of podocyte foot processes

The charge barrier is lost in nephrotic syndrome, resulting in albuminuria, hypoproteinemia, generalized edema, and hyperlipidemia.

Glomerular filtration rate	$GFR = U_{inulin} \times V/P_{inulin} = C_{inulin}$ $= K_f [(P_{GC} - P_{BS}) - (\pi_{GC} - \pi_{BS})].$ (GC = glomerular capillary; BS = Bowman's space.) π_{BS} normally equals zero.	Inulin is freely filtered and is neither reabsorbed nor secreted. Clinically, creatinine clearance is a good measure of GFR.
PAH	Secreted in proximal tubule. 2° active transport. Mediated by a carrier system for organic acids; competitively inhibited by probenecid.	
Effective renal plasma flow	$ERPF = U_{PAH} \times V/P_{PAH} = C_{PAH}.$ $RBF = RPF/1 - Hct.$	PAH is filtered and secreted (all PAH entering kidney is excreted).
Filtration fraction		$FF = GFR/RPF.$ $GFR = C_{inulin} \approx C_{creatinine}.$ $RPF = C_{PAH}.$

Free water clearance	Given urine flow rate, urine osmolarity, and plasma osmolarity, be able to calculate free water clearance: $C_{H_2O} = V - C_{osm}.$ V = urine flow rate; $C_{osm} = U_{osm}V/P_{osm}.$	
Glucose clearance	Glucose at a normal level is completely reabsorbed in proximal tubule. At plasma glucose of 200 mg/dL, glucosuria begins (threshold). At 350 mg/dL, transport mechanism is saturated (T_m).	Glucosuria is an important clinical clue to diabetes mellitus.
Amino acid clearance	Reabsorption by at least 3 distinct carrier systems, with competitive inhibition within each group. 2° active transport occurs in proximal tubule and is saturable.	

Nephron physiology

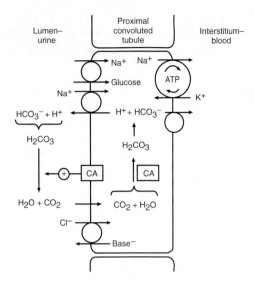

A. Early proximal convoluted tubule—"workhorse of the nephron." Reabsorbs all of the glucose and amino acids and most of the bicarbonate, sodium, and water. Secretes ammonia, which acts as a buffer for secreted H^+.

B. Thin descending loop of Henle—passively reabsorbs water via medullary hypertonicity (impermeable to sodium).

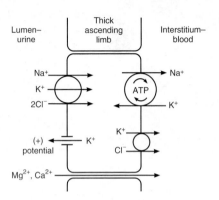

C. Thick ascending loop of Henle—actively reabsorbs Na^+, K^+, and Cl^- and indirectly induces the reabsorption of Mg^{2+} and Ca^{2+}. Impermeable to H_2O.

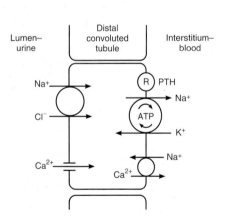

D. Early distal convoluted tubule—actively reabsorbs Na^+, Cl^-. Reabsorption of Ca^{2+} is under the control of PTH.

E. Collecting tubules—reabsorb Na^+ in exchange for secreting K^+ or H^+ (regulated by aldosterone). Reabsorption of water is regulated by ADH (vasopressin). Osmolarity of medulla can reach 1200 mOsm.

HIGH-YIELD FACTS

Physiology

Relative concentrations along renal tubule

$$\frac{TF}{P} = \frac{[\text{Tubular fluid}]}{[\text{Plasma}]}$$

Percent distance along proximal tubule

* Neither secreted nor reabsorbed; concentration increases as water is reabsorbed.

(Adapted, with permission, from Ganong WF. *Review of Medical Physiology*, 20th ed. New York: McGraw-Hill, 2001.)

Renin-angiotensin system

Mechanism	Renin is released by the kidneys upon sensing ↓ BP and cleaves angiotensinogen to angiotensin I (a decapeptide). Angiotensin I is then cleaved by angiotensin-converting enzyme (ACE), primarily in the lung capillaries, to angiotensin II (an octapeptide).
Actions of angiotensin II	1. Potent vasoconstriction
	2. Release of aldosterone from the adrenal cortex
	3. Release of ADH from posterior pituitary
	4. Stimulates hypothalamus → ↑ thirst

Overall, angiotensin II serves to ↑ intravascular volume and ↑ BP.

ANP released from atria may act as a "check" on the renin-angiotensin system (e.g., in heart failure).

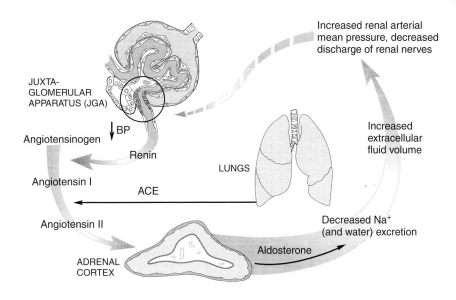

(Adapted, with permission, from Ganong WF. *Review of Medical Physiology*, 20th ed. New York: McGraw-Hill, 2001.)

Kidney endocrine functions

Endocrine functions of the kidney:

1. Endothelial cells of peritubular capillaries secrete erythropoietin in response to hypoxia
2. Conversion of 25-OH vitamin D to 1,25-$(OH)_2$ vitamin D by 1α-hydroxylase, which is activated by PTH
3. JG cells secrete renin in response to $\downarrow$ renal arterial pressure and $\uparrow$ renal sympathetic discharge (β_1 effect)
4. Secretion of prostaglandins that vasodilate the afferent arterioles to increase GFR

NSAIDs can cause acute renal failure in high vascoconstrictive states by inhibiting the renal production of prostaglandins which keep the afferent arterioles vasodilated to maintain GFR.

Hormones acting on kidney

	Stimulus for secretion	Action on kidneys
Vasopressin (ADH)	$\uparrow$ plasma osmolarity $\downarrow\downarrow$ blood volume	$\uparrow$ H_2O permeability of principal cells in collecting ducts $\uparrow$ urea absorption in collecting duct $\uparrow$ $Na^+/K^+/2Cl^-$ transporter in thick ascending limb
Aldosterone	$\downarrow$ blood volume (via angiotensin II) $\uparrow$ plasma [K^+]	$\uparrow$ Na^+ reabsorption, $\uparrow$ K^+ secretion, $\uparrow$ H^+ secretion in distal tubule
Angiotensin II	$\downarrow$ blood volume (via renin)	Contraction of efferent arteriole $\rightarrow$ $\uparrow$ GFR $\uparrow$ Na^+ and HCO_3^- reabsorption in proximal tubule
Atrial natriuretic peptide (ANP)	$\uparrow$ atrial pressure	$\downarrow$ Na^+ reabsorption, $\uparrow$ GFR
PTH	$\downarrow$ plasma [Ca^{2+}]	$\uparrow$ Ca^{2+} reabsorption, $\downarrow$ $(PO_4)^{3-}$ reabsorption, $\uparrow$ 1,25-$(OH)_2$ vitamin D production

Pituitary gland

Posterior pituitary $\rightarrow$ vasopressin and oxytocin, made in the hypothalamus and shipped to pituitary. Derived from neuroectoderm.

Anterior pituitary $\rightarrow$ FSH, LH, ACTH, GH, TSH, melanotropin (MSH), prolactin. Derived from oral ectoderm.

α subunit—common subunit to TSH, LH, FSH, and hCG.

β subunit—determines hormone specificity.

Acidophils—GH, prolactin.

BFLAT Major:
  Basophilic
  FSH
  LH
  ACTH
  TSH
  MSH
T.S.H. and **TSH** = The Sex Hormones and **TSH.**

PTH

Source	Chief cells of parathyroid.
Function	1. ↑ bone resorption of calcium and phosphate
	2. ↑ kidney reabsorption of calcium in distal convoluted tubule
	3. ↓ kidney reabsorption of phosphate
	4. ↑ 1,25-(OH)$_2$ vitamin D (cholecalciferol) production by stimulating kidney 1α-hydroxylase
Regulation	↓ in free serum Ca^{2+} ↑ PTH secretion.

PTH ↑ serum Ca^{2+}, ↓ serum (PO$_4$)$^{3-}$, ↑ urine (PO$_4$)$^{3-}$.
PTH stimulates both osteoclasts and osteoblasts.
PTH = **P**hosphate **T**rashing **H**ormone.

(Adapted, with permission, from Chandrasoma P et al. *Concise Pathology*, 3rd ed. Stamford, CT: Appleton & Lange, 1998:857.)

Shown above are the main actions of PTH and 1,25-(OH)$_2$D in the maintenance of calcium (**A**) and phosphate (**B**) homeostasis.

HIGH-YIELD FACTS

Physiology

Vitamin D

Source	Vitamin D_3 from sun exposure in skin. D_2 from plants. Both converted to 25-OH vitamin D in liver and to 1,25-$(OH)_2$ vitamin D (active form) in kidney.	If you do not get vitamin D, you get rickets (kids) or osteomalacia (adults).
Function	1. ↑ absorption of dietary calcium 2. ↑ absorption of dietary phosphate 3. ↑ bone resorption of Ca^{2+} and $(PO_4)^{3-}$	24,25-$(OH)_2$ vitamin D is an inactive form of vitamin D.
Regulation	↑ PTH causes ↑ 1,25-$(OH)_2$ vitamin D formation. ↓ $[Ca^{2+}]$ ↑ 1,25-$(OH)_2$ vitamin D production. ↓ phosphate causes ↑ 1,25-$(OH)_2$ vitamin D conversion. 1,25-$(OH)_2$ vitamin D feedback inhibits its own production.	

Calcium, phosphate, and alkaline phosphatase levels

	Ca^{2+}	Phosphate	Alkaline phosphatase	Common causes of hypercalcemia—**MISHAP:**
Hyperparathyroidism	↑	↓	↑	**M**alignancy
Paget's disease of bone	N/↑	N	↑↑↑	**I**ntoxication with vitamin D
Vitamin D intoxication	↑	↑	N/↑	
Osteoporosis	N	N	N	**S**arcoidosis
Renal insufficiency	↓	↑	N	**H**yperparathyroidism
				Alkali syndrome
	N = no change.			**P**aget's disease of bone

Calcitonin

Source	Parafollicular cells (C cells) of thyroid.	Calcitonin opposes actions of PTH. It is probably not important in normal calcium homeostasis.
Function	↓ bone resorption of calcium.	
Regulation	↑ in serum Ca^{2+} ↑ secretion.	

Thyroid hormones (T₃/T₄)

Iodine-containing hormones that control the body's metabolic rate.

Source   Follicles of thyroid.

Function

1. Bone growth (synergism with GH)
2. CNS maturation
3. β-adrenergic effects
4. ↑ basal metabolic rate via ↑ Na^+/K^+ ATPase activity = ↑ O_2 consumption, ↑ body temperature
5. ↑ glycogenolysis, gluconeogenesis, lipolysis
6. CV— ↑ CO, HR, SV, contractility, RR

T_3 functions—**4 B's**:

  Brain maturation
  Bone growth
  Beta-adrenergic effects
  BMR ↑

Regulation   TRH (hypothalamus) stimulates TSH (pituitary), which stimulates follicular cells. Negative feedback by T_3 to anterior pituitary ↓ sensitivity to TRH. TSI, like TSH, stimulates follicular cells (Graves' disease).

Steroid/thyroid hormone mechanism

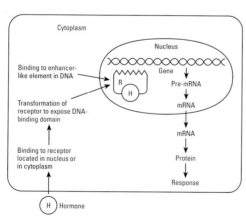

(Adapted, with permission, from Ganong WF. *Review of Medical Physiology*, 20th ed. New York: McGraw-Hill, 2001.)

The need for gene transcription and protein synthesis delays the onset of action of these hormones.

Steroid/thyroid hormones—

PET CAT:

  Progesterone
  Estrogen
  Testosterone
  Cortisol
  Aldosterone
  Thyroxine

Steroid hormones are lipophilic and insoluble in plasma; therefore, they must circulate bound to specific binding globulins, which ↑ solubility and allows for ↑ delivery of steroid to the target organ.

Adrenal steroids

Mineralocorticoids
C21

Glucocorticoids
21C

Androgens
C19

Estrogens
C18

Congenital adrenal hyperplasias

A = **17α-hydroxylase deficiency.** ↓ sex hormones, ↓ cortisol, ↑ mineralocorticoids. Cx = **HYPER**tension, hypokalemia; phenotypically female but no maturation.

B = **21ß-hydroxylase deficiency.** Most common form. ↓ cortisol (increased ACTH), ↓ mineralocorticoids, ↑ sex hormones. Cx = masculinization, female pseudohermaphroditism, **HYPO**tension, hyponatremia, hyperkalemia, ↑ plasma renin activity, and volume depletion. Salt wasting can lead to hypovolemic shock in the newborn.

C = **11ß-hydroxylase deficiency.** ↓ cortisol, ↓ aldosterone and corticosterone, ↑ sex hormones. Cx = masculinization, **HYPER**tension (11-deoxycorticosterone acts as a weak mineralocorticoid).

| **Insulin-dependent organs** | Muscle and adipose tissue depend on insulin for ↑ glucose uptake. Brain and RBCs take up glucose independent of insulin levels (GLUT-1). | Brain and RBCs depend on glucose for metabolism under normal circumstances. Brain uses ketone bodies in starvation. |

Prolactin regulation

Prolactin ↑ dopamine synthesis and secretion from the hypothalamus. Dopamine subsequently **inhibits** prolactin secretion. Dopamine agonists (e.g., bromocriptine) therefore **inhibit** prolactin secretion, whereas dopamine antagonists stimulate prolactin secretion. In females, prolactin inhibits GnRH synthesis and release, which inhibits ovulation. Amenorrhea is commonly seen in prolactinomas.

Prolactin regulation

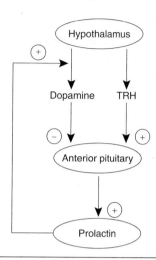

Estrogen

Source
Ovary (estradiol), placenta (estriol), blood (aromatization), testes.

Function
1. Growth of follicle
2. Endometrial proliferation, myometrial excitability
3. Development of genitalia
4. Stromal development of breast
5. Female fat distribution
6. Hepatic synthesis of transport proteins
7. Feedback inhibition of FSH
8. LH surge (estrogen feedback on LH secretion switches to positive from negative just before LH surge)
9. ↑ myometrial excitability

Potency—estradiol > estrone > estriol.

Estrogen hormone replacement therapy after menopause → ↓ hot flashes and ↓ postmenopausal bone loss.

Unopposed estrogen therapy— ↑ risk of endometrial cancer; use of progesterone with estrogen ↓ this risk.

Progesterone

Source
Corpus luteum, placenta, adrenal cortex, testes.

Function
1. Stimulation of endometrial glandular secretions and spiral artery development
2. Maintenance of pregnancy
3. ↓ myometrial excitability
4. Production of thick cervical mucus, which inhibits sperm entry into the uterus
5. ↑ body temperature
6. Inhibition of gonadotropins (LH, FSH)
7. Uterine smooth muscle relaxation

Elevation of progesterone is indicative of ovulation.

Menstrual cycle

Follicular growth is fastest during 2nd week of proliferative phase.

---

hCG

Source	Syncytiotrophoblast of placenta.
Function	1. Maintains the corpus luteum for the 1st trimester by acting like LH. In the 2nd and 3rd trimester, the placenta synthesizes its own estrogen and progesterone and the corpus luteum degenerates.
	2. Used to detect pregnancy because it appears in the urine 8 days after successful fertilization (blood and urine tests available).
	3. Elevated hCG in women with hydatidiform moles or choriocarcinoma.

Menopause

Cessation of estrogen production with age-linked decline in number of ovarian follicles. Average age of onset is 51 years (earlier in smokers).

Hormonal changes:
↓ estrogen, ↑↑ FSH, ↑ LH (no surge), ↑ GnRH.
Menopause causes **HAVOC**:
Hot flashes, **A**trophy of the **V**agina, **O**steoporosis, **C**oronary artery disease.

Androgens

	Testosterone, dihydrotestosterone (DHT), androstenedione.
Source	DHT testosterone (testis, adrenal), androstenedione (adrenal).
Targets	Skin, prostate, seminal vesicles, epididymis, liver, muscle, brain.
Function	1. Differentiation of wolffian duct system into internal gonadal structures 2. 2° sexual characteristics and growth spurt during puberty 3. Required for normal spermatogenesis 4. Anabolic effects— ↑ muscle size, ↑ RBC production 5. ↑ libido

Potency—DHT > testosterone > androstenedione.

Testosterone is converted to DHT by the enzyme 5α-reductase, which is inhibited by finasteride.

Testosterone and androstenedione are converted to estrogen in adipose tissue by enzyme aromatase.

Male spermatogenesis

PRODUCTS	FUNCTIONS OF PRODUCTS
Androgen-binding protein (ABP)	Ensures that testosterone in seminiferous tubule is high
Inhibin	Inhibits FSH
Testosterone	Differentiates male genitalia, has anabolic effects on protein metabolism, maintains gametogenesis, maintains libido, inhibits GnRH, and fuses epiphyseal plates in bone.

FSH → **S**ertoli cells → **S**perm production
LH → **L**eydig cell

Response to high altitude

1. Acute ↑ in ventilation
2. Chronic ↑ in ventilation
3. ↑ erythropoietin → ↑ hematocrit and hemoglobin (chronic hypoxia)
4. ↑ 2,3-DPG (binds to hemoglobin so that hemoglobin releases more O_2)
5. Cellular changes (↑ mitochondria)
6. ↑ renal excretion of bicarbonate (e.g., use of acetazolamide) to compensate for the respiratory alkalosis
7. Chronic hypoxic pulmonary vasoconstriction results in RVH

Important lung products

1. Surfactant—produced by type II pneumocytes, ↓ alveolar surface tension, ↑ compliance
2. Prostaglandins
3. Histamine
4. Angiotensin-converting enzyme (ACE)— angiotensin I → angiotensin II; inactivates bradykinin (ACE inhibitors ↑ bradykinin and cause cough, angioedema)
5. Kallikrein—activates bradykinin

Surfactant—dipalmitoyl phosphatidylcholine (lecithin) deficient in neonatal RDS.

Collapsing pressure =

$$\frac{2 \text{ (tension)}}{\text{radius}}$$

Lung volumes

1. Residual volume (RV)—air in lung at maximal expiration
2. Expiratory reserve volume (ERV)—air that can still be breathed out after normal expiration
3. Tidal volume (TV)—air that moves into lung with each quiet inspiration, typically 500 mL
4. Inspiratory reserve volume (IRV)—air in excess of tidal volume that moves into lung on maximum inspiration
5. Vital capacity (VC)—TV + IRV + ERV
6. Functional reserve capacity (FRC)—RV + ERV (volume in lungs after normal expiration)
7. Inspiratory capacity (IC)—IRV + TV
8. Total lung capacity—TLC = IRV + TV + ERV + RV

Vital capacity is everything but the residual volume.

A capacity is a sum of ≥ 2 volumes.

Oxygen-hemoglobin dissociation curve

When curve shifts to the right, ↓ affinity of hemoglobin for O_2 (facilitates unloading of O_2 to tissue).

An ↑ in all factors (except pH) causes a shift of the curve to the right.

A ↓ in all factors (except pH) causes a shift of the curve to the left.

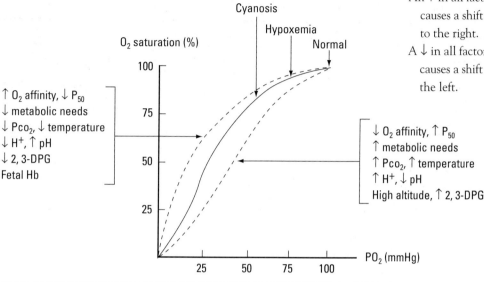

↑ O_2 affinity, ↓ P_{50}
↓ metabolic needs
↓ Pco_2, ↓ temperature
↓ H^+, ↑ pH
↓ 2, 3-DPG
Fetal Hb

↓ O_2 affinity, ↑ P_{50}
↑ metabolic needs
↑ Pco_2, ↑ temperature
↑ H^+, ↓ pH
High altitude, ↑ 2, 3-DPG

Pulmonary circulation

Normally a low-resistance, high-compliance system. Pco_2 exert opposite effects on pulmonary and systemic circulation. A ↓ in Pao_2 causes a hypoxic vasoconstriction that shifts blood away from poorly ventilated regions of lung to well-ventilated regions of lung.

1. Perfusion limited—O_2 (normal health), CO_2, N_2O. Gas equilibrates early along the length of the capillary. Diffusion can be ↑ only if blood flow ↑.
2. Diffusion limited—O_2 (exercise, emphysema, fibrosis), CO. Gas does not equilibrate by the time blood reaches the end of the capillary.

A consequence of pulmonary hypertension is cor pulmonale and subsequent right ventricular failure (jugular venous distention, edema, hepatomegaly).

Determination of physiologic dead space

$$V_D = V_T \times \frac{(Paco_2 - Peco_2)}{Paco_2}$$

$Paco_2$ = arterial Pco_2, $Peco_2$ = expired air Pco_2.

V/Q mismatch

Zone 1 — $P_A > P_a > P_v$

Zone 2 — $P_a > P_A > P_v$

Zone 3 — $P_a > P_v > P_A$

Ideally, ventilation is matched to perfusion (i.e., V/Q = 1) in order for adequate oxygenation to occur efficiently.

Lung zones:
1. Apex of the lung—V/Q = 3 (wasted ventilation)
2. Base of the lung—V/Q = 0.6 (wasted perfusion)

Both ventilation and perfusion are greater at the base of the lung than at the apex of the lung.

With exercise (↑ cardiac output), there is vasodilation of apical capillaries, resulting in a V/Q ratio that approaches 1.

Certain organisms that thrive in high O_2 (e.g., TB) flourish in the apex.

V/Q → 0 = airway obstruction (shunt).

V/Q → ∞ = blood flow obstruction (physiologic dead space).

CO_2 transport

Carbon dioxide is transported from tissues to the lungs in 3 forms:

1. **Bicarbonate (90%)**

CO_2 from peripheral tissue

$CO_2 + H_2O \rightleftarrows H_2CO_3 \rightleftarrows H^+ + HCO_3^-$

Carbonic anhydrase

$HHb \rightleftarrows H^+ + Hb^-$

Cl^-

2. Bound to hemoglobin as carbaminohemoglobin (5%)
3. Dissolved CO_2 (5%)

In lungs, oxygenation of hemoglobin promotes dissociation of CO_2 from hemoglobin (Haldane effect).

In peripheral tissue, ↑ H^+ shifts curve to right, unloading O_2 (Bohr effect).

(Adapted, with permission, from Ganong WF. *Review of Medical Physiology,* 20th ed. New York: McGraw-Hill, 2001.)

Salivary secretion

Source — Parotid, submandibular, and sublingual glands.

Function —
1. α-amylase (ptyalin) begins starch digestion
2. Bicarbonate neutralizes oral bacterial acids, maintains dental health
3. Mucins (glycoproteins) lubricate food

Salivary secretion is stimulated by both sympathetic and parasympathetic activity.

Stomach secretions

	Function	Source
Mucus	Lubricant, protects surface from H^+	Mucous cell
Intrinsic factor	Vitamin B_{12} absorption (in small intestine)	Parietal cell
H^+	Kills bacteria, breaks down food, activates pepsinogen to pepsin	Parietal cell
Pepsinogen	Broken down to pepsin (a protease)	Chief cell
Gastrin	Stimulates acid secretion	G cell

GI secretory products

Product	Source	Function	Regulation	Notes
Intrinsic factor	Parietal cells (stomach)	Vitamin B_{12} binding protein required for vitamin's uptake in terminal ileum		Autoimmune destruction of parietal cells → chronic gastritis → pernicious anemia
Gastric acid	Parietal cells	Lowers pH to optimal range for pepsin function; sterilizes chyme	Stimulated by histamine, ACh, gastrin; inhibited by prostaglandin, somatostatin, and GIP	Not essential for digestion; inadequate acid → ↑ risk of *Salmonella* infections
Pepsin	Chief cells (stomach)	Begins protein digestion; optimal function at pH 1.0–3.0	Stimulated by vagal input, local acid	Inactive pepsinogen converted to pepsin by H^+
Gastrin	G cells of antrum and duodenum	1. Stimulates secretion of HCl, IF, and pepsinogen 2. Stimulates gastric motility	Stimulated by stomach distention, amino acids, peptides, vagus (via GRP); inhibited by secretin and stomach acid pH < 1.5	Hypersecreted in Zollinger-Ellison syndrome → peptic ulcers; phenylalanine and tryptophan are potent stimulators
Bicarbonate	Surface mucosal cells of stomach and duodenum	Neutralizes acid; present in unstirred layer with mucus on luminal surface, preventing autodigestion	Stimulated by secretin (potentiated by vagal input, CCK)	
Cholecystokinin (CCK)	I cells of duodenum and jejunum	1. Stimulates gallbladder contraction 2. Stimulates pancreatic enzyme secretion 3. Inhibits gastric emptying	Stimulated by fatty acids, amino acids	In cholelithiasis, pain worsens after eating fatty foods due to CCK release
Secretin	S cells of duodenum	Nature's antacid: 1. Stimulates pancreatic HCO_3^- secretion 2. Inhibits gastric acid secretion	Stimulated by acid and fatty acids in lumen of duodenum	Alkaline pancreatic juice in duodenum neutralizes gastric acid, allowing pancreatic enzymes to function
Somatostatin	D cells in pancreatic islets, gastrointestinal mucosa	Inhibits: 1. Gastric acid and pepsinogen secretion 2. Pancreatic and small intestine fluid secretion 3. Gallbladder contraction 4. Release of both insulin and glucagon	Stimulated by acid; inhibited by vagus	Highly inhibitory hormone; anti-GH effects (↓ digestion and ↓ absorption of substances needed for growth)

GI secretory products (continued)

Nitric oxide
Causes smooth muscle relaxation (e.g., lower esophageal sphincter [LES] relaxation).

Retroperitoneal
Partially peritonealized
Completely peritonealized

Gastrin
Secreted in response to gastric distention, vagal stimulation, and amino acid entering the stomach; causes gastric H^+ secretion.

Cholecystokinin (CCK)
Secreted in response to amino acids and fatty acids entering the duodenum; causes contraction of gallbladder, relaxation of sphincter of Oddi, and pancreatic secretion of enzymes and HCO_3^-.

Gallbladder

Pancreas

Duodenum

Secretin
Secreted in response to H^+ and fatty acids entering the duodenum; causes pancreatic secretion of HCO_3^- and inhibits gastric H^+ secretion.

Parasympathetic (ACh)
Increases production of saliva; increases gastric H^+ secretion; increases pancreatic enzyme and HCO_3^- secretion; stimulates enteric nervous system to create intestinal peristalsis; relaxes sphincters.

Vasoactive intestinal peptide (VIP)
Secreted by smooth muscle and nerves of intestines; relaxes intestinal smooth muscle; causes pancreatic HCO_3^- secretion and inhibits gastric H^+ secretion.

Sympathetic (NE)
Increases production of saliva; decreases splanchnic blood flow in fight-or-flight response; decreases motility; constricts sphincters.

Cecum

Rectum

(Adapted, with permission, from Mehta S et al. *Step-Up: A High-Yield, Systems-Based Review for the USMLE Step I Examination*. Baltimore: Lippincott Williams & Wilkins, 2000:83.)

HIGH-YIELD FACTS

Physiology

Regulation of gastric acid secretion

Glucose absorption

Occurs at duodenum and proximal jejunum.

Absorbed across cell membrane by sodium-glucose cotransporter.

Pancreatic exocrine secretion

Secretory acini synthesize and secrete zymogens, stimulated by ACh and CCK.

Pancreatic ducts secrete mucus and alkaline fluid when stimulated by secretin.

Pancreatic enzymes

α-amylase—starch digestion, secreted in active form.

Lipase, phospholipase A, colipase—fat digestion.

Proteases (trypsin, chymotrypsin, elastase, carboxypeptidases)—protein digestion, secreted as proenzymes.

Trypsinogen is converted to active enzyme trypsin by enterokinase, a duodenal brush-border enzyme. Trypsin then activates the other proenzymes and can also activate trypsinogen (positive feedback loop).

Pancreatic insufficiency is seen in cystic fibrosis and other conditions. Patients present with malabsorption, steatorrhea (greasy, malodorous stool). Limit fat intake, monitor for signs of fat-soluble vitamin (A, D, E, K) deficiency.

Stimulation of pancreatic functions

Secretin	Stimulates ductal cells to secrete bicarbonate-rich fluid.
Cholecystokinin	Major stimulus for secretion of enzyme-rich fluid by pancreatic acinar cells.
ACh	Major stimulus for zymogen release, poor stimulus for bicarbonate secretion.
Somatostatin	Inhibits the release of gastrin and secretin.

Carbohydrate digestion	Only monosaccharides are absorbed.
Salivary amylase	Starts digestion, hydrolyzes α-1,4 linkages to give maltose, maltotriose, and α-limit dextrans.
Pancreatic amylase	Highest concentration in duodenal lumen, hydrolyzes starch to oligosaccharides, maltose, and maltotriose.
Oligosaccharide hydrolases	At brush border of intestine, the rate-limiting step in carbohydrate digestion, produce monosaccharides (glucose, galactose, fructose).

Bilirubin	Product of heme metabolism, actively taken up by hepatocytes. Conjugated version is water soluble. Jaundice (yellow skin, sclerae) results from elevated bilirubin levels.

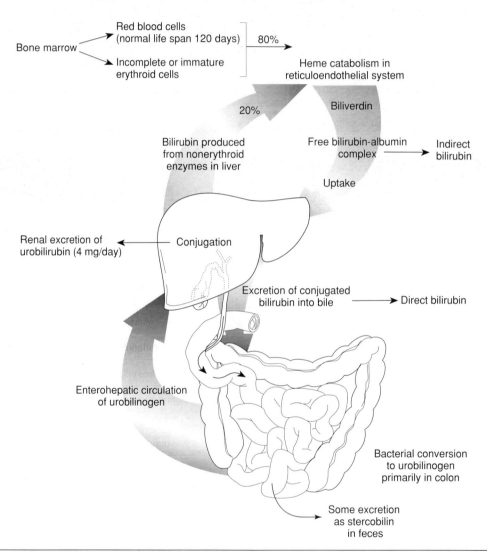

Bone marrow → Red blood cells (normal life span 120 days) / Incomplete or immature erythroid cells — 80% → Heme catabolism in reticuloendothelial system

Biliverdin

20%

Bilirubin produced from nonerythroid enzymes in liver

Free bilirubin-albumin complex → Indirect bilirubin

Uptake

Renal excretion of urobilirubin (4 mg/day) ← Conjugation

Excretion of conjugated bilirubin into bile → Direct bilirubin

Enterohepatic circulation of urobilinogen

Bacterial conversion to urobilinogen primarily in colon

Some excretion as stercobilin in feces

HIGH-YIELD FACTS

Physiology

Bile   Apical surface of hepatocytes faces bile canaliculi. Basolateral surface faces sinusoids.

Rapid Review

The following tables represent a collection of high-yield associations of diseases, "buzzwords," findings, and associated pathologies that may be useful for quick review right before the exam.

Classic Findings
**Most Common
    Associations**
Equation Review

Disease/Finding	Association
Actinic keratosis	Often precedes squamous cell carcinoma
Addison's disease	1° adrenocortical deficiency
Albright's syndrome	Polyostotic fibrous dysplasia, precocious puberty, café-au-lait spots, short stature, young girls
Albuminocytologic dissociation	Guillain-Barré (↑ protein in CSF with only modest ↑ in cell count)
Alport's syndrome	Hereditary nephritis with nerve deafness
Anti–basement membrane	Goodpasture's syndrome
Anticentromere antibodies	Scleroderma (CREST)
Anti-double-stranded DNA antibodies (ANA antibodies)	SLE (type III hypersensitivity)
Anti–epithelial cell	Pemphigus vulgaris
Antigliadin antibodies	Celiac disease
Antihistone antibodies	Drug-induced SLE
Anti-IgG antibodies	Rheumatoid arthritis
Antimitochondrial antibodies	1° biliary cirrhosis
Antineutrophil antibodies	Vasculitis
Antiplatelet antibodies	Idiopathic thrombocytopenic purpura
Arachnodactyly	Marfan's syndrome
Argyll Robertson pupil	Neurosyphilis
Arnold-Chiari malformation	Cerebellar tonsillar herniation
Aschoff bodies	Rheumatic fever
Atrophy of the mammillary bodies	Wernicke's encephalopathy
Auer rods	Acute myelogenous leukemia (especially the promyelocytic type)
Autosplenectomy	Sickle cell anemia
Babinski's sign	UMN lesion
Baker's cyst in popliteal fossa	Rheumatoid arthritis
"Bamboo spine" on x-ray	Ankylosing spondylitis
Bartter's syndrome	Hyperreninemia
Basophilic stippling of RBCs	Lead poisoning
Becker's muscular dystrophy	Defective dystrophin; less severe than Duchenne's
Bell's palsy	LMN CN VII palsy
Bence Jones proteins	Multiple myeloma (kappa or lambda Ig light chains in urine), Waldenström's macroglobulinemia (IgM)

Berger's disease	IgA nephropathy
Bernard-Soulier disease	Defect in platelet adhesion
Bilateral hilar adenopathy, uveitis	Sarcoidosis
Birbeck granules on EM	Histiocytosis X (eosinophilic granuloma)
Bloody tap on LP	Subarachnoid hemorrhage
"Blue bloater"	Chronic bronchitis
Blue-domed cysts	Fibrocystic change of the breast
Blue sclera	Osteogenesis imperfecta
Boot-shaped heart on x-ray	Tetralogy of Fallot; RVH
Bouchard's nodes	Osteoarthritis (PIP swelling 2° to osteophytes)
Boutonnière deformity	Rheumatoid arthritis
Branching rods in oral infection	*Actinomyces israelii*
"Brown tumor" of bone	Hemorrhage causes brown color of osteolytic cysts: 1. Hyperparathyroidism 2. Osteitis fibrosa cystica (von Recklinghausen's disease)
Brushfield's spots	Down syndrome
Bruton's disease	X-linked agammaglobulinemia
Budd-Chiari syndrome	Posthepatic venous thrombosis
Buerger's disease	Small/medium-artery vasculitis
Burkitt's lymphoma	8:14 translocation; associated with EBV
Burton's lines	Lead poisoning
C-ANCA, P-ANCA	Wegener's granulomatosis, polyarteritis nodosa
Café-au-lait spots on skin	Neurofibromatosis
Caisson disease	Gas emboli
Calf pseudohypertrophy	Duchenne's muscular dystrophy
Call-Exner bodies	Granulosa-theca cell tumor of the ovary
Cardiomegaly with apical atrophy	Chagas' disease
Cerebriform nuclei	Mycosis fungoides (cutaneous T-cell lymphoma)
Chagas' disease	Trypanosome infection
Chancre	1° syphilis (not painful)
Chancroid	*Haemophilus ducreyi* (painful)
Charcot's triad	Multiple sclerosis (nystagmus, intention tremor, scanning speech), cholangitis (jaundice, RUQ pain, fever)
Charcot-Leyden crystals	Bronchial asthma (eosinophil membranes)
Chédiak-Higashi disease	Phagocyte deficiency

Cherry-red spot on macula	Tay-Sachs, Niemann-Pick disease, central retinal artery occlusion
Cheyne-Stokes respirations	Central apnea in CHF and ↑ intracranial pressure
"Chocolate cysts"	Endometriosis (frequently involve both ovaries)
Chronic atrophic gastritis	Predisposition to gastric carcinoma
Chvostek's sign	Hypocalcemia (facial muscle spasm upon tapping)
Clear cell adenocarcinoma of the vagina	DES exposure in utero
Clue cells	*Gardnerella* vaginitis
Codman's triangle on x-ray	Osteosarcoma
Cold agglutinins	*Mycoplasma pneumoniae,* infectious mononucleosis
Cold intolerance	Hypothyroidism
Condylomata lata	2° syphilis
Continuous machinery murmur	Patent ductus arteriosus
Cori's disease	Debranching enzyme deficiency
Cotton-wool spots	Chronic hypertension
Cough, conjunctivitis, coryza + fever	Measles
Councilman bodies	Toxic or viral hepatitis
Cowdry type A bodies	Herpesvirus
Crescents in Bowman's capsule	Rapidly progressive crescentic glomerulonephritis
Crigler-Najjar syndrome	Congenital unconjugated hyperbilirubinemia
Curling's ulcer	Acute gastric ulcer associated with severe burns
Currant-jelly sputum	*Klebsiella*
Curschmann's spirals	Bronchial asthma (whorled mucous plugs)
Cushing's ulcer	Acute gastric ulcer associated with CNS injury
D dimers	DIC
Depigmentation of neurons in substantia nigra	Parkinson's disease (basal ganglia disorder—rigidity, resting tremor, bradykinesia)
Dermatitis, dementia, diarrhea	Pellagra (niacin, vitamin B_3 deficiency)
Diabetes insipidus + exophthalmos + lesions of skull	Hand-Schüller-Christian disease
Dog or cat bite	*Pasteurella multocida*
Donovan bodies	Granuloma inguinale
Dressler's syndrome	Post-MI fibrinous pericarditis

Dubin-Johnson syndrome	Congenital conjugated hyperbilirubinemia (black liver)
Duchenne's muscular dystrophy	Deleted dystrophin gene (X-linked recessive)
Eburnation	Osteoarthritis (polished, ivory-like appearance of bone)
Edwards' syndrome	Trisomy 18 associated with rocker-bottom feet, low-set ears, heart disease
Eisenmenger's complex	Late cyanosis shunt (uncorrected L → R shunt becomes R → L shunt)
Elastic skin	Ehlers-Danlos syndrome
Erb-Duchenne palsy	Superior trunk brachial plexus injury ("waiter's tip")
Erythema chronicum migrans	Lyme disease
Fanconi's syndrome	Proximal tubular reabsorption defect
"Fat, female, forty, and fertile"	Acute cholecystitis
Fatty liver	Alcoholism
Ferruginous bodies	Asbestosis
Gardner's syndrome	Colon polyps with osteomas and soft tissue tumors
Gaucher's disease	Glucocerebrosidase deficiency
Ghon focus	Primary TB
Gilbert's syndrome	Benign congenital unconjugated hyperbilirubinemia
Glanzmann's thrombasthenia	Defect in platelet aggregation
Goodpasture's syndrome	Autoantibodies against alveolar and glomerular basement membrane proteins
Gowers' maneuver	Duchenne's (use of patient's arms to help legs pick self off the floor)
Guillain-Barré syndrome	Idiopathic polyneuritis
"Hair-on-end" appearance on x-ray	β-thalassemia, sickle cell anemia (extramedullary hematopoiesis)
Hampton's hump on x-ray	Pulmonary embolism
Hand-Schüller-Christian disease	Chronic progressive histiocytosis
HbS	Sickle cell anemia
hCG elevated	Choriocarcinoma, hyadatidiform mole (occurs with and without embryo)
Heberden's nodes	Osteoarthritis (DIP swelling 2° to osteophytes)
Heinz bodies	G6PD deficiency
Henoch-Schönlein purpura	Hypersensitivity vasculitis associated with hemorrhagic urticaria and URIs
Heterophil antibodies	Infectious mononucleosis (EBV)
HbF	Thalassemia major
High-output cardiac failure (dilated cardiomyopathy)	Wet beriberi (thiamine, vitamin B_1 deficiency)
HLA-B27	Reiter's syndrome, ankylosing spondylitis
HLA-DR3 or -DR4	Diabetes mellitus type 1 (caused by autoimmune destruction of β cells)
Homer Wright rosettes	Neuroblastoma

Honeycomb lung on x-ray	Interstitial fibrosis
Horner's syndrome	Ptosis, miosis, and anhidrosis
Howell-Jolly bodies	Splenectomy (or nonfunctional spleen)
Huntington's disease	Caudate degeneration (autosomal dominant)
Hyperphagia + hypersexuality + hyperorality + hyperdocility	Klüver-Bucy syndrome (amygdala)
Hyperpigmentation of skin	1° adrenal insufficiency (Addison's disease)
Hypersegmented neutrophils	Macrocytic anemia
Hypertension + hypokalemia	Conn's syndrome
Hypochromic microcytosis	Iron deficiency anemia, lead poisoning
Increased α-fetoprotein in amniotic fluid/maternal serum	Anencephaly, spina bifida (neural tube defects)
Increased uric acid levels	Gout, Lesch-Nyhan syndrome, myeloproliferative disorders, loop and thiazide diuretics
Intussusception	Adenovirus (causes hyperplasia of Peyer's patches)
Janeway lesions	Endocarditis
Jarisch-Herxheimer reaction	Syphilis—overaggressive treatment of an asymptomatic patient that causes symptoms due to rapid lysis
Job's syndrome	Neutrophil chemotaxis abnormality
Kaposi's sarcoma	AIDS in MSM (men who have sex with men)
Kartagener's syndrome	Dynein defect
Kayser-Fleischer rings	Wilson's disease
Keratin pearls	Squamous cell carcinoma
Kimmelstiel-Wilson nodules	Diabetic nephropathy
Klüver-Bucy syndrome	Bilateral amygdala lesions
Koilocytes	HPV
Koplik spots	Measles
Krukenberg tumor	Gastric adenocarcinoma with ovarian metastases
Kussmaul hyperpnea	Diabetic ketoacidosis
Lens dislocation + aortic dissection + joint hyperflexibility	Marfan's syndrome (fibrillin deficit)
Lesch-Nyhan syndrome	HGPRT deficiency
Letterer-Siwe disease	Langerhans cell histiocytosis
Lewy bodies	Parkinson's disease
Libman-Sacks disease	Endocarditis associated with SLE

Lines of Zahn	Arterial thrombus
Lisch nodules	Neurofibromatosis (von Recklinghausen's disease)
Low serum ceruloplasmin	Wilson's disease
Lucid interval	Epidural hematoma
"Lumpy-bumpy" appearance of glomeruli on immunofluorescence	Poststreptococcal glomerulonephritis
Lytic bone lesions on x-ray	Multiple myeloma
Mallory bodies	Alcoholic liver disease
Mallory-Weiss syndrome	Esophagogastric lacerations
McArdle's disease	Muscle phosphorylase deficiency
McBurney's sign	Appendicitis
MLF syndrome (INO)	Multiple sclerosis
Monoclonal antibody spike	Multiple myeloma (called the M protein; usually IgG or IgA), MGUS (monoclonal gammopathy of undetermined significance), Waldenström's (M protein = IgM) macroglobulinemia
Myxedema	Hypothyroidism
Necrotizing vasculitis (lungs) and necrotizing glomerulonephritis	Wegener's and Goodpasture's (hemoptysis and glomerular disease)
Needle-shaped, negatively bifringent crystals	Gout
Negri bodies	Rabies
Nephritis + cataracts + hearing loss	Alport's syndrome
Neurofibrillary tangles	Alzheimer's disease
Niemann-Pick disease	Sphingomyelinase deficiency
No lactation postpartum	Sheehan's syndrome (pituitary infarction)
Nutmeg liver	CHF
Occupational exposure to asbestos	Malignant mesothelioma
"Orphan Annie" nuclei	Papillary carcinoma of the thyroid
Osler's nodes	Endocarditis
Owl's eye	CMV
Painless jaundice	Pancreatic cancer (head)
Palpable purpura on legs and buttocks	Henoch-Schönlein purpura
Pancoast's tumor	Bronchogenic apical tumor associated with Horner's syndrome
Pannus	Rheumatoid arthritis
Parkinson's disease	Nigrostriatal dopamine depletion
Periosteal elevation on x-ray	Pyogenic osteomyelitis

Peutz-Jeghers syndrome	Benign polyposis
Peyronie's disease	Penile fibrosis
Philadelphia chromosome (*bcr-abl*)	CML (may sometimes be associated with AML)
Pick bodies	Pick's disease
Pick's disease	Progressive dementia, similar to Alzheimer's
"Pink puffer"	Emphysema (centroacinar [smoking], panacinar [α_1-antitrypsin deficiency])
Plummer-Vinson syndrome	Esophageal webs with iron deficiency anemia
Podagra	Gout (MP joint of hallux)
Podocyte fusion	Minimal change disease
Polyneuropathy, cardiac pathology, and edema	Dry beriberi (thiamine, vitamin B_1 deficiency)
Polyneuropathy preceded by GI or respiratory infection	Guillain-Barré syndrome
Pompe's disease	Lysosomal glucosidase deficiency associated with cardiomegaly
Port-wine stain	Hemangioma
Positive anterior "drawer sign"	Anterior cruciate ligament injury
Pott's disease	Vertebral tuberculosis
Pseudopalisade tumor cell arrangement	Glioblastoma multiforme
Pseudorosettes	Ewing's sarcoma
Ptosis, miosis, anhidrosis	Horner's syndrome (Pancoast's tumor)
Rash on palms and soles	2° syphilis, Rocky Mountain spotted fever
Raynaud's syndrome	Recurrent vasospasm in extremities
RBC casts in urine	Acute glomerulonephritis
Recurrent pulmonary *Pseudomonas* and *S. aureus* infections	Cystic fibrosis
Red urine in the morning	Paroxysmal nocturnal hemoglobinuria
Reed-Sternberg cells	Hodgkin's lymphoma
Reid index (increased)	Chronic bronchitis
Reinke crystals	Leydig cell tumor
Reiter's syndrome	Urethritis, conjunctivitis, arthritis
Renal cell carcinoma + cavernous hemangiomas + adenomas	Von Hippel–Lindau disease

Renal epithelial casts in urine	Acute toxic/viral nephrosis
Rhomboid crystals, positively bifringent	Pseudogout
Rib notching	Coarctation of aorta
Roth's spots in retina	Endocarditis
Rotor's syndrome	Congenital conjugated hyperbilirubinemia
Rouleaux formation (RBCs)	Multiple myeloma
Russell bodies	Multiple myeloma
S3	Left-to-right shunt (VSD, PDA, ASD), mitral regurgitation, LV failure (CHF)
S4	Aortic stenosis, hypertrophic subaortic stenosis
Schiller-Duval bodies	Yolk sac tumor
Senile plaques	Alzheimer's disease
Sézary syndrome	Cutaneous T-cell lymphoma
Sheehan's syndrome	Postpartum pituitary necrosis
Shwartzman reaction	*Neisseria meningitidis*
Signet-ring cells	Gastric carcinoma
Simian crease	Down syndrome
Sipple's syndrome	MEN type IIa
Sjögren's syndrome	Dry eyes, dry mouth, arthritis
Skip lesions	Crohn's
Slapped cheeks	Erythema infectiosum (fifth disease)
Smith antigen	SLE
"Smudge cell"	CLL
Soap bubble on x-ray	Giant cell tumor of bone
Spike and dome on EM	Membranous glomerulonephritis
Spitz nevus	Benign juvenile melanoma
Splinter hemorrhages in fingernails	Endocarditis
Starry-sky pattern	Burkitt's lymphoma
"Strawberry tongue"	Scarlet fever
Streaky ovaries	Turner's syndrome
String sign on x-ray	Crohn's disease
Subepithelial humps on EM	Poststreptococcal glomerulonephritis
Suboccipital lymphadenopathy	Rubella
Sulfur granules	*Actinomyces israelii*

HIGH-YIELD FACTS

Rapid Review

Swollen gums, bruising, poor wound healing, anemia	Scurvy (ascorbic acid, vitamin C deficiency)—vitamin C is necessary for hydroxylation of proline and lysine in collagen synthesis
Systolic ejection murmur (crescendo-decrescendo)	Aortic valve stenosis
t(8;14)	Burkitt's lymphoma (c-*myc* activation)
t(9;22)	Philadelphia chromosome, CML (*bcr-abl* hybrid)
t(14;18)	Follicular lymphomas (*bcl*-2 activation)
Tabes dorsalis	3° syphilis
Tendon xanthomas (classically Achilles)	Familial hypercholesterolemia
Thumb sign on lateral x-ray	Epiglottitis (*Haemophilus influenzae*)
Thyroidization of kidney	Chronic bacterial pyelonephritis
Tophi	Gout
"Tram-track" appearance on LM	Membranoproliferative glomerulonephritis
Trousseau's sign	Visceral cancer, pancreatic adenocarcinoma (migratory thrombophlebitis), hypocalcemia (carpal spasm)
Virchow's node	Left supraclavicular node enlargement from metastatic carcinoma of the stomach
Virchow's triad	Pulmonary embolism (triad = blood stasis, endothelial damage, hypercoagulation)
von Recklinghausen's disease	Neurofibromatosis with café-au-lait spots
von Recklinghausen's disease of bone	Osteitis fibrosa cystica ("brown tumor")
Wallenberg's syndrome	PICA thrombosis
Waterhouse-Friderichsen syndrome	Adrenal hemorrhage associated with meningococcemia
Waxy casts	Chronic end-stage renal disease
WBC casts in urine	Acute pyelonephritis
WBCs in urine	Acute cystitis
Wermer's syndrome	MEN type I
Whipple's disease	Malabsorption syndrome caused by *Tropheryma whippelii*
Wilson's disease	Hepatolenticular degeneration
"Wire loop" appearance on LM	Lupus nephropathy
"Worst headache of my life"	Berry aneurysm—associated with adult polycystic kidney disease
Xanthochromia (CSF)	Subarachnoid hemorrhage
Xerostomia + arthritis + keratoconjunctivitis sicca	Sjögren's syndrome

Zenker's diverticulum	Upper GI diverticulum
Zollinger-Ellison syndrome	Gastrin-secreting tumor associated with ulcers

MOST COMMON ASSOCIATIONS

Most Common ...	
Bacteremia/pneumonia (IVDA)	*S. aureus*
Bacteria associated with cancer	*H. pylori*
Bacteria found in GI tract	*Bacteroides* (second most common is *E. coli*)
Brain tumor (adults)	Mets > astrocytoma (including glioblastoma multiforme) > meningioma > schwannoma
Brain tumor (kids)	Medulloblastoma (cerebellum)
Brain tumor—supratentorial (kids)	Craniopharyngioma
Breast cancer	Infiltrating ductal carcinoma (in the United States, 1 in 9 women will develop breast cancer)
Breast mass	Fibrocystic change (in postmenopausal women, carcinoma is the most common)
Breast tumor (benign)	Fibroadenoma
Bug in debilitated, hospitalized pneumonia patient	*Klebsiella*
Cardiac 1° tumor (adults)	Myxoma (4:1 left to right atrium; "ball and valve")
Cardiac 1° tumor (kids)	Rhabdomyoma
Cardiac tumor (adults)	Mets
Cardiomyopathy	Dilated cardiomyopathy
Chromosomal disorder	Down syndrome (associated with ALL, Alzheimer's dementia, and endocardial cushion defects)
Chronic arrhythmia	Atrial fibrillation (associated with high risk of emboli)
Congenital cardiac anomaly	VSD
Constrictive pericarditis	Tuberculosis
Coronary artery involved in thrombosis	LAD > RCA > LCA
Cyanosis (early; less common)	Tetralogy of Fallot, transposition of great vessels, truncus arteriosus
Cyanosis (late; more common)	VSD, ASD, PDA (close with indomethacin; open with misoprostol)
Demyelinating disease	Multiple sclerosis
Dietary deficit	Iron
Epiglottitis	*Haemophilus influenzae* type B
Esophageal cancer	Squamous cell carcinoma

Gene involved in cancer	p53 tumor suppressor gene
Group affected by cystic fibrosis	Caucasians (fat-soluble vitamin deficiencies, mucous plugs/lung infections)
Gynecologic malignancy	Endometrial carcinoma
Heart murmur	Mitral valve prolapse
Heart valve in bacterial endocarditis	Mitral
Heart valve in bacterial endocarditis in IVDA	Tricuspid
Heart valve (rheumatic fever)	Mitral valve (aortic is 2nd)
Helminth infection (U.S.)	*Enterobius vermicularis* (*Ascaris lumbricoides* is 2nd most common)
Hereditary bleeding disorder	Von Willebrand's
Kidney stones	Calcium = radiopaque (2nd most common is ammonium = radiopaque; formed by urease-positive organisms such as *Proteus vulgaris* or *Staphylococcus*)
Liver disease	Alcoholic liver disease
Location of brain tumors (adults)	Supratentorial
Location of brain tumors (kids)	Infratentorial
Lysosomal storage disease	Gaucher's disease
Male cancer	Prostatic carcinoma
Malignancy associated with noninfectious fever	Hodgkin's disease
Malignant skin tumor	Basal cell carcinoma (rarely metastasizes)
Mets to bone	Breast, lung, thyroid, testes, prostate, kidney
Mets to brain	Lung, breast, skin (melanoma), kidney (renal cell carcinoma), GI
Mets to liver	Colon, gastric, pancreatic, breast, and lung carcinomas
Motor neuron disease	ALS
Neoplasm (kids)	ALL (2nd most common is cerebellar medulloblastoma)
Nephrotic syndrome	Membranous glomerulonephritis
Obstruction of male urinary tract	BPH
Opportunistic infection in AIDS	*Pneumocystis carinii* pneumonia
Organ receiving mets	Adrenal glands (due to rich blood supply)
Organ sending mets	Lung > breast, stomach
Ovarian tumor (benign)	Serous cystadenoma
Ovarian tumor (malignant)	Serous cystadenocarcinoma
Pancreatic tumor	Adenocarcinoma (head of pancreas)
Patient with ALL/CLL/AML/CML	ALL—child, CLL—adult > 60, AML—adult > 60, CML—adult 35–50

Patient with Hodgkin's	Young male (except nodular sclerosis type—female)
Patient with minimal change disease	Young child
Patient with Reiter's	Male
Pituitary tumor	Prolactinoma (2nd—somatotropic "acidophilic" adenoma)
Preventable cancer	Lung cancer
Primary bone tumor (adults)	Multiple myeloma
Primary hyperparathyroidism	Adenomas (followed by hyperplasia, then carcinoma)
Primary liver tumor	Hepatoma
Renal tumor	Renal cell carcinoma—associated with von Hippel–Lindau and acquired polycystic kidney disease; paraneoplastic syndromes (erythropoietin, renin, PTH, ACTH)
Secondary hyperparathyroidism	Hypocalcemia of chronic renal failure
Sexually transmitted disease	*Chlamydia*
Site of diverticula	Sigmoid colon
Site of metastasis	Regional lymph nodes
Site of metastasis (2nd most common)	Liver
Sites of atherosclerosis	Abdominal aorta > coronary > popliteal > carotid
Skin cancer	Basal cell carcinoma
Stomach cancer	Adenocarcinoma
Testicular tumor	Seminoma
Thyroid cancer	Papillary carcinoma
Tracheoesophageal fistula	Lower esophagus joins trachea/upper esophagus—blind pouch
Tumor in men	Prostate carcinoma
Tumor in women	Leiomyoma (estrogen dependent)
Tumor of infancy	Hemangioma
Tumor of the adrenal medulla (adults)	Pheochromocytoma (benign)
Tumor of the adrenal medulla (kids)	Neuroblastoma (malignant)
Type of Hodgkin's	Nodular sclerosis (vs. mixed cellularity, lymphocytic predominance, lymphocytic depletion)
Type of non-Hodgkin's	Follicular, small cleaved
Type of pituitary adenoma	Prolactinoma
Vasculitis	Temporal arteritis (risk of ipsilateral blindness due to thrombosis of ophthalmic artery)
Viral encephalitis	HSV
Vitamin deficiency (U.S.)	Folic acid (pregnant women are at high risk; body stores only 3- to 4-month supply)

HIGH-YIELD FACTS

Rapid Review

Most Frequent Cause of ...	
Addison's	Autoimmune (infection is the 2nd most common cause)
Aneurysm, dissecting	Hypertension
Aortic aneurysm, abdominal and descending aorta	Atherosclerosis
Aortic aneurysm, ascending	3° syphilis
Bacterial meningitis (adults)	*Neisseria meningitidis*
Bacterial meningitis (elderly)	*Streptococcus pneumoniae*
Bacterial meningitis (kids)	*Haemophilus influenzae* type B
Bacterial meningitis (newborns)	*E. coli*
Cancer associated with AIDS	Kaposi's sarcoma
Congenital adrenal hyperplasia	21-hydroxylase deficiency
Cretinism	Iodine deficit/hypothyroidism
Cushing's syndrome	Corticosteroid therapy (2nd most common cause is excess ACTH secretion by pituitary)
Death in CML	Blast crisis
Death in SLE	Lupus nephropathy
Dementia	Alzheimer's (2nd most common is multi-infarct)
DIC	Gram-negative sepsis, obstetric complications, cancer, burn trauma
Ejection click	Aortic/pulmonic stenosis
Food poisoning	*S. aureus*
Glomerulonephritis (adults)	IgA nephropathy (Berger's disease)
Hematoma—epidural	Rupture of middle meningeal artery (arterial bleeding is fast)
Hematoma—subdural	Rupture of bridging veins (trauma; venous bleeding is slow)
Hemochromatosis	Multiple blood transfusions (can result in CHF and ↑ risk of hepatocellular carcinoma)
Hepatic cirrhosis	EtOH
Hepatocellular carcinoma	Cirrhotic liver (often associated with hepatitis B and C)
Holosystolic murmur	VSD, tricuspid regurgitation, mitral regurgitation
Hypertension, 2°	Renal disease
Hypoparathyroidism	Thyroidectomy
Hypopituitarism	Adenoma
Infection in blood transfusion	Hepatitis C

Infection in burn victims	*Pseudomonas*
Leukemia (adults)	AML
"Machine-like" murmur	PDA
Mental retardation	Down syndrome (fragile X is the second most common cause)
MI	Atherosclerosis
Mitral valve stenosis	Rheumatic heart disease
Myocarditis	Coxsackie B
Nephrotic syndrome (adults)	Membranous glomerulonephritis
Nephrotic syndrome (kids)	Minimal change disease (associated with infections/vaccinations; treat with corticosteroids)
Opening snap	Mitral stenosis
Osteomyelitis	*S. aureus*
Osteomyelitis in patients with sickle cell disease	*Salmonella*
Osteomyelitis with IVDA	*Pseudomonas*
Pancreatitis (acute)	EtOH and gallstones
Pancreatitis (chronic)	EtOH (adults), cystic fibrosis (kids)
Peau d'orange	Carcinoma of the breast
PID	*Neisseria gonorrhoeae* (monoarticular arthritis)
Pneumonia, hospital-acquired	*Klebsiella*
Pneumonia in cystic fibrosis, burn infection	*Pseudomonas aeruginosa*
Preventable blindness	*Chlamydia*
Primary amenorrhea	Turner's (XO)
Primary hyperaldosteronism	Adenoma of adrenal cortex
Primary hyperparathyroidism	Adenoma
Pulmonary hypertension	COPD
Right heart failure due to a pulmonary cause	Cor pulmonale
Right-sided heart failure	Left-sided heart failure
Sheehan's syndrome	Postpartum pituitary infarction 2° to hemorrhage
SIADH	Small cell carcinoma of the lung
UTI	*E. coli*
UTI (young women)	*E. coli* and *Staphylococcus saprophyticus*

Topic	Equation	Page
Sensitivity	$\text{Sensitivity} = \dfrac{a}{a + c}$	116
Specificity	$\text{Specificity} = \dfrac{d}{b + d}$	116
Positive predictive value	$PPV = \dfrac{a}{a + b}$	116
Negative predictive value	$NPV = \dfrac{d}{c + d}$	116
Relative risk	$RR = \dfrac{\left[\dfrac{a}{a + b}\right]}{\left[\dfrac{c}{c + d}\right]}$	116
Attributable risk	$AR = \left[\dfrac{a}{a + b}\right] - \left[\dfrac{c}{c + d}\right]$	116
Hardy-Weinberg equilibrium	$p^2 + 2pq + q^2 = 1$ $p + q = 1$	145
Henderson-Hasselbalch equation	$pH = pKa + \log \dfrac{[HCO_3^-]}{0.03\ P_{CO_2}}$	276
Volume of distribution	$V_d = \dfrac{\text{amount of drug in the body}}{\text{plasma drug concentration}}$	288
Clearance	$CL = \dfrac{\text{rate of elimination of drug}}{\text{plasma drug concentration}}$	288
Half-life	$t_{1/2} = \dfrac{0.7 \times V_d}{CL}$	288
Loading dose	$LD = C_p \times \dfrac{V_d}{F}$	288
Maintenance dose	$MD = C_p \times \dfrac{CL}{F}$	288
Cardiac output	$CO = \dfrac{\text{rate of } O_2 \text{ consumption}}{\text{arterial } O_2 \text{ content} - \text{venous } O_2 \text{ content}}$	345
Cardiac output	$CO = \text{stroke volume} \times \text{heart rate}$	345
Mean arterial pressure	$MAP = \text{cardiac output} \times \text{total peripheral resistance}$	345
Mean arterial pressure	$MAP = \tfrac{1}{3}\text{ systolic} + \tfrac{2}{3}\text{ diastolic}$	345
Stroke volume	$SV = \text{end diastolic volume} - \text{end systolic volume}$	345
Ejection fraction	$EF = \dfrac{\text{stroke volume}}{\text{end diastolic volume}} \times 100$	345
Resistance	$R = \dfrac{\text{driving pressure}}{\text{flow}} = \dfrac{8\eta\ (\text{viscosity}) \times \text{length}}{\pi\ r^4}$	346
Net filtration pressure	$P_{net} = \left[(P_c - P_i) - (\pi_c - \pi_i)\right]$	356

Glomerular filtration rate	$GFR = U_{inulin} \times \dfrac{V}{P_{inulin}} = C_{inulin}$	357
Glomerular filtration rate	$GFR = K_f[(P_{GC} - P_{BS}) - (\pi_{GC} - \pi_{BS})]$	357
Effective renal plasma flow	$ERPF = U_{PAH} \times \dfrac{V}{P_{PAH}} = C_{PAH}$	357
Renal blood flow	$RBF = \dfrac{RPF}{1 - Hct}$	357
Filtration fraction	$FF = \dfrac{GFR}{RPF}$	357
Free water clearance	$C_{H_2O} = V - C_{osm}$	357
Physiologic dead space	$V_D = V_T \times \dfrac{(Paco_2 - Peco_2)}{Paco_2}$	369

Database of Recommended Review Resources

This section is a database of current basic science review books, sample examination books, software, Web sites, and commercial review courses that have been **recommended by** medical students studying for the USMLE Step 1. At the end of the section is a list of publishers and independent bookstores with addresses and phone numbers. For each book, we list the Title of the book, the First Author (or editor), the Series Name (where applicable), the Current Publisher, the Copyright Year, the Number of Pages, the ISBN Code, the Approximate List Price, the Format of the book, and the Number of Test Questions. The entries for most books also include Summary Comments that describe their style and overall utility for studying. Finally, each book receives a Rating. Books are sorted into a comprehensive section as well as into sections corresponding to the seven traditional basic medical science disciplines (anatomy, behavioral science, biochemistry, microbiology, pathology, pharmacology, and physiology). Within each section, books are arranged first by Rating and then alphabetically by First Author within each Rating group.

For the 2004 edition of *First Aid for the USMLE Step 1*, the database of rated review books has been reorganized and updated with the addition of many new books and software and with the removal of some older, outdated items. A letter rating scale with six different grades reflects the detailed student evaluations for **Rated Resources.** Each rated resource receives a rating as follows:

A+	Excellent for boards review.
A A–	Very good for boards review; choose among the group.
B+ B	Good, but use only after exhausting better sources.
B–	Fair, but there are many better books in the discipline; or low-yield subject material.

The Rating is meant to reflect the overall usefulness of the resource in preparing for the USMLE Step 1 examination. This is based on a number of factors, including:

- The cost
- The readability of the text
- The appropriateness and accuracy of the material
- The quality and number of sample questions
- The quality of written answers to sample questions
- The quality and appropriateness of the illustrations (e.g., graphs, diagrams, photographs)
- The length of the text (longer is not necessarily better)
- The quality and number of other resources available in the same discipline
- The importance of the discipline for the USMLE Step 1 examination

Please note that ratings do not reflect the quality of the resources for purposes other than reviewing for the USMLE Step 1 examination. Many books with lower ratings are well written and informative but are not ideal for boards preparation. We have not listed or commented on general textbooks available in the basic sciences.

Evaluations are based on the cumulative results of formal and informal surveys of thousands of medical students at many medical schools across the country. The summary comments and overall ratings represent a consensus opinion, but there may have been a broad range of opinion or limited student feedback on any particular resource.

Please note that the data listed are subject to change in that:

- Publishers' prices change frequently.
- Bookstores often charge an additional markup.
- New editions come out frequently, and the quality of updating varies.
- The same book may be reissued through another publisher.

We actively encourage medical students and faculty to submit their opinions and ratings of these basic science review materials so that we may update our database. (See p. xv, How to Contribute.) In addition, we ask that publishers and authors submit for evaluation review copies of basic science review books, including new editions and books not included in our database. We also solicit reviews of new books or suggestions for alternate modes of study that may be useful in preparing for the examination, such as flash cards, computer-based tutorials, commercial review courses, and World Wide Web sites.

Disclaimer/Conflict of Interest Statement

No material in this book, including the ratings, reflects the opinion or influence of the publisher. All errors and omissions will gladly be corrected if brought to the attention of the authors through the publisher. Please note that the entire Underground Clinical Vignette series are independent publications by the authors of this book; their ratings are based solely on data from the student survey and feedback forms.

TOP RATED RESOURCES

 Kaplan Medical (Qbank)   Test/2000+ q
Kaplan
www.kaplanmedical.com
Internet-based question bank providing tailored CBT-format exams. Test content and performance feedback are provided by organ system and discipline. Questions are representative in style and at times content to those on the actual exam. Reading the often detailed explanations is time well spent. There is a free online demonstration; costs vary with subscription period. Requires time commitment.

 WebPath: The Internet Pathology Laboratory   Review/290 q
Klatt
www-medlib.med.utah.edu/WebPath/webpath.html
Features a wealth of outstanding gross and microscopic illustrations, clinical vignette questions, and case studies. Contains many classic, high-quality illustrations. Includes 21 exams with more than 290 questions that reflect current boards format and difficulty level but are typically shorter. Online exams include illustrations and a timer. A WebPath CD-ROM is available for $60.00 and features the online Web site plan supplemented with 40% more material, including additional topics, tutorials, and radiology. The CD-ROM is ideal for computers with slow or no Internet access. May be ordered directly from the Web site.

 Digital Anatomist Interactive Atlases   Review
University of Washington
www9.biostr.washington.edu/da.html
Good site containing an interactive neuroanatomy course along with a three-dimensional atlas of the brain, thorax, and knee. Atlases have computer-generated images along with cadaver dissections. Each atlas also has a useful quiz in which users identify structures in the slide images. Excellent source for reviewing neuro images.

 Introduction to Clinical Microbiology   Review
http://medic.med.uth.tmc.edu/path/00001450.htm
Basic introduction to and review of the fundamentals of microbiology. Includes a useful review of the different types of culture media and lab tests. The information on bugs is a shallow but quick read.

REVIEW RESOURCES

World Wide Web Sites

B | The Whole Brain Atlas

Review

Johnson

www.med.harvard.edu/AANLIB/home.html

Collection of high-quality brain MR and CT images with views of normal, aging, and diseased brains (CVA, degenerative, neoplastic, and inflammatory diseases). The interface is technologically impressive but complex. Guided tours and image correlation to cases are especially useful. Although not all of the images are particularly high yield for the boards, this is an excellent introduction to neuroimaging.

B | Active Learning Centre

Test/100+ q

Turchin

www.med.jhu.edu/medcenter/quiz/home.cgi

Quiz engine site based on a large database with an extensive list of bugs, drugs, and vaccines. Questions generated test the basic characteristics of each element in the database in a multiple-choice, matching, or essay format that the user selects. Questions are not boards style but are useful for learning the memory-intensive subjects of microbiology and pharmacology.

B– | Blackwell's Step 1 Online Q&A

Review

www.blackwellmedstudent.com

Full-length, seven-block, 350-question practice exam in a format similar to the real exam. Questions are written by students who recently took Step 1. Questions do not come with explanations. Some students report multiple errors and an awkward interface. Limited student feedback.

B– | Medrevu.com (irevu)

Test/4500+ q

www.medrevu.com

Subscription-based site that is affiliated with Lippincott Williams & Wilkins and features more than 4500 USMLE-style questions. Questions vary in quality, and some are not in vignette style. Costs vary with subscription period. Includes a free 50-question demonstration. Site organization could be improved. Questions may be more difficult than those of Qbank. Less expensive than Qbank.

REVIEW RESOURCES

World Wide Web Sites

TOP RATED RESOURCES

 Pathophysiology for the Boards and Wards—USMLE Step 1
$32.95   Review only
Ayala
Blackwell Science, 2003, 352 pages, ISBN 1405103426
System-based outline with a focus on pathology. Superior organization with color glossy photos and excellent, concise tables. Includes clinical scenarios and a few questions at the end of each chapter. The appendix has a helpful overview of neurology, immunology, "zebras," syndromes, and pearls.

 Blackwell's Underground Clinical Vignettes Step 1 Bundle
$199.00   Review
Bhushan
Blackwell Science, 2002, 9 volumes, ISBN 0632045590
All nine volumes of the UCV Step 1 books bundled with a free, 50-plus-page *Basic Science Color Atlas* containing more than 250 full-color photographs linked to the vignette cases. Designed for easy quizzing. The atlas includes histology, gross pathology, hematology, and microbiology images. Case-based vignettes provide a good review supplement. Best if started early with coursework.

 Blueprints Step 1 Q&A
$28.95   Test
Clement
Blackwell Science, 2003, 160 pages, ISBN 140510323X
Contains one full-length exam of 350 questions split into blocks of 50. Written by students. Excellent for practicing the multistep questions that are becoming increasingly prevalent on the real thing. High yield.

 Rapid Review for USMLE Step 1
$33.95   Review/1400 q
Goljan
Mosby, 2002, 215 pages, ISBN 0323008410
Outline format with high-yield marginal notes, figures, and tables that highlight key content. Narrative clinical boxes illustrate clinical relevance. Practice exams provide clinically oriented questions. Includes a CD-ROM of questions. Represents the actual format of the exam.

A⁻ **Step Up: A High-Yield Systems-Based Review for the USMLE Step 1**

$34.95   Review only

Mehta

Lippincott Williams & Wilkins, 2003, 360 pages, ISBN 0781737931

Comprehensive and unique organ-system-based review text composed primarily of outlines, charts, tables, and diagrams. The appendix includes 38 clinical cases and an alphabetical section on pharmacology. The organ system format appeals to many students. Includes good "quick hit" factoids. Revised edition for 2003.

B⁺ **USMLE Step 1 (REA)**

$39.95   Review/1080 q

Cargan

REA, 2001, 1200 pages, ISBN 0878910743

Contains three full-length practice exams with more than 2100 questions covering the full range of USMLE topics. Similar in content to the actual exam, but somewhat outdated in its organization. Useful for quick study.

B⁺ **Board Simulator Series**

$25.95 (each)   Test/770 q

Gruber

Lippincott Williams & Wilkins

Body Systems Reviews I: 1997, 375 pages, ISBN 0683302981

Body Systems Reviews II: 1997, 375 pages, ISBN 068330299X

Body Systems Reviews III: 1997, 375 pages, ISBN 0683303007

General Principles in the Basic Sciences: 1997, 375 pages, ISBN 0683302965

Normal and Abnormal Processes in the Basic Sciences: 1997, 375 pages, ISBN 0683302973

USMLE Step 1 Board Simulator on CD-ROM for Windows (includes all volumes), 2000, ISBN 0781792657, $99.95

Four exams per book with approximately 160 questions each. Follows the USMLE content outline. Numerous vignettes reflect the clinical slant of the exam, but questions need updating. Includes good black-and-white photographs. The comprehensive systems-based approach is most effective if all three "Reviews" books are used. For the motivated student. Questions tend to be more picky than those of the actual USMLE exam. Explanations discuss important concepts. *General Principles* has some overlap with *Normal and Abnormal Processes*. *Normal and Abnormal Processes* can be used independently, as it covers all seven major subject areas. The CD-ROM for Windows allows customized testing and performance feedback.

B+ **Kaplan's Organ-Based Review Books**   **$499.00** Review/1200 q
Kaplan

Kaplan, 2002, Item 63410104, ISBN 0X63410101

Includes two organ-system-based review books, a test-taking and strategy guide, a Qbook of 850 questions, and a CD-ROM with 350 questions in one full-length simulation. Very dense and comprehensive. Useful only if started early, possibly with coursework. Excellent as a reference for studying. Somewhat expensive for the amount of material. The software is also available separately. Books and CD-ROMs can be purchased by calling 1-800-KAP-ITEM.

B+ **Appleton & Lange's Review for the USMLE Step 1**   **$39.95** Test/1200 q
King

McGraw-Hill, 2002, 481 pages, ISBN 0071377425

Features seven subject-based tests and three 100-question comprehensive exams. Good buy for the number of questions. Gives thorough explanations of right and wrong answers. Offers a reasonable, straightforward, question-based review to assess your strengths and weaknesses. Testing includes references to diagrams, images, and a few color plates. Revised and updated to current USMLE format.

B+ **NMS Review for USMLE Step 1 Examination, 6th ed.**   **$42.95** Test/1000+ q
Lazo

Lippincott Williams & Wilkins, 2002, 442 pages (plus CD-ROM), ISBN 0781732921

Good source of practice questions and answers. The newest edition features clinically based integrated content with an increased number of patient-based questions. Some questions are too picky or difficult. Includes good annotated explanations, but occasionally gives unnecessary detail. Organized as four 200-question booklets, making it good for simulating exam conditions, yet clinical vignettes with multiple questions per case description do not reflect current boards format. Color plates are helpful. The CD-ROM provides practice with the computer-based format but is disorganized. A good buy for the number of questions.

B+ **NMS USMLE Step 1**   **$49.95** Software/1000+ q
Lazo

Lippincott Williams & Wilkins, 1998, ISBN 0683300954

Windows/Mac-based testing software. Features questions from Lazo's *NMS Review for USMLE Step 1*. Organized as four comprehensive tests. Flexible test modes. Questions are well written and include frequent clinical vignettes. Illustrations are poorly reproduced. Does not accurately reflect the CBT format.

B+ **Clinical Vignettes for the USMLE** $24.95 Test/400 q
Step 1: PreTest
McGraw-Hill
McGraw-Hill, 2002, 332 pages, ISBN 0071373764
Clinical vignette–style questions with detailed explanations. Covers all
the basic sciences. Serves as a good self-evaluation tool, although ques-
tions may not mirror those on the actual USMLE exam.

B+ **Crashing the Boards: USMLE Step 1** $24.95 Review only
Yeh
Lippincott Williams & Wilkins, 1999, 184 pages, ISBN 0781719771
Brief coverage of high-yield topics. Great diagrams; exhibits a good sense
of humor. No photos. Good organization (bulleted facts and highlighted
boxing). Useful for supplementary, last-minute review. Incomplete and
outdated book reviews are included in the back. Retains outdated strategies for the paper-and-pencil exam. Compare with Carl's *Medical
Boards—Step 1 Made Ridiculously Simple*.

B **Blackwell's UCV Basic Science** $34.95 Review
Color Atlas
Bhushan
Blackwell, 2003, 160 pages, ISBN 1405103833
Supplement to the UCV series. Offers 250 clinical exam photographs cov-
ering gross pathology, microscopic pathology, hematology, and microbiol-
ogy. Excellent pictures, but difficult to locate specific images quickly. La-
beling and organization could be improved.

B **Integrated Basic Sciences: PreTest** $29.95 Review/453 q
Brown
McGraw-Hill, 1998, 304 pages, ISBN 007052551X
Great clinical review questions. Each of the 151 vignettes is followed by a
group of three questions testing anatomy and normal and abnormal function. Answers are discussed in detail. Covers many core diseases, organized
by system. Time-consuming; for the motivated student.

B **Medical Boards—Step 1 Made** $29.95 Review only
Ridiculously Simple
Carl
MedMaster, 2003, 367 pages, ISBN 0940780593
Quick and easy reading. The table and chart format is organized by sub-
ject. Mixed reviews. Some charts are poorly labeled. Consider as an ad-
junct. Compare with Yeh's *Crashing the Boards: USMLE Step 1*.

Rapid Preparation for USMLE Step 1

$36.00   Test/926 q

Johnson

J&S Publishing, 1997, 406 pages, ISBN 1888308028

A "best of J&S" compendium. Questions are organized by subject and are drawn as exact duplicates from other books in the series. Includes thorough explanations with key concepts in boldface; however, some are incomplete or inaccurate. Also features high-quality black-and-white MR and CT images, line drawings, histology, and gross photo illustrations. Clinical vignette–based questions.

B **Gold Standard Prep Set for USMLE Step 1**

$265.00   Audiotapes

Knouse

Gold Standard, 2001

Set of 48 approximately 90-minute audiotapes covering USMLE Step 1 material. Limited but positive feedback on updated and expanded set of audiotapes. Popular among some students as a way to review while driving, while working out, and during down time. Contains some inaccuracies. Available only by mail order; call (740) 592-4124, fax (740) 592-4045, or visit www.boardprep.net.

B **Cracking the Boards: USMLE Step 1**

$34.95   Review/400 q

Princeton Review

Random House, 2000, 832 pages, ISBN 0375761632

Comprehensive text review based on the USMLE content outline, written by past and present medical students. The style is wordy and broad spectrum but offers few details. The organ-based format appeals to some students. Includes many labeled illustrations, charts, and photos. Student opinion varies widely.

B **USMLE Step 1 Recall: Buzzwords for the Boards**

$32.95   Review only

Reinheimer

Lippincott Williams & Wilkins, 1999, 304 pages, ISBN 0683306391

Quizzes on main topics and key points in a two-column question-and-answer format. Good for self-testing, group study, and quick review. Use as a change of pace; hits many important clinical features but is not comprehensive or tightly organized. Sometimes focuses on obscure details and memorization rather than on the comprehension and integration that the real exam emphasizes.

B **USMLE Step 1 Recall PDA:**
Buzzwords for the Boards
Reinheimer

$32.95   Software/1000+ q

Lippincott Williams & Wilkins, 2001, ISBN 078173343X
Derived from the book of the same name, but for the PDA. Useful for
quick review.

B **Preparation for the USMLE Step 1 Basic**
Medical Sciences, Volumes A, B, C
Waintrub

$15.00   Test/315 q
(each)

Maval Publishing, 1999, 78 pages, ISBN 1884083137 (Vol. A),
1884083145 (Vol. B), 1884083153 (Vol. C)
Three tests with appropriate-format, straightforward questions and explanatory answers. Includes a suggested time frame for test simulation.
Moderate clinical orientation. Good color photographs. Moderately expensive for the number of questions.

B **Preparation for the USMLE Step 1 Basic**
Medical Sciences, Volumes D, E
Waintrub

$15.00   Test/210 q
(each)

Maval Publishing, 1995, 57 pages, ISBN 1884083161
Same format and comments as for Volumes A, B, and C, but even more
expensive for the number of questions.

B **Preparation for the USMLE Step 1 Basic**
Medical Sciences, Volume F
Waintrub

$18.00   Test/540 q

Maval Publishing, 1997, 150 pages, ISBN 1884083080
Six practice tests and answers; otherwise same comments as for Volumes
A through E. Free with the purchase of the *USMLE Review Book* (listed
separately) from the Maval Publishing Web site.

B **USMLE Step 1 Simulated Test 1 & 2**
Walling

$18.00   Test/515 q
(each)

Maval Publishing, 1999, 87 pages, ISBN 1884083188 (Test 1), ISBN
1884083196 (Test 2)
Two 90-question simulated exams in each booklet covering all the basic
science topics. Clinically oriented, but questions are simplistic. Good images. Moderately expensive for the amount of material.

Exam Master Step 1   **$149.00**   Software/8000 q
Exam Master
Exam Master Corporation, 2001, ISBN 1581290683
Windows/Mac-based testing software with access to up to 8000 Step 1
questions. Questions are relatively simple, but some are obscure. Offers
the ability to hide multiple-choice options. The new version eliminates K-
type, nonclinical questions and provides compatibility with Windows 98.

 Rypins' Basic Sciences Review, Vol. I   **$39.95**   Review/1000+ q
Frohlich
Lippincott Williams & Wilkins, 2001, 832 pages, ISBN 0781725186
Multitopic textbook with few figures and tables. A good general reference,
but should be used with other subject-specific sources. Well priced for the
number of pages and questions. Requires extensive time commitment. Includes good pathology/pharmacology coverage.

 Rypins' Questions and Answers   **$34.95**   Test/1600+ q
for Basic Sciences Review
Frohlich
Lippincott Williams & Wilkins, 2001, 288 pages, ISBN 0781725208
Questions with answers to supplement *Rypins' Basic Sciences Review*. De-
cent overall question-based review of all subjects. Good-quality questions,
but answers lack detail. Requires time commitment. Includes a CD-ROM.

 USMLE Step 1: The Stanford Solutions   **$18.95**   Answers
to the NBME Computer-Based Sample
Test Questions
Kush
Planet Med Publishing, 1999, 110 pages, ISBN 1893730077
Explanations, with references, of the NBME practice CD-ROM. Expen-
sive for the amount of material.

 Laughing Your Way to Passing the USMLE   **$19.95**   Review only
Volume 1: Basic Sciences
Silverstein
MedHumor Publications, 2001, 200 pages, ISBN 0970028733
USMLE review–oriented crossword puzzle book containing more than 750
frequently tested facts, concepts, and key disease associations, presented in
a way that facilitates learning. Organized by the traditional basic sciences.
Style may not work for most students. Limited student feedback. Also
available at www.passtheboards.com.

B- **USMLE Review Book, Step 1**
Basic Medical Sciences

$18.00   Review only

Walling

Maval Publishing, 1999, 290 pages, ISBN 1884083218

Detailed summaries of important information, organized by USMLE content outline. Consists primarily of text, with some tables, photos, and diagrams. Requires time commitment; not for quick review. Limited student feedback.

TOP RATED RESOURCES

 High-Yield Embryology — $24.95 — Review only

Dudek

Lippincott Williams & Wilkins, 2000, 192 pages, ISBN 0781721326
Excellent, concise review of embryology for the USMLE. Features superior organization with clinical correlations. Includes a high-yield list of embryologic origins of tissues. Expensive for the amount of material. No index or review questions.

 High-Yield Gross Anatomy — $24.95 — Review only

Dudek

Lippincott Williams & Wilkins, 2001, 200 pages, ISBN 0781730430
Excellent, concise review with clinical correlations. Contains well-labeled, high-yield radiologic images, but may be useful to supplement with an atlas. No index.

 High-Yield Neuroanatomy — $24.95 — Review only

Fix

Lippincott Williams & Wilkins, 2000, 168 pages, ISBN 0683307215
Clean, easy-to-read outline format. Straightforward text with excellent diagrams and illustrations. The first several chapters are particularly good. Compare with Goldberg's *Clinical Neuroanatomy Made Ridiculously Simple*. No index.

B⁺ Underground Clinical Vignettes: Anatomy — $22.95 — Review only

Bhushan

Blackwell Science, 2002, 144 pages, ISBN 0632045418
Concise clinical cases illustrating approximately 100 frequently tested diseases with an anatomic basis. Cardinal signs, symptoms, and buzzwords are highlighted. Use as a supplement to other sources of review.

B⁺ Liebman's Neuroanatomy Made Easy & Understandable — $31.00 — Review/Few q

Gertz

Aspen, 1999, 210 pages, ISBN 0834216329
Easy-to-read text containing excellent diagrams. Offers a fast, straightforward, high-yield review. Some humor and interesting facts help the student remember pathways. Expensive. Incomplete, but more thorough than Goldberg's *Clinical Neuroanatomy Made Ridiculously Simple*.

B+ **Clinical Neuroanatomy Made Ridiculously Simple** $13.95   Review/Few q

Goldberg

MedMaster, 2000, 97 pages, ISBN 0940780461

Easy to read, memorable, and simplified, with clever hand-drawn diagrams. Offers a quick, high-yield review of clinical neuroanatomy. Good emphasis on clinically relevant pathways, cranial nerves, and neurologic diseases. Offers only spotty coverage of some key boards topics, and includes no CT or MR images. Format is somewhat difficult to follow. Compare with Fix's *High-Yield Neuroanatomy*.

B+ **Anatomy: Review for USMLE Step 1** $25.00   Test/560 q

Johnson

J&S Publishing, 1998, 275 pages, ISBN 1888308036

Easy-to-read text offering clinical case-based questions with detailed explanations. Offers a good superficial overview of cell biology, histology, gross anatomy, embryology, and neuroanatomy. Discusses clinically relevant anatomic science with good explanations, illustrations, and pictures; also covers many clinically relevant genetic diseases. Some key topics are not covered. Includes good photomicrographs, cross-sectional imaging-based questions, and patient photos.

B+ **Wheater's Functional Histology** $59.95   Review only

Young

Churchill Livingstone, 2000, 424 pages, ISBN 0443056129

Color atlas with pictures of normal histology and accompanying text. Useful as a text for coursework; skim through photomicrographs for USMLE review. Image captions provide an excellent source for review of basic cell biology.

B **Cell Biology: Review for New National Boards** $25.00   Review/524 q

Adelman

J&S Publishing, 1995, 203 pages, ISBN 0963287389

Question-based review format like that of other J&S books. Covers classic topics in cell biology. Contains some high-quality micrographs. Recycles some questions and illustrations from J&S's *Anatomy*. Not as useful as other books in the series.

B **Color Atlas of Embryology** $36.00   Review only

Drews

Thieme, 1996, 421 pages, ISBN 0865775443

Embryology presented through use of 176 color plates. Topics range from the basics of reproductive biology to general embryology and subjects related to cellular and molecular biology.

B ## BRS Embryology   **$29.95**   Review/500 q
Dudek
Lippincott Williams & Wilkins, 1998, 293 pages, ISBN 0683302728
Outline-based review of embryology that is typical for books in this series.
Good review of important embryology, but too detailed. A good discussion
of congenital malformations is included at the end of each chapter along
with questions. A comprehensive exam at the end of the book is the most
high-yield part of the book.

B ## High-Yield Histology   **$24.95**   Review only
Dudek
Lippincott Williams & Wilkins, 2000, 232 pages, ISBN 0781721342
Quick and easy review of a relatively low-yield subject. Tables include
some high-yield information. Good pictures. The appendix contains clas-
sic electron micrographs.

B ## BRS Neuroanatomy   **$32.95**   Review/500 q
Fix
Lippincott Williams & Wilkins, 2001, 528 pages, ISBN 0781728290
Updated text covers anatomy and embryology of the nervous system.
Complete but lengthy; requires time commitment. Compare with *High-
Yield Neuroanatomy* by the same author.

B ## Clinical Anatomy Made Ridiculously Simple   **$19.95**   Review only
Goldberg
MedMaster, 2002, 175 pages, ISBN 0940780534
Easy reading, simple diagrams, and lots of mnemonics and amusing associations. Incomplete. Humorous style has variable appeal to students, so
browse before buying. Offers good coverage of selected topics. Best if used
during coursework.

B ## Netter's Atlas of Human Physiology   **$39.95**   Review only
Hansen
Icon Learning Systems, 2002, 250 pages, ISBN 1929007019
Organ-system-based text with more than 250 of Dr. Netter's classic illus-
trations. Offers a clear, concise, "big picture" view of physiology. May be
too detailed for boards review. Limited student feedback.

B **Clinical Anatomy** $30.95 Review/264 q

Monkhouse

Churchill Livingstone, 2001, 336 pages, ISBN 0443063958
Reviews core concepts in human clinical anatomy, integrating systemic
and regional anatomical description with text boxes highlighting clinical
applications. Self-assessment questions are included at the end of each
section. Nicely illustrated and well written. Limited student feedback.

B **Review Questions for Neuroanatomy:** $24.95 Test/965 q
Structural and Functional

Mosenthal

CRC Press–Parthenon, 1996, 134 pages, ISBN 1850706530
Good, non-boards-style questions with explanations. Some diagrams with
questions on lesions are included throughout. Includes embryology of the
nervous system. Best of series. Some clinical vignettes.

B **Clinical Neuroanatomy: A Review** $32.00 Review/440 q
with Questions and Explanations

Snell

Lippincott Williams & Wilkins, 2001, 336 pages, ISBN 0781729890
Comprehensive review book requiring time commitment. Features frequent clinical correlations and many clear diagrams. Reorganized to integrate structure with function in a systems format.

B **Digging Up the Bones: Neuroscience** $21.95 Review only

Yarzagaray

McGraw-Hill, 1999, 197 pages, ISBN 0070383693
Dense text with few figures and tables. Limited student feedback.

B⁻ **Anatomy Recall** $32.95 Review only

Blackbourne

Lippincott Williams & Wilkins, 2000, 368 pages, ISBN 0683304364
Q&A format. Good for quick review, but may be too detailed for boards
review.

B⁻ **Neuroanatomy: Review for USMLE** $25.00 Review/524 q
Step 1

Brown

J&S Publishing, 2001, 235 pages, ISBN 1888308117
Twelve chapters covering various areas of neuroanatomy. Contains general
questions, short clinical scenarios followed by questions related to the
clinical case, and anatomical matching sections. Figures are crudely
drawn. Questions are not in current USMLE format.

B– **Oklahoma Notes Neuropathology and Basic Neuroscience**

$29.95 Review/101 q

Brumback

Springer-Verlag, 1996, 186 pages, ISBN 0387946357

Uses an organ system approach by integrating CNS anatomy, pathology, physiology, and some pharmacology. Easy to read. Includes high-quality line drawings. Use either with an organ system review or as a supplement to a subject review. Limited student feedback.

B– **BRS Gross Anatomy**

$32.95 Review/500 q

Chung

Lippincott Williams & Wilkins, 2000, 468 pages, ISBN 0683307274

Detailed, lengthy text in outline format with illustrations and tables. Better for coursework than for quick boards review. Good clinical correlation section.

B– **Neuroanatomy: Illustrated**

$42.95 Review only

Crossman

Churchill Livingstone, 2000, 202 pages, ISBN 0443062161

Offers illustrations of neuroanatomical structures using colored line drawings, scanning electron micrographs, confocal micrographs, photographs of cadaveric specimens, MRI, cross sections of the brain and spinal cord, and angiograms to highlight the descriptive text. Significant content may have been sacrificed for brevity.

B– **Embryology: Review for New National Boards**

$25.00 Test/569 q

Gasser

J&S Publishing, 1997, 221 pages, ISBN 188830801X

Typical format for this series. Occasional vignettes reflect the clinical slant of the USMLE. The question format does not reflect the format of the USMLE; however, pictures are of high quality. Too long for boards review for such a low-yield topic. Limited student feedback.

B– **Essentials of Clinical Neuroanatomy and Neurophysiology**

$29.95 Review only

Gilman

F. A. Davis, 2003, 281 pages, ISBN 0803607725

Discussions of neuroanatomy, neurophysiology, and neuropharmacology with illustrations and images. Well organized, but too dense for boards review.

B- Color Atlas of Neuroscience

$37.00   Review only

Greenstein

Thieme, 2000, 448 pages, ISBN 0865777101

Visual approach to the anatomy, physiology, and pharmacology of neuroscience with 193 color plates and concise text. Requires considerable time commitment. Use to supplement larger texts.

B- Netter's Anatomy Flash Cards

$29.95   Cards

Hansen

Icon Learning Systems, 2002, ISBN 1929007086

Flash-card format using Dr. Netter's timeless illustrations. Extremely detailed. Useful as an adjunct to other sources. Limited student feedback.

B- Anatomy, Histology & Cell Biology: PreTest

$24.95   Test/500 q

Klein

McGraw-Hill, 2002, 497 pages, ISBN 0071370870

Difficult questions with detailed answers. Some illustrations. Requires extensive time commitment. Includes a high-yield section that highlights clinically relevant relationships and lessons.

B- Basic Concepts in Cell Biology and Histology

$29.95   Review only

McKenzie

McGraw-Hill, 2000, 427 pages, ISBN 0070369305

Divided by tissue type and organ system. Lots of diagrams. Overly detailed for boards review of a low-yield topic.

B- Basic Concepts in Neuroscience

$29.95   Review only

Slaughter

McGraw-Hill, 2002, 312 pages, ISBN 0071360468

Detailed description of many aspects of neuroscience. More suitable for coursework than for quick review.

B- Clinical Anatomy: An Illustrated Review with Questions and Explanations

$32.00   Review/500+ q

Snell

Lippincott Williams & Wilkins, 2001, 272 pages, ISBN 0781729890

Well-organized summary of Snell's major book. Includes excellent diagrams and tables. Questions incorporate radiographs, CT scans, and MRIs. Does not cover neuroanatomy or embryology. Neither text nor questions are as clinical as the title implies. Only some answers have explanations, and most are too short.

Basic Concepts in Embryology   **$29.95**   Review only
Sweeney
McGraw-Hill, 1998, 480 pages, ISBN 0070633088
Thorough examination of a low-yield topic. Use as a reference and not for
boards review.

REVIEW RESOURCES

Anatomy

TOP RATED RESOURCES

A⁻ **Underground Clinical Vignettes: Behavioral Science** **$22.95** Review only

Bhushan

Blackwell Science, 2002, 120 pages, ISBN 0632045434
Concise clinical cases illustrating commonly tested diseases in behavioral science. Cardinal signs, symptoms, and buzzwords are highlighted. Use as a supplement to other sources of review. Some cases lack details.

A⁻ **BRS Behavioral Science** **$32.95** Review/500 q

Fadem

Lippincott Williams & Wilkins, 1999, 312 pages, ISBN 0683306812
Easy-to-read outline format with boldfacing of key terms. Good, detailed coverage of high-yield topics. Lengthy; gives more information than may be needed for the USMLE. Includes excellent tables and charts as well as a short but complete statistics chapter. Offers great coverage of ethics and patient communication topics. Good review questions.

A⁻ **High-Yield Behavioral Science** **$19.95** Review only

Fadem

Lippincott Williams & Wilkins, 2001, 144 pages, ISBN 0781730848
Clear, concise, quick review of behavioral science. Logical presentation with crammable charts, graphs, and tables. Features a short but adequate statistics chapter. No index.

B⁺ **High-Yield Biostatistics** **$24.95** Review only

Glaser

Lippincott Williams & Wilkins, 2001, 112 pages, ISBN 078172242X
Well-written book with extensive coverage of biostatistics. Includes good review questions and tables. Still a low-yield topic. For the motivated student; not for last-minute cramming. Suitable as a course companion. Some explanations are confusing.

B⁺ **USMLE Behavioral Science Made Ridiculously Simple** **$16.95** Review only

Sierles

MedMaster, 1998, 171 pages, ISBN 0940780348
Easy reading; reasonable yield for the amount of text. Includes medical sociology; strong on psychopathology with illustrative examples. No biostatistics. At times offers too much detail on low-yield topics.

B **Behavioral Science/Psychiatry: Review**   **$25.00**   Test/500+ q
for New National Boards
Frank
J&S Publishing, 1998, 248 pages, ISBN 1888308001
Answers given in text format with additional information to help teach
and expand on concepts.

B **Appleton & Lange's Review of Epidemiology**   **$24.95**   Review/100 q
and Biostatistics
Hanrahan
McGraw-Hill, 1994, 109 pages, ISBN 083850244X
Excellent, concise overview of epidemiology with complete explanations
and diagrams. Does not include other behavioral science subtopics. Expensive and limited yield. Good for the motivated student.

B **Digging Up the Bones: Biostatistics**   **$21.95**   Review only
and Epidemiology
Linardakis
McGraw-Hill, 1998, 350 pages, ISBN 0070382220
Fairly concise review with clinical applications. Most effective as a quick re-
fresher. Heavy on low-yield equations. Offers no self-testing opportunities.

B⁻ **Behavioral Science: PreTest**   **$24.95**   Test/500 q
Ebert
McGraw-Hill, 2002, 358 pages, ISBN 0071374701
Detailed answers cross-referenced with other resources. Good test ques-
tions. Requires time commitment. Includes a brief high-yield section.

B⁻ **Oklahoma Notes Behavioral Sciences**   **$14.95**   Review/169 q
Krug
Springer-Verlag, 1995, 311 pages, ISBN 0387943935
Typewritten; easy reading. Presented in outline format. Questions are of
mixed quality. Good tables. For the motivated student.

B⁻ **Digging Up the Bones: Behavioral Sciences**   **$21.95**   Review only
Linardakis
McGraw-Hill, 1998, 88 pages, ISBN 0070382182
Concise narrative review of behavioral sciences; disorganized format cov-
ers some high-yield topics. Choppy style.

TOP RATED RESOURCES

A⁻ **Underground Clinical Vignettes: Biochemistry** $22.95   Review only
Bhushan
Blackwell Science, 2002, 120 pages, ISBN 0632045450
Concise clinical cases illustrating approximately 100 frequently tested diseases with a biochemical basis. Cardinal signs, symptoms, and buzzwords are highlighted. Useful supplement to other sources of review.

A⁻ **High-Yield Biochemistry** $24.95   Review only
Wilcox
Lippincott Williams & Wilkins, 2003, 128 pages, ISBN 0781743141
Concise and crammable text in outline format with good clinical correlations at the end of each chapter. Features many diagrams and tables. Good as a study supplement.

B⁺ **Lippincott's Illustrated Reviews: Biochemistry** $35.95   Review/250+ q
Champe
Lippincott Williams & Wilkins, 1994, 420 pages, ISBN 0397510918
Excellent book, but requires time commitment, so an early start is necessary. Best used while taking the course. Excellent diagrams. Emphasizes "big picture" concepts. Good clinical correlations. Comprehensive review of biochemistry, including low-yield topics. Skim high-yield diagrams to maximize USMLE review.

B **Biochemistry Illustrated** $45.95   Review only
Campbell
Churchill Livingstone, 2000, 240 pages, ISBN 044306217X
Excellent diagrams with explanations but no questions. Good for students who prefer learning by diagrams. Readable but expensive; requires time commitment.

B **IMS Metabolism** $25.95   Review/170+ q
Coffee
Fence Creek, 1998, 434 pages, ISBN 1889325260
Detailed coverage of general metabolic functions. Good diagrams, tables, and clinical correlations. Most chapters begin with a relevant clinical case and end with its resolution. Review questions are included after every chapter. Very readable. Compare with *Lippincott's Illustrated Reviews: Biochemistry*.

REVIEW RESOURCES

Biochemistry

B High-Yield Cell & Molecular Biology $24.95 Review only
Dudek
Lippincott Williams & Wilkins, 1999, 128 pages, ISBN 0683303597
Cellular and molecular biology presented in outline format, with good diagrams and clinical correlations. Brief but complete. Includes descriptions of laboratory techniques and genetic disorders. No questions or vignettes.

B Clinical Biochemistry $36.95 Review only
Gaw
Churchill Livingstone, 1999, 176 pages, ISBN 0443061831
Biochemistry and physiology presented in a clinical framework. Visually pleasing. Focuses on adult medicine; skimpy on inherited disorders, genetics, and molecular biochemistry. Case studies are included throughout, but no standard question-and-answer exercises are given. May be more wards than boards oriented.

B Clinical Biochemistry Made Ridiculously Simple $22.95 Review
Goldberg
MedMaster, 1999, 95 pages, ISBN 0940780305
Conceptual approach to clinical biochemistry, with humor. Casual style does not appeal to all students. Mnemonics tend to be somewhat complicated. Offers a good overview and integration of all metabolic pathways. Includes a 23-page clinical review that is very high yield and crammable. Also contains a unique foldout "road map" of metabolism. For students with a firm biochemistry background.

B Medical Genetics $46.95 Review
Jorde
Mosby , 2003, 384 pages, ISBN 0323020259
Intended as an up-to-date introductory text on medical genetics. Contains numerous well-integrated photographs, diagrams, and drawings. "Clinical commentaries" on specific diseases are used to further illustrate or reinforce the text. Includes study questions. Great for use during coursework and as a reference for boards review.

B Biochemistry: Review for USMLE Step 1 $25.00 Test/533 q
Kumar
J&S Publishing, 2001, 265 pages, ISBN 1888308109
Quick question-based review of biochemistry. Includes clinical vignettes and extended matching questions but few diagrams. Use in conjunction with other resources.

B BRS Biochemistry

$32.95 Review/500 q

Marks

Lippincott Williams & Wilkins, 1998, 350 pages, ISBN 0683304917
Easy-to-read outline with good boldfaced chapter summaries. Very thorough; at times too detailed. Features mixed-quality diagrams. High-yield clinical correlations are given at the end of each chapter. Includes questions with short answers.

B Molecular Biology Series

$99.95 Software/500+ q

MedTech

MedTech Publishing, 1995, ISBN 1889185019
Many good questions with clear explanations. Expensive for student purchase; a discount is available directly through the publisher (800-260-2600 or www.medtech.com). Limited student feedback. Available for either Windows or Macintosh.

B STARS Biochemistry Review

$27.50 Review/600 q

Roskoski

W. B. Saunders, 1996, 242 pages, ISBN 0721651755
Content review in dense outline format with small type. Chapters are short and include only relevant pathways. Good for students who prefer an outline-based review. Parallels core text by the same authors. A comprehensive exam at the end of the book has some questions with a clinical slant.

B Biochemistry and Genetics: PreTest

$24.95 Test/500 q

Wilson

McGraw-Hill, 2002, 300 pages, ISBN 0071375783
Difficult questions with detailed, referenced explanations. Best for the motivated student who uses with a review book. Contains some questions on biochemical disorders but no clinical vignettes. Features six pages of high-yield facts focusing on genetically based diseases.

B- Oklahoma Notes Biochemistry

$14.95 Review/549+ q

Briggs

Springer-Verlag, 1995, 287 pages, ISBN 0387943986
Dense text with many hand-drawn diagrams. Includes a good chapter on medical genetics. Non–clinically oriented questions with brief explanations in the margin. Multiple authors; inconsistent style. Easy reading, but not thorough.

IMS Medical Molecular Genetics   **$27.95**   Review/150+ q
Hoffee
Fence Creek, 1998, 384 pages, ISBN 1889325287
Detailed coverage of molecular biology and medical genetics. Includes
photographs. Easy reading with good explanations and diagrams. Chapters
begin and end with clinical cases. Highly clinical, but lengthy for boards
review; focus on chapter outline and review questions.

 Basic Concepts in Medical Genetics   **$29.95**   Review only
Horwitz
McGraw-Hill, 2000, 149 pages, ISBN 0071345000
Presents concise summaries of medical genetic concepts with clinical ap-
plications and anecdotes. Better suited for a specialized genetics course
than for boards review.

 Digging Up the Bones: Biochemistry   **$21.95**   Review only
Linardakis
McGraw-Hill, 1998, 115 pages, ISBN 0070382174
Collection of high-yield biochemistry facts. Use for last-minute review or
in conjunction with another review book. Some lists are helpful. Few clin-
ical correlations. Limited student feedback.

TOP RATED RESOURCES

Underground Clinical Vignettes: Microbiology

$22.95 (each)   Review only

Bhushan

Blackwell Science

Microbiology, Vol. I: 2002, 128 pages, ISBN 0632045477

Microbiology, Vol. II: 2002, 105 pages, ISBN 0632045493

Concise clinical cases illustrating approximately 100 frequently tested diseases in microbiology and immunology. Cardinal signs, symptoms, and buzzwords are highlighted. Use as a supplement to other sources of review.

Clinical Microbiology Made Ridiculously Simple

$25.95   Review only

Gladwin

MedMaster, 2003, 272 pages, ISBN 0940780496

Very good chart-based review of microbiology. Includes clever and humorous mnemonics. Best of this series. Text is easy to read. An excellent antibiotic review helps for pharmacology as well. "Ridiculous" style does not appeal to everyone. Requires a supplemental source for immunology. Excellent if you have limited time or are "burning out."

Cases in Medical Microbiology and Infectious Disease

$39.95   Review/200 q

Gilligan

ASM Press, 1997, 350 pages, ISBN 155581106X

Presents and discusses 70 cases in detail. Cases test pathogenesis and lab diagnosis of organisms, clinical presentations, epidemiology, and treatment. More than 100 full-color images demonstrate laboratory and clinical diagnosis of disease. Excellent for integrating basic and clinical concepts.

High-Yield Immunology

$19.95   Review only

Johnson

Lippincott Williams & Wilkins, 1999, 68 pages, ISBN 0683306146

Format typical of high-yield series. Accurately covers high-yield details within the topic in proportion to boards coverage of immunology. Good for quick review. Some illustrations and diagrams could be improved. Some sections may not be detailed enough.

REVIEW RESOURCES

Microbiology

A⁻ **Medical Microbiology and Immunology:**   **$39.95**   Review/654 q
Examination and Board Review
Levinson
McGraw-Hill, 2002, 614 pages, ISBN 0071382178
Clear, concise writing with excellent diagrams and tables. Includes an excellent immunology section. The "Summary of Medically Important Organisms" is highly crammable. Requires time commitment. Can be detailed and dense; best if started early with the course. Covers all topics, including low-yield ones. Good practice questions and comprehensive exam, but questions have letter answers only. Compare with *Lippincott's Illustrated Reviews: Microbiology*.

B⁺ **Medical MicroCards**   **$19.95**   150 cards
Orlando
Medfiles, 1996, 150 pages, ISBN 0965537307
Concise flash cards cover bacteriology, virology, mycology, and parasitology. Designed for fast review; no extraneous information is given. Covers disease characteristics, treatment, prevention, and clinical findings. Mixed reviews. Compare with Topf's *Microbiology Companion*.

B⁺ **Case Studies in Immunology:**   **$33.95**   Review/100 q
A Clinical Companion
Rosen
Garland, 2001, 250 pages, ISBN 0815340508
Originally designed as a clinical companion to Janeway's *Immunobiology*, this text provides an excellent synopsis of the major disorders of immunity in a clinical vignette format. Integrates basic and clinical science. Wonderful images, illustrations, questions, and discussion.

B⁺ **How the Immune System Works**   **$24.95**   Review only
Sompayrac
Blackwell Science, 2002, 144 pages, ISBN 063204702X
Concise overview of immunology. Attempts to place complicated concepts into a simple but not simplistic "big picture." Includes a good general introduction, but best used as a companion to other, more detailed resources. Weak in clinical immunology. Limited student feedback.

B⁺ **Microbiology Companion**   **$27.95**   Review/Cards
Topf
Alert and Oriented, 1997, 243 pages, ISBN 0964012413
Chart format is well organized; spiral binding makes it easy to read and carry. Most relevant to microbiology topics. Ties in relevant drugs. Very little immunology. Needs updating. High-yield flash cards (180) are a plus.

B+ **STARS Microbiology Review**   **$21.95**   Review/600 q
Walker
W. B. Saunders, 1998, 255 pages, ISBN 0721646425
Parallels the core text by the same authors. Learning objectives are clearly
defined. Includes numerous questions throughout as well as a 160-question
comprehensive exam with answers and a detailed discussion. Immunology
is not included.

B+ **Clinical Microbiology Review**   **$36.95**   Review only
Warinner
Wysteria, 2001, 152 pages, ISBN 0967783933
Concise yet comprehensive review in chart form with some clinical correlations. Each page is devoted to a single organism with ample space for
adding notes during class. No immunology. Spatial organization, color
coding, and bulleting of facts facilitate subject review. A great cross-refer-
ence section groups organisms by general characteristics. The new edition
includes color plates of significant microbes. Limited but positive student
feedback. Compare with Topf's *Microbiology Companion*.

B+ **Appleton & Lange's Review of**   **$34.95**   Test/995 q
Microbiology and Immunology
Yotis
McGraw-Hill, 2001, 288 pages, ISBN 0071362657
Large number of questions with detailed answers. Well referenced. Inade-
quate as a primary source, but a very good supplement. For the motivated
student. Good diagrams, figures, and tables. Includes a good immunology
section but weak coverage of immune disorders.

B **IMS Immunology**   **$27.95**   Review/170 q
Anderson
Fence Creek, 1999, 194 pages, ISBN 1889325341
Integrates clinical cases and questions into each chapter. Answers and ex-
planations are provided. Some chapters contain more detail than neces-
sary for boards preparation.

B **Concepts in Microbiology, Immunology,**   **$17.95**   Review/100+ q
and Infectious Disease
Gupta
Parthenon, 1997, 150 pages, ISBN 1850707979
Brief paragraphs in outline form on each disease cover most important
points. Good clinical questions are included at the end of each section.
Features a good section on immunologic disorders. No illustrations. Format may not appeal to all students; best for the well-prepared student. For
quick review. Many answers are not sufficiently explained.

B Buzzwords in Microbiology

$19.95   Review only

Hurst

Bryan Edwards, 1997, 240 pages, ISBN 1878576089

Spiral-bound flash cards containing important facts about the most medically relevant bacteria and fungi. Directed toward boards review. Bullet presentation of information affords easy and quick review. Features good pictures and buzzwords. Does not cover virology, parasitology, or immunology.

B Oklahoma Notes Microbiology and Immunology

$14.95   Review/312+ q

Hyde

Springer-Verlag, 1995, 229 pages, ISBN 0387943927

Easy to read, but not adequate as a sole study source. Good summary statements are given at the end of each chapter. Features extended matching questions. Poor typeface and diagrams. Unequal coverage.

B BRS Microbiology and Immunology

$32.95   Review/500 q

Johnson

Lippincott Williams & Wilkins, 2001, 300 pages, ISBN 0781727707

Concise outline format with good questions and illustrations. The immunology section is especially useful. For the motivated student.

B Bugcards: The Complete Microbiology Review for Class, the Boards, and the Wards

$26.50   Cards

Levine

BL Publishing, 1998, 154 flash cards, ISBN 0967165504

High-quality flash cards (similar to "Pharm Cards") designed for rapid class and USMLE microbiology review. Cover all medically relevant bacteria, viruses, fungi, and parasites. Include important buzzwords, mnemonics, and clinical vignettes to aid in recall. Unique "disease process cards" summarize all organisms for a particular disease (e.g., UTI or pneumonia). Useful for quick review of facts, but not recommended as a comprehensive primary review source.

B Digging Up the Bones: Microbiology and Immunology

$21.95   Review

Linardakis

McGraw-Hill, 1998, 107 pages and flash cards, ISBN 0070382158

Brief, easy-to-read collection of phrases and associations. Includes a few tables and simple diagrams. Expensive for the amount of material given. Features detachable flash cards. Limited student feedback.

B **Basic Immunology**   **$32.95**   Review/150 q
Sharon
Lippincott Williams & Wilkins, 1998, 303 pages, ISBN 0683077295
Well-organized text with many figures and tables. Features unique images
of clinical presentations. Includes a section on organ transplantation.
Comprehensive, but may be better suited to coursework than to boards re-
view. Limited student feedback.

B **Microbiology: Review for USMLE Step 1**   **$19.95**   Test/573 q
Stokes
J&S Publishing, 2002, 266 pages, ISBN 1888308125
Easy reading. Covers many high-yield topics and includes case-based questions and extended matching questions. Includes a very good question-
and-answer-based review of clinically relevant microbiology and immunology, but lacking somewhat in detailed information. Helpful as a
supplement to a review book.

B **Lippincott's Illustrated Reviews:**   **$35.95**   Review/Few q
Microbiology
Strohl
Lippincott Williams & Wilkins, 2001, 528 pages, ISBN 0397515685
Comprehensive, highly illustrated review of microbiology similar in style
to Champe's *Lippincott's Illustrated Reviews: Biochemistry*. Includes a 50-
page color section with more than 150 clinical and laboratory pho-
tographs. Compare with Levinson's *Medical Microbiology and Immunology*.

B **NMS Microbiology and Infectious Disease**   **$35.95**   Review/500 q
Virella
Lippincott Williams & Wilkins, 1996, 575 pages, ISBN 0683062352
Outline format. Too detailed in some areas. Insufficient immunology;
NMS has a separate immunology book. Lacks a good explanation of bac-
terial genetics. Features updated material on AIDS. Useful only if previ-
ously used as a textbook. Limited student feedback.

B **STARS Microbiology**   **$32.00**   Review
Walker
W. B. Saunders, 1998, 513 pages, ISBN 0721646417
Presents pathogens in a consistent outline format, from pathogenicity to
treatment. Features numerous multicolor tables and illustrations. No ques-
tions. Requires time commitment. Consider as a course supplement.

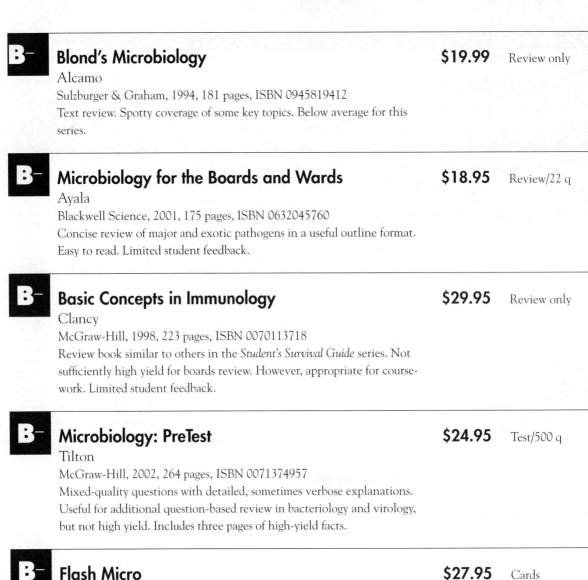

B⁻ Blond's Microbiology
$19.99 Review only

Alcamo

Sulzburger & Graham, 1994, 181 pages, ISBN 0945819412

Text review. Spotty coverage of some key topics. Below average for this series.

B⁻ Microbiology for the Boards and Wards
$18.95 Review/22 q

Ayala

Blackwell Science, 2001, 175 pages, ISBN 0632045760

Concise review of major and exotic pathogens in a useful outline format. Easy to read. Limited student feedback.

B⁻ Basic Concepts in Immunology
$29.95 Review only

Clancy

McGraw-Hill, 1998, 223 pages, ISBN 0070113718

Review book similar to others in the *Student's Survival Guide* series. Not sufficiently high yield for boards review. However, appropriate for course-work. Limited student feedback.

B⁻ Microbiology: PreTest
$24.95 Test/500 q

Tilton

McGraw-Hill, 2002, 264 pages, ISBN 0071374957

Mixed-quality questions with detailed, sometimes verbose explanations. Useful for additional question-based review in bacteriology and virology, but not high yield. Includes three pages of high-yield facts.

B⁻ Flash Micro
$27.95 Cards

Ting

Stanford Ink, 1999, 131 cards, ISBN 0967231809

Concise flash cards designed for boards review. Include 190 pathogens but no immunology. Color coded. Compare with Orlando's *Medical Micro-Cards*. Mixed student feedback.

TOP RATED RESOURCES

BRS Pathology   **$32.95**   Review/500 q

Schneider

Lippincott Williams & Wilkins, 2001, 488 pages, ISBN 0683302655
Concise review with appropriate content emphasis. Features outline-format chapters with boldfacing of key facts. Includes excellent questions with explanations at the end of each chapter and a comprehensive exam at the end of the book. Offers well-organized tables and diagrams as well as some good black-and-white photographs representative of classic pathology. Correlate with color photographs from an atlas. The latest edition contains a new chapter on laboratory testing and "key associations" with each disease. Short on clinical details for vignette questions. Consistently high student recommendations. Worthwhile to master this book. Most effective if started early and then reviewed during study periods.

Underground Clinical Vignettes: **$22.95**   Review only
Pathophysiology   **(each)**

Bhushan

Blackwell Science
Pathophysiology, Vol. I: 2002, 128 pages, ISBN 0632045515
Pathophysiology, Vol. II: 2002, 116 pages, ISBN 0632045531
Pathophysiology, Vol. III: 2002, 120 pages, ISBN 0632045558
Concise clinical cases illustrating approximately 100 frequently tested pathology and physiology cases in each book. Cardinal signs, symptoms, and buzzwords are highlighted. Use as a supplement to other sources of review.

BrainChip for Pathology   **$19.95**   Review only

Garcia

Blackwell Science, 2002, 144 pages, ISBN 0632046392
More than 160 clinical cases and color photographs. Excellent pictures and relevant text.

Robbins Review of Pathology   **$34.95**   Review/1100+ q

Goljan

W. B. Saunders, 2000, 310 pages, ISBN 0721682596
Question book of pathology with answer explanations. Questions are almost entirely clinically based and are accompanied by a number of high-quality histologic and gross images as well as by references to the *Robbins Pathologic Basis of Disease* and *Basic Pathology* textbooks. Questions can be difficult or picky. Answer explanations are brief but well written. Very good review resource.

REVIEW RESOURCES

Pathology

Pathology: PreTest $24.95   Test/500 q
Brown
McGraw-Hill, 2002, 530 pages, ISBN 0071372237
Picky, difficult questions with detailed, complete answers. Questions are
often obscure or esoteric. Features high-quality black-and-white photographs but no color photographs. Can be used as a supplement to other
review books. For the motivated student who desires exposure to a variety
of photographs. Thirty-five pages of high-yield facts are useful for concept
summaries.

 STARS Pathology $34.00   Review only
Goljan
W. B. Saunders, 1998, 528 pages, ISBN 0721670237
Well-organized, concise, and easy-to-read explanations of pathology. Illus-
trated with diagrams; lacks photos and imaging. Excellent charts and ta-
bles. Some students use as a primary source.

 STARS Pathology Review $24.95   Review/500+ q
Goljan
W. B. Saunders, 1998, 352 pages, ISBN 0721670245
Companion book to *STARS Pathology*. Uses a concise outline to summarize key concepts. Includes chapter questions with answers and detailed
explanations as well as a comprehensive 150-question practice exam. Features more than 100 illustrations, including photos and histologic images.

 Interactive Case Study Companion $49.95   Software/
to Robbins Pathologic Basis of Disease   Case studies
Kumar
W. B. Saunders, 1999, ISBN 0721684629
Ninety-nine clinical cases with 1500 images covering a full range of topics
in general and systemic pathology. Great learning supplement. Can be
time-consuming. For the motivated student.

 Pathophysiology of Heart Disease $34.95   Review only
Lilly
Lippincott Williams & Wilkins, 2002, 448 pages, ISBN 0781740274
Collaborative project by medical students and faculty at Harvard. Well organized, easy to read, and concise; offers comprehensive coverage of cardiovascular pathophysiology from the medical student's perspective. An
excellent bridge between the basic and clinical sciences. Very good for review of this subject, but does not cover other areas of pathology tested on
the boards. May be too detailed for boards review.

B+ **Pathophysiology of Disease: Introduction to Clinical Medicine**   **$44.95**   Review/Few q

McPhee

McGraw-Hill, 2000, 662 pages, ISBN 0838581609

Interdisciplinary course text useful for understanding the pathophysiology of clinical symptoms. Offers excellent integration of basic sciences with mechanisms of disease. Great graphs, diagrams, and tables. Most helpful if used during coursework owing to its length. Few non-boards-style questions. Clinical emphasis nicely complements *BRS Pathology*.

B+ **Pathology: Review for New National Boards**   **$25.00**   Test/509 q

Miller

J&S Publishing, 1993, 222 pages, ISBN 0963287338

Question-and-answer-based review of pathology. Includes many case-based questions. Focuses on high-yield topics. Features good black-and-white photographs. Includes some picky questions with incomplete answers. Inadequate as a sole source of review. Expensive for the number of questions.

B+ **Pathophysiology: PreTest**   **$24.95**   Test/500 q

Mufson

McGraw-Hill, 2002, 200 pages, ISBN 0071375074

Includes 500 questions and answers with detailed explanations. Questions may be more difficult than those on the boards. Features a brief section of high-yield topics.

B+ **Pocket Companion to Robbins Pathologic Basis of Disease**   **$29.95**   Review only

Robbins

W. B. Saunders, 1999, 800 pages, ISBN 0721678599

Good for reviewing associations between keywords and specific diseases. Highly condensed, complete, and easy to understand. Explains most important diseases and pathologic processes. No photographs or illustrations. Useful as a quick reference.

B **Appleton & Lange's Review of General Pathology**   **$34.95**   Test/1300+ q

Catalano

McGraw-Hill, 2003, 352 pages, ISBN 0071389954

Short text sections followed by numerous questions with answers. Some useful high-yield tables are included at the beginning of each section. Good photomicrographs. Covers only general pathology (i.e., no organ-based pathology). Can be used as a supplement to more detailed texts. Good review when time is short.

B **Colour Atlas of Anatomical Pathology** $65.95   Review only

Cooke

Churchill Livingstone, 2004, 300 pages, ISBN 0443073600

Beautifully photographed atlas of gross pathology. Easy-to-read, clinically
relevant content.

B **Lange Smart Charts** $24.95   Review only

Groysman

McGraw-Hill, 2001, 356 pages, ISBN 0838581757

Flip chart of tables with information grouped together for ease of recall.
Organized by body systems with mnemonics. Best used as a summary reference for fast review.

B **USMLE Pathology Review: The Study Guide** $47.95   Review/300+ q

Hassanein

Sage, 1998, 416 pages, ISBN 0761905170

Key pathology concepts presented in an outline format. Numerous questions with answers and explanations. Includes a comprehensive 184-ques-
tion exam. No index.

B **EBS Essentials of Pathophysiology** $39.95   Review/69 q

Kaufman

Lippincott Williams & Wilkins, 1996, 816 pages, ISBN 0316484059

Review book with few questions. Features clinical descriptions of important diseases, but too detailed for high-yield review. Good diagrams, tables,
and black-and-white photographs. More appropriate as a course text and
reference. For the highly motivated student. Limited student feedback.

B **NMS Pathology** $32.95   Review/500 q

LiVolsi

Lippincott Williams & Wilkins, 1993, 525 pages, ISBN 0683062433

Outline form. Comprehensive review of a large amount of material. Sometimes too detailed for boards review. Slow reading. Best if used with
course.

B **Pathology: Examination and Board Review** $39.95   Review/Few q

Newland

McGraw-Hill, 1995, 360 pages, ISBN 0838577199

Concise text review with some high-quality charts and photomicrographs.
Includes non-boards-style questions at the end of each chapter with letter
answers only.

B **Renal Pathophysiology: The Essentials**   **$28.00**   Review only

Rose

Lippincott Williams & Wilkins, 1993, 344 pages, ISBN 0683073540
Excellent review and explanations of various disease processes of the kidney. Includes review questions within the text for comprehension; not boards style. Good reference during boards review.

B **Color Atlas of Pathophysiology**   **$39.00**   Review only

Silbernagl

Thieme, 2000, 380 pages, ISBN 0865778663
More than 180 high-quality illustrations that demonstrate disturbed physiologic processes that lead to dysfunction. Limited student feedback.

B **Case Studies in General
and Systemic Pathology**   **$30.00**   Review/300+ q

Underwood

Churchill-Livingstone, 1996, 172 pages, ISBN 0443050961
Presents 60 cases with excellent images and integrated questions/answers. Full-color images include gross specimens, histology, and MRIs. Closely linked to Underwood's *General and Systemic Pathology*.

B‒ **Basic Concepts in Pathology**   **$29.95**   Review only

Brown

McGraw-Hill, 1998, 456 pages, ISBN 0070083215
Good review of basic concepts. No images. Not entirely suitable for USMLE review.

B‒ **Wheater's Basic Histopathology**   **$52.95**   Review only

Burkitt

Churchill-Livingstone, 1996, 252 pages, ISBN 0443050880
Color atlas with text. Contains excellent pictures of pathologic histology. Not directed toward boards-type review. May be more useful for photomicrograph-based questions.

B‒ **Rypins' Intensive Reviews: Pathology**   **$21.95**   Review/220+ q

Damjanov

Lippincott Williams & Wilkins, 1998, 432 pages, ISBN 0397515553
Typical of this series. Includes a comprehensive exam with answers and explanations. Illustrated with simple diagrams; no photos included.

Review Questions for Human Pathology $19.95 Test/1300+ q

Jones

Parthenon, 1999, 322 pages, ISBN 1850705992

Includes more than 1300 questions with answers and discussions. Many questions are in outdated USMLE format. Step 1–level questions are interspersed with questions at the level of Step 2 and Step 3. Good value for the price.

TOP RATED RESOURCES

B+ **Pharmacology: Review for New National Boards**   **$25.00**   Test/539 q

Billingsley

J&S Publishing, 1995, 186 pages, ISBN 0963287370

Question-and-answer book typical for this series. Includes clinical vignettes. Good explanations cover many high-yield pharmacology topics. Easy, fast reading. Questions about drug structures are probably low yield. Useful adjunct to a review book. Limited student feedback.

B+ **Lippincott's Illustrated Reviews: Pharmacology**   **$35.95**   Review/230+ q

Harvey

Lippincott Williams & Wilkins, 1999, 528 pages, ISBN 0781724139

Outline format with practice questions and many excellent and memorable illustrations and tables. Cross-referenced to *Lippincott's Illustrated Reviews: Biochemistry*. Good for the "big picture." Good pathophysiologic approach. Detailed, so use with coursework and review for the USMLE. For the motivated student. Includes ten illustrated case studies with questions and answers in the appendix. The revised printing edition includes a "special millennium update" that covers all new drugs introduced since 1996.

B+ **Pharm Recall**   **$32.95**   Test

Ramachandran

Lippincott Williams & Wilkins, 1999, 512 pages, ISBN 068330285X

Approach to pharmacology review in a question-and-answer "recall" format. A high-yield drug summary is included. Good for cramming and memorization.

B+ **Basic Concepts in Pharmacology**   **$29.95**   Review only

Stringer

McGraw-Hill, 2001, 285 pages, ISBN 0071356991

Presents summaries of "elusive" concepts in pharmacology, from simple to complex. Good for basic concepts. No questions. Limited student feedback.

B⁺ **Katzung and Trevor's Pharmacology: Examination and Board Review**

$39.95   Review/1000 q

Trevor

McGraw-Hill, 2002, 662 pages, ISBN 0838581471

Well-organized text in narrative format with concise explanations. Features good charts and tables. Good for drug interactions and toxicities. Offers two practice exams and 17 case studies with questions and detailed answers. Includes some low-yield/obscure drugs. The 40-page crammable list of "top boards drugs" is especially high yield. Compare closely with *Lippincott's Illustrated Reviews: Pharmacology*.

B **Underground Clinical Vignettes: Pharmacology**

$22.95   Review only

Bhushan

Blackwell Science, 2002, 136 pages, ISBN 0632045574

Concise clinical cases illustrating approximately 100 frequently tested pharmacology concepts. Cardinal signs, symptoms, and buzzwords are highlighted. Clinical vignette style is less effective for pharmacology. Use as a supplement to other sources of review.

B **NMS Pharmacology**

$32.95   Review/450+ q

Dworkin

Lippincott Williams & Wilkins, 1996, 385 pages, ISBN 0683062514

Outline format. More tables and diagrams are included in the new edition. Often too detailed, and lacks emphasis on high-yield material. Features a lengthy USMLE-type exam. Requires time commitment. Typical for this series.

B **Pharmacology Companion**

$27.95   Review/Cards

Gallia

Alert and Oriented, 1997, 339 pages, ISBN 096401243X

Spiral bound with high-yield flash cards. Chart format illustrates mechanisms, uses, and side effects of each drug or class of drugs. Includes few diagrams, and the format does not seem to work as well as it does in Topf's *Microbiology Companion*. Needs updating. Limited student feedback.

B **Pharm Cards: A Review for Medical Students**

$32.95   Cards

Johannsen

Lippincott Williams & Wilkins, 2002, 228 cards, ISBN 0781734010

Updated edition highlights important features of major drugs/drug classes. Good for class review; also offers a quick, focused review for the USMLE. Lacks pharmacokinetics. Good charts and diagrams. Highly rated by students who enjoy flash-card-based review. Bulky to carry around.

B **Blond's Pharmacology** $19.99 Review only
Kostrzewa
Sulzburger & Graham, 1995, 398 pages, ISBN 094581948X
Concise review of pharmacology. Features many good diagrams. Some key
topics are inadequately covered.

B **Digging Up the Bones: Pharmacology** $21.95 Review/Cards
Linardakis
McGraw-Hill, 1998, 99 pages and 100+ flash cards, ISBN 007038214X
Brief, easy-to-read collection of phrases and drug associations. Contains
more than 100 flash cards of top drugs with clinical use, mechanisms, and
side effects. Use as a supplement.

B **Color Atlas of Pharmacology** $39.00 Review only
Luellmann
Thieme, 386 pages, 2000, ISBN 0865778434
Highly visual approach to pharmacology. No questions. Includes 149 color
plates accompanied by brief descriptions.

B **Clinical Pharmacology Made Ridiculously Simple** $20.95 Review only
Olson
MedMaster, 2001, 164 pages, ISBN 094078050X
Includes general principles and many drug summary charts. Particularly
strong in cardiovascular drugs and antimicrobials; incomplete in other areas. Consists primarily of tables; lacks the humorous illustrations and
mnemonics typical of this series. Well organized, but occasionally too detailed. Effective as a chart-based review book but not as a sole study
source. Must be supplemented with a more detailed text.

B **Quick Look Medicine: Pharmacology** $21.95 Review/100+ q
Raffa
Fence Creek, 1999, 204 pages, ISBN 1889325384
Covers essential facts and concepts using diagrams. Includes numerous
questions, answers, and explanations. Limited student feedback.

B **Instant Pharmacology** $39.99 Review/130 q
Saeb-Parsy
John Wiley & Sons, 1999, 349 pages, ISBN 0471976393
Text divided into several parts, the first addressing basic mechanisms
found in pharmacology. Drugs encountered in this section are summarized
in the "Dictionary of Drugs." Ends with a comprehensive exam. Includes
answers but no explanations.

Pharmacology: PreTest   **$24.95**   Test/500 q
Stern
McGraw-Hill, 2002, 294 pages, ISBN 0071367047
Picky, difficult questions with detailed answers. A new high-yield chapter
is a comparison chart intended only as a sample learning tool.

 STARS Pharmacology Review   **$22.95**   Review/Some q
Brenner
W. B. Saunders, 2000, 271 pages, ISBN 0721677584
Focuses on prototypical drugs and their mechanisms and clinical uses. Emphasizes application of basic science concepts to everyday clinical problem
solving. Includes section examinations and a comprehensive exam of
USMLE-style questions based on clinical vignettes. Very detailed. Best
used with other sources. Answers and detailed rationales for each question
are provided.

 High-Yield Pharmacology   **$24.95**   Review only
Christ
Lippincott Williams & Wilkins, 2003, 144 pages, ISBN 0781745128
Pharmacology review in an easy-to-follow outline format. No questions or
index. Offers a good summary. Best used with a more extensive text.

TOP RATED RESOURCES

 BRS Physiology $32.95 Review/400 q

Costanzo

Lippincott Williams & Wilkins, 2003, 352 pages, ISBN 0781739195

Clear, concise review of physiology. Fast, easy reading; comprehensive and efficient. Includes great charts and tables. Good practice questions with explanations and a clinically oriented final exam. Excellent review book, but may not be enough for in-depth coursework. Comparatively weak respiratory and acid-base sections.

 Physiology $36.95 Review only

Costanzo

W. B. Saunders, 2002, 395 pages, ISBN 0721695493

Comprehensive coverage of concepts outlined in *BRS Physiology*. Excellent diagrams and charts. Each systems-based chapter includes a detailed summary of objectives and a boards-relevant clinical case. Requires time.

 Physiology Cases and Problems (Board Review Series) $32.95 Review/Many q

Costanzo

Lippincott Williams & Wilkins, 2001, 352 pages, ISBN 0781724821

Roughly 50 cases in vignette format with several questions per case. Includes detailed answers with explanations. For the motivated student.

 Hematology at a Glance $29.95 Review only

Mehta

Blackwell Science, 2000, 128 pages, ISBN 0632047933

Covers common blood issues. Includes color illustrations. Presented in a logical sequence that is easy to read. Good for class use as well.

B+ High-Yield Acid Base $18.95 Review only

Longnecker

Lippincott Williams & Wilkins, 1998, 100 pages, ISBN 0683303937

Concise and well-written description of acid-base disorders. Includes chapters discussing differential diagnosis and 12 clinical cases. Introduces a multistep approach to the material. A bookmark with useful factoids is included with the text. No index or questions.

REVIEW RESOURCES

Physiology

B⁺ **Appleton & Lange's Review of Physiology** $32.95   Test/700+ q
Penney
McGraw-Hill, 1998, 277 pages, ISBN 0838502741
Boards-style questions with letter answers and explanations. Includes no
vignettes. Questions are somewhat picky. Limited review.

B⁺ **Respiratory Physiology: The Essentials** $31.00   Review/100+ q
West
Lippincott Williams & Wilkins, 1999, 192 pages, ISBN 0683307347
Comprehensive coverage of respiratory physiology. Clearly organized with
useful charts and diagrams. The new edition includes appendices with
more than 100 questions and answers with explanations. Best used as a
course supplement. Limited student feedback.

B **NMS Physiology** $32.95   Review/300 q
Bullock
Lippincott Williams & Wilkins, 2001, 872 pages, ISBN 0683306030
Very complete text in outline form. Often too detailed, but some good diagrams. Moderately difficult questions with detailed answers. Provides
some pathophysiology and clinical correlations. More useful if used as a
course text and reference; too long as a review text. Inexpensive for the
amount of material. For the motivated student.

B **Color Atlas of Physiology** $35.00   Review only
Despopoulos
Thieme, 2003, 448 pages, ISBN 1588900614
Compact, with more than 150 colorful but complicated diagrams on the
right and dense explanatory text on the left. Some translation problems.
A unique, highly visual approach worthy of consideration. Useful as an
adjunct to other review books.

B **Clinical Physiology Made Ridiculously Simple** $19.95   Review only
Goldberg
MedMaster, 2001, 160 pages, ISBN 0940780216
Easy reading with many amusing associations. Style does not work for
everyone. Not as well illustrated as the rest of the series. Use as a supple-
ment to other review books.

B **Blond's Physiology** $20.00   Review only
Grossman
Sulzburger & Graham, 1995, 439 pages, ISBN 0945819420
Comprehensive but easy-to-read review text of physiology. Clear and sim-
ple classic diagrams and charts. Better than average for this series. Strong
endocrine chapter; good hormone list.

B | **Concepts in Physiology** | **$17.95** | Review/100+ q

Gupta

Parthenon, 1996, 135 pages, ISBN 1850707308

Systems-based review in paragraph form. Some sections have clinical questions at the end of the chapter with explanations. Format may not appeal to all students. Limited student feedback.

B | **Physiology: Review for New National Boards** | **$25.00** | Test/506 q

Jakoi

J&S Publishing, 1994, 214 pages, ISBN 0963287346

Good review book, but inadequate as a sole source of review. Quick reading. Below-average question quality for this series. Answer discussions cover many important topics.

B | **Quick Look Medicine: Cardiopulmonary System** | **$19.95** | Review/117 q

Richardson

Fence Creek, 1999, 164 pages, ISBN 1889325422

Presents concepts in diagram format. Includes questions, answers, and detailed explanations for self-assessment. Discussion covers cardiovascular and pulmonary physiology as well as cardiopulmonary pathophysiology.

B | **Memorix Physiology** | **$35.25** | Review

Schmidt

Chapman & Hall, 1997, 281 pages, ISBN 041271440X

Systems-based coverage of key concepts in an easy-to-carry handbook. Similar in format to the *Color Atlas of Physiology*. Contains more than 200 color illustrations and tables. Expensive for the amount of material.

B– | **Digging Up the Bones: Physiology** | **$21.95** | Review only

Linardakis

McGraw-Hill, 1998, 350 pages, ISBN 0070382212

Organ-based collection of facts. Text includes tables, graphs, and some illustrations. Clinical vignettes accompany each topic.

B– | **Linardakis' Illustrated Review of Physiology** | **$37.95** | Review/200 q

Linardakis

Michaelis Medical, 1998, 340 pages, ISBN 1884084176

Comprehensive, illustration-based review of medical physiology. Color illustrations are integrated into text.

Review Questions for Physiology　　　　　　$24.95　Test/700 q

Pasley

CRC Press-Parthenon, 1998, 142 pages, ISBN 1850706018

Few clinical vignette-type questions. Answers are on the same page as questions, making it easy to move through questions and check answers at the same time.

 Physiology: PreTest　　　　　　　　　　$24.95　Test/500 q

Ryan

McGraw-Hill, 2002, 322 pages, ISBN 0071371990

Questions with detailed, well-written explanations. Some questions are too difficult or picky. May be useful for the motivated student following extensive review from other sources. Includes 34 pages of high-yield facts.

Commercial Review Courses

Kaplan Medical

Northwestern Medical
  Review

Postgraduate Medical
  Review Education

The Princeton Review

Youel's Prep, Inc.

Commercial preparation courses can be helpful for some students, but such courses are expensive and require significant time commitment. They are usually effective in organizing study material for students who feel overwhelmed by the volume of material. Note that the multiweek courses may be quite intense and may thus leave limited time for independent study. Also note that some commercial courses are designed for first-time test takers while others focus on students who are repeating the examination. Some courses focus on IMGs who want to take all three Steps in a limited amount of time. Student experience and satisfaction with review courses are highly variable. We suggest that you discuss options with recent graduates of review courses you are considering. Course content and structure can evolve rapidly. Some student opinions can be found in discussion groups on the World Wide Web.

Kaplan Medical

Kaplan Medical offers a wide range of options for USMLE preparation, including live lectures, video lectures, and online products. All of its courses and products focus on providing the most exam-relevant information available.

Live Lectures. Kaplan's IntensePrep™ offers a highly structured, interactive live review led by expert faculty. Designed for medical students with little time to prepare, it includes approximately 15 days of live lectures during which faculty members cover the material students need to know to master the Step 1 exam. IntensePrep students also receive six months of access to Kaplan's WebPrep course, which offers more than 80 hours of high-yield, audio-streamed lectures plus an online diagnostic exam that generates a personalized study plan. This course features seven volumes of lecture notes and a question book that includes 850 practice questions.

Kaplan also offers longer live-lecture courses, including LivePrep (6 weeks) and Extended LivePrep (14 weeks), which are aimed at students who are repeating the exam or at students and physicians seeking more time to prepare.

Center Study. MedPass, Kaplan's center-based lecture course, is designed for medical students seeking flexibility. It is offered at more than 120 Kaplan Centers across the United States and includes 30 visits to local Kaplan Centers, where students are given access to approximately 175 hours of video lecture review. This course also includes seven volumes of lecture notes, a question book that contains 850 practice questions, and a full-length simulated exam with full performance analysis and detailed explanations.

For those who would like more center access, Kaplan offers CenterPrep, which includes a personalized study plan and three months of access to Kaplan Centers.

Online Resources. Kaplan Medical offers several options for online question review. Its popular online question bank, Qbank, includes 2100 exam-style questions with detailed explanations. With Qbank, students can customize practice tests by discipline and organ system, receive instant on-screen feedback, and track their cumulative performance. Students can purchase one month or three months of access.

Another Step 1 resource is Kaplan's new Integrated Vignettes Qbank, an online clinical case question bank that allows users to practice answering case-based, USMLE-style vignettes that are organized by symptom. Each vignette contains multidisciplinary questions covering different ways the underlying basic science concepts could be tested. IV Qbank includes 1200 questions and is available in one-month or three-month increments.

For students who would like to use both Step 1 Qbank and IV Qbank to prepare for the exam, Kaplan offers Qreview, which contains more than 3500 questions and provides six months of simultaneous access to both Qbanks. Qreview provides students with collective reporting of their results across both Qbanks. Qbank demos are available at kaplanmedical.com.

More information on Kaplan courses can be obtained at (800) 533-8850 or at www.kaplanmedical.com.

Northwestern Medical Review

Northwestern Medical Review offers live-lecture review courses for both the COMLEX Level I and USMLE Step 1 examinations. Three courses (Plans) are available for each exam: NBI 100—a three-day course; NBI 200—a 5-day course; and NBI 300—a 10- or 15-day course. All courses are in live-lecture format, and most are taught by the authors of the Northwestern Review Books. In addition to organized lecture notes and books for each subject, courses include Web-based CBT test bank access and a large pool of practice questions and simulated exams. All plans are available in a customized, on-site format for groups of second-year students from individual U.S. medical schools. Additionally, public sites are frequently offered in East Lansing and Ann Arbor, Michigan; Philadelphia, Pennsylvania; St. Louis, Missouri; San Antonio, Texas; Los Angeles, California; and Long Island, New York. International sites may also be offered at the request of groups of students and international educational organizations.

Tuition for NBI 100 ranges from $160 to $290; NBI 200 from $250 to $390; and NBI 300 from $550 to $980. Tuition is based on group size, program duration, and early-enrollment discounts. Home-study materials, CBT question bank access, and DVD materials are also available for purchase independent of the live-lecture plans. Northwestern offers a retake option as well as a liberal cancellation policy. Contact:

Northwestern Medical Review
P.O. Box 22174
Lansing, MI 48909-2174
Phone: 1-866-MedPass
Fax: (517) 347-7005
E-mail: registrar@northwesternmedicalreview.com
www.northwesternmedicalreview.com

Postgraduate Medical Review Education

Postgraduate Medical Review Education (PMRE) has 27 years of experience with medical licensing exam preparation.

PMRE offers complete home-study courses for the USMLE Step 1 in the form of audio cassettes and books. Package A has 66 hours of live classes on audio tapes for $998. It includes a transcript book and a 2003 update book with graphs, tables, and professor handouts. Package E has 9000 questions and answers on 20 hours of audio tape for $250.

PMRE uses professors who write questions for USMLE exams and professionally recorded materials. For more information, contact:

PMRE
1909 Tyler Street, #305
Hollywood, FL 33020
Phone: 1-800-ECFMG-30
E-mail: usmlepmre@aol.com
www.PMRE.com

The Princeton Review

The Princeton Review offers three flexible preparation options for the USMLE Step 1: the USMLE Online Course, the USMLE Classroom Course, and the USMLE Online Workout. In selected cities, The Princeton Review also offers a more intensive preparation course for IMGs.

USMLE Online Course. The USMLE Online Course offers comprehensive, self-paced preparation, including the following:

- Seventy-five hours of online review, including lessons, vignettes, and drills
- Three full-length diagnostic tests with detailed score reports
- Seven comprehensive review manuals consisting of more than 1500 pages
- Seven mini-tests to gauge students' knowledge in each subject
- Twenty-four-hour e-mail support from Princeton Review Online instructors
- Three months of online access

USMLE Classroom Course. The USMLE Classroom Course for American Medical Students (available in selected cities) includes the following:

- Expert live instruction to complement online resources
- Twenty-seven hours of live classroom instruction from a medical resident
- Seventy-five hours of online review, including lessons, vignettes, and drills
- Three full-length diagnostic tests with detailed score reports
- Seven comprehensive review manuals consisting of more than 1500 pages
- Seven mini-tests to gauge students' knowledge in each subject

USMLE Online Workout. The USMLE Online Workout offers the following:

- Two thousand USMLE-style questions presented in the CBT format
- Three full-length diagnostic exams
- Seven mini-tests: Anatomy, Behavioral Science, Biochemistry, Microbiology and Immunology, Pathology, Pharmacology, and Physiology
- More than 40 subject-specific drills
- High-yield slide review for Anatomy and Pathology

- Complete explanations of all questions and answers
- Three months of access

More information can be found on The Princeton Review's Web site at www.PrincetonReview.com.

Youel's Prep, Inc.

Youel's Prep, Inc., has specialized in medical boards preparation for 25 years. Youel's Prep provides Web casts (*Youel's WebPrep™*), videotapes (*VideoPrep™*), audiotapes (*AudioPrep™*), books (*BookPrep™*), live lectures (*Youel's LivePrep™*), and tutorials for small groups and for individuals (*TutorialPrep™*). All Web casts, videotapes, audiotapes, live lectures, and tutorials are correlated with a three-book set consisting of Prep Notes©; two textbooks, *Youel's Jewels I©* and *Youel's Jewels II©* (984 pages); and a question-and-answer book, *Case Studies*.

FastTrac for the Basic Sciences©, available in audiotape and book form, offers 984 questions, answers, and explanations and is designed for both a HeadStart and FastFinish for the boards.

ClinicalSkillsAssesmentPrep™ (*C-SAPPrep™*), available in videotape (24 hours), audiotape (24 hours), and book form, provides a concise summary of the symptoms, signs, and syndromes essential to taking a focused history and physical and preparing proper patient notes. *ClerkPrep©*, available in videotape, audiotape, and book form, provides a HeadStart for clinical clerkships. *ClerkPrep™* is offered in 24-hour and 40-hour programs. *Q-Prep* consists of two books with 1854 questions, answers, and explanations.

All Youel's Prep courses are physician taught and written, reflecting the clinical slant of the boards. In addition, all programs are updated continuously. Accordingly, books are not printed until the order is received. Delivery in the United States is usually within one week. Optional express delivery is available.

Youel's Prep Home Study Program™—consisting of *Youel's Web Prep™*, *VideoPrep™*, *AudioPrep™*, and *BookPrep™*—allows students to own their materials and to use them for repetitive study in the convenience of their homes. Purchasers of any of the Youel's Prep programs are enrolled as members of the Youel's Prep Family of Students™. This provides free telephone tutoring by Youel.

Youel's Prep live lectures are held at select medical schools, at the invitation of the school and students. Programs are customized to meet individual and school needs and can be custom-designed for 16 to 56 hours. First-year students are urged to call early to arrange live lecture programs at their schools for next year. Youel's Prep-India and Nepal offers on-site programs in selected cities.

For more information, contact:

Youel's Prep, Inc.
P.O. Box 4605
West Palm Beach, FL 33402
Phone: (800) 645-3985
Fax: (561) 366-8628
E-mail: info@youelsprep.com
www.youelsprep.com

Publisher Contacts

If you do not have convenient access to a medical bookstore, consider ordering directly from the publisher.

Appleton & Lange
(see McGraw-Hill)

BL Publishing
3614 North Raven Wash Drive
Tucson, Arizona 85745
(520) 743-1711
blpublishing@hotmail.com

Blackwell Publishing
AIDC
P.O. Box 20
Williston, VT 05495-9957
(800) 216-2522
Fax: (802) 864-7626
www.blackwellpublishing.com

Churchill Livingstone
(see Elsevier Science)

Elsevier Science
Order Fulfillment
11830 Westline Industrial Drive
St. Louis, MO 63146
(800) 545-2522
www.us.elsevierhealth.com

Gold Standard Board Prep
2619 West Loughlin Drive
Chandler, AZ 85224
(480) 699-0152
Fax: (740) 592-4045
www.boardprep.net

J&S Publishing
1300 Bishop Lane
Alexandria, VA 22302
(703) 823-9833
Fax: (703) 823-9834
jandspub@hotmail.com
www.jandspub.com

Lippincott Williams & Wilkins
P.O. Box 1600
Hagerstown, MD 21740
(800) 777-2295
Fax: (301) 223-2400
orders@lww.com
www.lww.com

Maval Publishing, Inc.
567 Harrison Street
Denver, CO 80206
(303) 338 8725
Fax: (303) 745 6215
maval@maval.com
www.maval.com

McGraw-Hill/Appleton & Lange Customer Service
P.O. Box 545
Blacklick, OH 43004-0545
(800) 338-3987
Fax: (614) 755-5645
www.mghmedical.com

MedMaster, Inc.
P.O. Box 640028
Miami, FL 33164
(800) 335-3480
(305) 653-3480
Fax: (954) 962-4508
mmbks@aol.com
www.medmaster.net

MedTech USA
6310 San Vicente Boulevard,
    Suite 404
Los Angeles, CA 90048
(800) 640-8000
Fax: (323) 964-1001
mail@medtech.com
www.medtech.com

Mosby-Year Book
(see Elsevier Science)

Parthenon Publishing
29 W. 35th Street, 7th Floor
New York, NY 10001
(917) 351-7148
Fax: (917) 212-947-3027
usa@parthpub.com
www.parthpub.com

Springer-Verlag, NY Inc.
175 Fifth Avenue
New York, NY 10010
(212) 460-1500
(800) SPRINGER (1-800-777-4643)
Main fax: (212) 473-6272
Order fax: (201) 348-4505
orders@Springer-NY.com
www.Springer-NY.com

W. B. Saunders
(see Elsevier Science)

Sulzburger & Graham
83 Woodmere Boulevard
Woodmere, NY 11598
(800) 366-7086
(212) 947-0100.
Fax: (516) 569-4654
orders@sgpublishing.com
www.sgpublishing.com

Abbreviations and Symbols

Abbreviation	Meaning
1°	primary
2°	secondary
3°	tertiary
AA	amino acid
AAV	adeno-associated virus
Ab	antibody
ABP	androgen-binding protein
Ac-CoA	acetylcoenzyme A
ACE	angiotensin-converting enzyme
ACh	acetylcholine
AChE	acetylcholinesterase
ACL	anterior cruciate ligament
ACTH	adrenocorticotropic hormone
ADA	adenosine deaminase, Americans with Disabilities Act
ADH	antidiuretic hormone
ADHD	attention-deficit hyperactivity disorder
ADP	adenosine diphosphate
Ag	antigen
AICA	anterior inferior cerebellar artery
AIDS	acquired immunodeficiency syndrome
ALA	aminolevulinic acid
ALL	acute lymphocytic leukemia
ALS	amyotrophic lateral sclerosis
ALT	alanine transaminase
AML	acute myelocytic leukemia
AMP	adenosine monophosphate
ANA	antinuclear antibody
ANOVA	analysis of variance
ANP	atrial natriuretic peptide
ANS	autonomic nervous system
AOA	American Osteopathic Association
AP	action potential
APC	antigen-presenting cell
APSAC	anistreplase
ARC	Appalachian Regional Commission
ARDS	adult respiratory distress syndrome
Arg	arginine
ASD	atrial septal defect
ASO	antistreptolysin O
Asp	aspartic acid
AST	aspartate transaminase
ATP	adenosine triphosphate
ATPase	adenosine triphosphatase
AV	atrioventricular
AVM	arteriovenous malformation
AZT	azidothymidine
BAL	British anti-Lewisite [dimercaprol]
BMI	body-mass index
BMR	basal metabolic rate
BP	blood pressure
BPG	bis-phosphoglycerate
BPH	benign prostatic hyperplasia
BUN	blood urea nitrogen
CAD	coronary artery disease

Abbreviation	Meaning
cAMP	cyclic adenosine monophosphate
C-ANCA	cytoplasmic antineutrophil cytoplasmic antibody
CBT	computer-based testing
CCK	cholecystokinin
CCl_4	carbon tetrachloride
CCT	cortical collecting tubule
CD	cluster of differentiation
CDP	cytidine diphosphate
CE	cholesterol ester
CEA	carcinoembryonic antigen
CETP	cholesterol-ester transfer protein
CFU	colony-forming unit
CFX	circumflex [artery]
cGMP	cyclic guanosine monophosphate
ChAT	choline acetyltransferase
CHF	congestive heart failure
CIN	candidate identification number, cervical intraepithelial neoplasia
CJD	Creutzfeldt-Jakob disease
CK-MB	creatine kinase, MB fraction
CL	clearance
CLL	chronic lymphocytic leukemia
CM	chylomicron
CML	chronic myeloid leukemia
CMT	Computerized Mastery Test
CMV	cytomegalovirus
CN	cranial nerve
CNS	central nervous system
CO	cardiac output
CoA	coenzyme A
COGME	Council on Graduate Medical Education
COMLEX	Comprehensive Osteopathic Medical Licensing Examination
COPD	chronic obstructive pulmonary disease
COX	cyclooxygenase
CPAP	continuous positive airway pressure
CPK	creatine phosphokinase
CRH	corticotropin-releasing hormone
CSA	Clinical Skills Assessment
CSF	cerebrospinal fluid, colony-stimulating factor
CT	computed tomography
CVA	cardiovascular accident, costovertebral angle
Cx	complication
Cys	cysteine
d4T	didehydrodeoxythymidine [stavudine]
DAF	decay-accelerating factor
DAG	diacylglycerol
dATP	deoxyadenosine triphosphate
ddC	dideoxycytidine
ddI	didanosine
DES	diethylstilbestrol
DHAP	dihydroxyacetone phosphate

Abbreviation	Meaning
DHB	dihydrobiopterin
DHEA	dehydroepiandrosterone
DHPG	dihydroxy-2-propoxymethyl guanine
DHS	Department of Homeland Security
DHT	dihydrotestosterone
DI	diabetes insipidus
DIC	disseminated intravascular coagulation
DIP	distal interphalangeal [joint]
DIT	diiodotyrosine
DKA	diabetic ketoacidosis
DNA	deoxyribonucleic acid
2,4-DNP	2,4-dinitrophenol
DO	doctor of osteopathy
DOPA	dihydroxyphenylalanine (methyldopa)
2,3-DPG	2,3-diphosphoglycerate
DPM	doctor of podiatric medicine
DPPC	dipalmitoyl phosphatidylcholine
DS	double stranded
dsDNA	double-stranded deoxyribonucleic acid
dsRNA	double-stranded ribonucleic acid
dTMP	deoxythymidine monophosphate
DTR	deep tendon reflex
DTs	delirium tremens
DVT	deep venous thrombosis
EBV	Epstein-Barr virus
EC_{50}	median effective concentration
ECF	extracellular fluid
ECFMG	Educational Commission for Foreign Medical Graduates
ECG	electrocardiogram
ECT	electroconvulsive therapy
EDTA	ethylenediamine tetra-acetic acid
EDV	end-diastolic volume
EEG	electroencephalogram
EF	ejection fraction, elongation factor
ELISA	enzyme-linked immunosorbent assay
EM	electron micrograph, electron microscopic, electron microscopy
EMB	eosin–methylene blue
EOM	extraocular muscle
epi	epinephrine
EPO	erythropoietin
EPS	extrapyramidal system
ER	endoplasmic reticulum
ERAS	Electronic Residency Application Service
ERCP	endoscopic retrograde cholangiopancreatography
ERP	effective refractory period
ERPF	effective renal plasma flow
ERV	expiratory reserve volume
ESR	erythrocyte sedimentation rate
ESV	end-systolic volume
EtOH	ethyl alcohol
FAD	oxidized flavin adenine dinucleotide
$FADH_2$	reduced flavin adenine dinucleotide
FAP	familial adenomatous polyposis
5f-dUMP	5-fluorodeoxyuridine monophosphate
FE_{Na}	excreted fraction of filtered sodium
FEV_1	forced expiratory volume in 1 second
FF	filtration fraction
FFA	free fatty acid
FGF	fibroblast growth factor
f-met	formylmethionine
FMG	foreign medical graduate

Abbreviation	Meaning
FMN	flavin mononucleotide
FRC	functional residual capacity
FSH	follicle-stimulating hormone
FSMB	Federation of State Medical Boards
FTA-ABS	fluorescent treponemal antibody—absorbed
5-FU	5-fluorouracil
FVC	forced vital capacity
G3P	glucose-3-phosphate
G6P	glucose-6-phosphate
G6PD	glucose-6-phospate dehydrogenase
GABA	γ-aminobutyric acid
GBM	glomerular basement membrane
G-CSF	granulocyte colony-stimulating factor
GFAP	glial fibrillary acid protein
GFR	glomerular filtration rate
GGT	γ-glutamyl transpeptidase
GH	growth hormone
GI	gastrointestinal
GIP	gastric inhibitory peptide
Glu	glutamic acid
GM-CSF	granulocyte-macrophage colony-stimulating factor
GMP	guanosine monophosphate
GN	glomerulonephritis
GnRH	gonadotropin-releasing hormone
GPe	globus pallidus externa
GPi	globus pallidus interna
GRP	gastrin-releasing peptide
GSH	reduced glutathione
GSSG	oxidized glutathione
GTP	guanosine triphosphate
GU	genitourinary
HAART	highly active antiretroviral therapy
HAV	hepatitis A virus
Hb	hemoglobin
HBcAb	hepatitis B core antibody
HBcAg	hepatitis B core antigen
HBeAb	hepatitis B early antibody
HBeAg	hepatitis B early antigen
HBsAb	hepatitis B surface antibody
HBsAg	hepatitis B surface antigen
HBV	hepatitis B virus
hCG	human chorionic gonadotropin
HCV	hepatitis C virus
HDL	high-density lipoprotein
HDV	hepatitis D virus
HEV	hepatitis E virus
HGPRTase	hypoxanthine-guanine phosphoribosyltransferase
HHS	[Department of] Health and Human Services
HHV	human herpesvirus
5-HIAA	5-hydroxyindoleacetic acid
His	histidine
HIV	human immunodeficiency virus
HLA	human leukocyte antigen
HMG-CoA	hydroxymethylglutaryl-coenzyme A
HMP	hexose monophosphate
HMWK	high-molecular-weight kininogen
HNPCC	hereditary nonpolyposis colorectal cancer
HPA	hypothalamic-pituitary-adrenal [axis]
HPSA	Health Professional Shortage Area
HPV	human papillomavirus

Abbreviation	Meaning
HR	heart rate
HSV	herpes simplex virus
HSV-1	herpes simplex virus 1
HSV-2	herpes simplex virus 2
5-HT	5-hydroxytryptamine (serotonin)
HTLV	human T-cell leukemia virus
HUS	hemolytic-uremic syndrome
IBD	inflammatory bowel disease
IC	inspiratory capacity
ICA	internal carotid artery
ICF	intracellular fluid
ICP	intracranial pressure
ID$_{50}$	median infectious dose
IDDM	insulin-dependent diabetes mellitus
IDL	intermediate-density lipoprotein
I/E	inspiratory/expiratory [ratio]
IF	immunofluorescence
IFN	interferon
Ig	immunoglobulin
IHSS	idiopathic hypertrophic subaortic stenosis
IL	interleukin
Ile	isoleucine
IMA	inferior mesenteric artery
IMED	International Medical Education Directory
IMG	international medical graduate
IMP	inosine monophosphate
INH	isonicotine hydrazine [isoniazid]
IP$_3$	inositol triphosphate
IRV	inspiratory reserve volume
ITP	idiopathic thrombocytopenic purpura
IV	intravenous
IVC	inferior vena cava
JG	juxtaglomerular [cells]
JGA	juxtaglomerular apparatus
KSHV	Kaposi's sarcoma–associated herpesvirus
LA	left atrial
LAD	left anterior descending [artery]
LCA	left coronary artery
LCAT	lecithin-cholesterol acyltransferase
LCL	lateral collateral ligament
LCME	Liaison Committee on Medical Education
LCV	lymphocytic choriomeningitis virus
LD	lymphocyte depleted [Hodgkin's]
LDH	lactate dehydrogenase
LDL	low-density lipoprotein
LES	lower esophageal sphincter
Leu	leucine
LFA-1	leukocyte function–associated antigen 1
LFT	liver function test
LGN	lateral geniculate nucleus
LH	luteinizing hormone
LLQ	left lower quadrant
LM	light microscopy
LMN	lower motor neuron
LP	lymphocyte predominant [Hodgkin's]
LSE	Libman-Sacks endocarditis
LT	leukotriene
LV	left ventricle, left ventricular
Lys	lysine
MAC	membrane attack complex
MAO	monoamine oxidase
MAP	mean arterial pressure

Abbreviation	Meaning
MC	mixed cellularity [Hodgkin's]
MCA	middle cerebral artery
MCHC	mean corpuscular hemoglobin concentration
MCL	medial collateral ligament
MCP	metacarpophalangeal [joint]
MCV	mean corpuscular volume
MEN	multiple endocrine neoplasia
MEOS	microsomal ethanol oxidizing system
Met	methionine
MGN	medial geniculate nucleus
MHC	major histocompatibility complex
MHPSA	Mental Health Professional Shortage Area
MI	myocardial infarction
MIT	monoiodotyrosine
MLF	medial longitudinal fasciculus
MMR	measles, mumps, rubella [vaccine]
6-MP	6-mercaptopurine
MPO	myeloperoxidase
MPTP	1-methyl-4-phenyl-1,2,3,6-tetrahydropyridine
MRI	magnetic resonance imaging
mRNA	messenger ribonucleic acid
MS	multiple sclerosis
MSH	melanocyte-stimulating hormone
MUA/P	Medically Underserved Area and Population
MVO$_2$	myocardial oxygen consumption
NAD+	oxidized nicotinamide adenine dinucleotide
NADH	reduced nicotinamide adenine dinucleotide
NADP+	oxidized nicotinamide adenine dinucleotide phosphate
NADPH	reduced nicotinamide adenine dinucleotide phosphate
NBME	National Board of Medical Examiners
NBOME	National Board of Osteopathic Medicine Examiners
NBPME	National Board of Podiatric Medicine Examiners
NE	norepinephrine
NF	neurofibromatosis
NIDDM	non-insulin-dependent diabetes mellitus
NK	natural killer [cells]
NPV	negative predictive value
NS	nodular sclerosing [Hodgkin's]
NSAID	nonsteroidal anti-inflammatory drug
OAA	oxaloacetic acid
OCD	obsessive-compulsive disorder
OCP	oral contraceptive pill
OMT	osteopathic manipulative technique
OR	odds ratio
PA	posteroanterior
PABA	para-aminobenzoic acid
PAH	para-aminohippuric acid
PALS	periarterial lymphatic sheath
PAN	polyarteritis nodosa
P-ANCA	perinuclear antineutrophil cytoplasmic antibody
PAS	periodic acid Schiff
PCL	posterior cruciate ligament
PCP	phencyclidine hydrochloride, *Pneumocystis carinii* pneumonia
PCR	polymerase chain reaction

Abbreviation	Meaning
PCWP	pulmonary capillary wedge pressure
PD	posterior descending [artery]
PDA	patent ductus arteriosus
PDE	phosphodiesterase
PE	pulmonary embolism
PEP	phosphoenolpyruvate
PFK	phosphofructokinase
PFT	pulmonary function test
PG	prostaglandin
Phe	phenylalanine
PICA	posterior inferior cerebellar artery
PID	pelvic inflammatory disease
PIP	proximal interphalangeal [joint]
PIP$_2$	phosphatidylinositol 4,5-bisphosphate
PK	pyruvate kinase
PKU	phenylketonuria
PML	progressive multifocal leukoencephalopathy
PMN	polymorphonuclear [leukocyte]
PNET	primitive neuroectodermal tumor
PNH	paroxysmal nocturnal hemoglobinuria
PNS	peripheral nervous system
PPRF	paramedian pontine reticular formation
PPV	positive predictive value
PRPP	phosphoribosylpyrophosphate
PSA	prostate-specific antigen
PSS	progressive systemic sclerosis
PT	prothrombin time
PTH	parathyroid hormone
PTHrP	parathyroid hormone–related protein
PTSD	post-traumatic stress disorder
PTT	partial thromboplastin time
PV	plasma volume
RBC	red blood cell
RBF	renal blood flow
RCA	right coronary artery
RDS	respiratory distress syndrome
REM	rapid eye movement
RER	rough endoplasmic reticulum
RNA	ribonucleic acid
RPF	renal plasma flow
RPR	rapid plasma reagin
RR	relative risk, respiratory rate
rRNA	ribosomal ribonucleic acid
RS	Reed-Sternberg [cells]
RSV	respiratory syncytial virus
RUQ	right upper quadrant
RV	right ventricle, right ventricular, residual volume
RVH	right ventricular hypertrophy
SA	sinoatrial, subarachnoid
SAM	S-adenosylmethionine
SC	subcutaneous
SCID	severe combined immunodeficiency disease
SD	standard deviation, subdural
SEM	standard error of the mean
SERM	selective estrogen receptor modulator
SER	smooth endoplasmic reticulum
SEVIS	Student Exchange Visitor Information System
SEVP	Student Exchange Visitor Program
SGOT	serum glutamic oxaloacetic transaminase
SGPT	serum glutamic pyruvate transaminase
SIADH	syndrome of inappropriate antidiuretic hormone

Abbreviation	Meaning
SLE	systemic lupus erythematosus
SLL	small lymphocytic lymphoma
SMA	superior mesenteric artery
SMX	sulfamethoxazole
SNc	substantia nigra compacta
snRMP	small nuclear ribonucleoprotein
SOD	superoxide dismutase
SR	sarcoplasmic reticulum
SRP	sponsoring residency program
SRS-A	slow-reacting substance of anaphylaxis
SS	single stranded
ssDNA	single-stranded deoxyribonucleic acid
SSPE	subacute sclerosing panencephalitis
SSRI	selective serotonin reuptake inhibitor
ssRNA	single-stranded ribonucleic acid
STD	sexually transmitted disease
STN	subthalamic nucleus
SV	sinus venosus, stroke volume
SVC	superior vena cava
SVT	supraventricular tachycardia
$t_{1/2}$	half-life
T$_3$	triiodothyronine
T$_4$	thyroxine
TB	tuberculosis
TBW	total body water
3TC	dideoxythiacytidine [lamivudine]
TCA	tricarboxylic acid [cycle], tricyclic antidepressant
Tc cell	cytotoxic T cell
TCR	T-cell receptor
TFT	thyroid function test
TG	triglyceride
TGF	transforming growth factor
THB	tetrahydrobiopterin
Th cell	helper T cell
THF	tetrahydrofolate
Thr	threonine
TIBC	total iron-binding capacity
TLC	total lung capacity
TMP-SMX	trimethoprim-sulfamethoxazole
TN	trigeminal neuralgia
TNF	tumor necrosis factor
TNM	tumor, node, metastases [staging]
TOEFL	Test of English as a Foreign Language
tPA	tissue plasminogen activator
TPP	thiamine pyrophosphate
TPR	total peripheral resistance
TRH	thyrotropin-releasing hormone
tRNA	transfer ribonucleic acid
Trp	tryptophan
TSH	thyroid-stimulating hormone
TSI	thyroid-stimulating immunoglobulin
TSS	toxic shock syndrome
TSST	toxic shock syndrome toxin
TTP	thrombotic thrombocytopenic purpura
TV	tidal volume
TXA	thromboxane
UA	urinalysis
UCV	Underground Clinical Vignettes
UDP	uridine diphosphate
UMN	upper motor neuron
URI	upper respiratory infection
USDA	United States Department of Agriculture
USIA	United States Information Agency

Abbreviation	Meaning
USMLE	United States Medical Licensing Examination
UTI	urinary tract infection
UV	ultraviolet
VA	ventral anterior, Veterans Administration
Val	valine
VC	vital capacity
V_d	volume of distribution
VDRL	Venereal Disease Research Laboratory

Abbreviation	Meaning
VF	ventricular fibrillation
VIPoma	vasoactive intestinal polypeptide-secreting tumor
VLDL	very low density lipoprotein
VPM	ventral posterior nucleus, medial
VPN	ventral posterior nucleus
V/Q	ventilation/perfusion [ratio]
VSD	ventricular septal defect
VZV	varicella-zoster virus
WBC	white blood cell

Index

458

459

464

465

Gustatory hallucinations, 133
Gynecomastia, 318, 340

H

Haemophilus ducreyi, 206
Haemophilus influenzae, 179, 180,
　　182, 185, 204, 205, 252,
　　292, 296
Hair
　　adriamycin, 335
　　alopecia, 166, 167, 335
　　etoposide, 335
　　finasteride, 331
　　hyperthyroidism, 260
　　hypothyroidism, 260
Hairy cell leukemia, 233
Hallucinations
　　arylcyclohexylamines, 313
　　delirium tremens, 128
　　illusions and delusions *vs.,* 133
　　schizophrenia, 134
　　substance abuse
　　　alcohol, 128
　　　amphetamines, 128
　　　cocaine, 128
　　　LSD, 128
　　　marijuana, 128
　　tricyclic antidepressants, 311
　　types of, 133
Haloperidol, 310, 340, 341
Halothane, 304, 312, 340
Hands
　　acromegaly, 261
　　Edwards' syndrome, 226
　　Marfan's syndrome, 228
Hansen's disease, 187
Hardy-Weinberg population
　　genetics, 145
Hartnup disease, 167
Hashimoto's thyroiditis, 217, 261
Hb structure regulation, 165
HDL good cholesterol, 163, 324
Headache
　　ethosuximide, 309
　　feverfew, 342
　　fluoroquinolones, 295
　　griseofulvin, 298
　　hydralazine, 315
　　nitroglycerin, 319
　　ondansetron, 328
　　poliomyelitis, 254
　　polyarteritis nodosa, 274
　　prazosin, 306, 315
　　pregnancy-induced hypertension,
　　　265
　　quinidine, 321
　　rickettsiae, 188
　　Rocky Mountain spotted fever,
　　　188
　　sildenafil, 332

substance abuse
　　amphetamines, 128
　　caffeine, 128
　　nicotine, 128
　temporal arteritis, 274
　venlafaxine, 312
　vitamin A, 166
Health and Human Services,
　　Department of (HHS), 47–48
Heart. *See* Cardiovascular medicine
Heberden's nodes, 256
Heinz bodies, 156
Helicobacter pylori, 185, 245, 296
HELLP syndrome, 265
Helminths, medically important,
　　194
Hemagglutinin, 200
Hemangioblastomas, 228, 236
Hemarthroses, 240
Hematemesis, 280
Hematocrit, 368
Hematoma, intracranial, 253
Hematuria, 195, 228, 275
Heme catabolism, 165
Heme synthesis, 163, 165
Hemianopsia, 104, 107
Hemiballismus, 100
Hemidesmosome, 93
Hemochromatosis, 247, 249, 270
Hemoglobin, 156, 165, 368, 369
Hemoglobinopathies, 238
Hemolytic anemia
　　glycolytic enzyme deficiency, 153
　　hereditary spherocytosis, 228
　　NADPH, 156
　　normochromic anemia, 238
　　penicillin, 291
　　ribavirin, 299
Hemolytic bacteria, alpha/beta, 182,
　　183
Hemophilia, 240
Hemoptysis, 195, 250, 259, 274
Hemorrhage
　　Berry aneurysms, 254
　　cyclophosphamide, 335
　　disorders, 240
　　Duret, 107
　　Goodpasture's syndrome, 259
　　intracranial, 253
　　leiomyosarcoma, 266
　　normochromic anemia, 238
　　placenta accreta, 265
　　tumors, local effects of, 234
　　vitamin K, 169
Hemorrhagic shock syndrome, 200
Hemorrhoids, 129
Henderson-Hasslebalch equation,
　　276
Hepadenavirus, 195
Heparan sulfate, 93

Heparin
　　antidotes, 339
　　mast cells, 70
　　mechanism/clinical
　　　use/toxicity/note, 328
　　osteoporosis, 341
　　warfarin *vs.,* 329
Hepatitis
　　alcohol, 247, 280
　　clinical features, 206
　　cytokines, 337
　　drug reactions, 340
　　enzyme markers, 284
　　hepatocellular carcinoma, 249
　　heroin addiction, 129
　　interferons, 300
　　macrolides, 294
　　milk thistle, 342
　　nosocomial infections, 207
　　polyarteritis nodosa, 274
　　serologic markers, 202
　　transmission, 201
Hepatocellular carcinoma, 232, 233,
　　247, 249
Hepatomegaly, 272
Hepatosplenomegaly, 157, 201, 217,
　　242
Herbal therapy
　　clinical uses/toxicities, 342
Hereditary hyperbilirubinemias, 248
Hereditary nonpolyposis colorectal
　　cancer (HNPCC), 246
Hereditary spherocytosis, 228, 239,
　　346
Hermaphrodite, 227
Hernias, 86
Herniation syndromes, 107
Heroin, 129, 313
Herpes genitalis, 201
Herpes labialis, 201
Herpes simplex virus (HSV), 201,
　　204, 299
Herpesviruses, 195, 198, 199, 201,
　　254
Hesselbach's triangle, 86
Heterochromatin, 139
Heterocyclics, 312
Heterozygosity, loss of, 145
Hexamethonium, 303
Hexokinase, 152, 153
Hexosaminidase, 147
HGPRTase, 160
High-density lipoprotein (HDL),
　　163, 324
Hindgut, 88, 89
Hip dislocation, congenital, 224
Hirschsprung's disease, 246
Hirsutism, 266, 309
Histamine, 70, 71, 215, 368
Histidine, 158

Osteogenesis imperfecta, 151
  phenotype/genetic mechanism/
    prevalence, 146
Osteomalacia, 169
Osteomyelitis, 205
Osteopathic medical student. *See*
    Comprehensive Osteopathic
    Medical Licensing
    Examination (COMPLEX-
    USA)
Osteoporosis
  calcium/phosphate/alkaline
    phosphatase levels, 362
  drug reactions, 341
  glucocorticoids, 332
  homocystinuria, 159
  type I and II, 264
Osteosarcoma, 233, 235
Otitis media, 185, 274
Ototoxicity, 315, 340
Ouabain, 149
Ovaries
  cancer, 233, 335, 336
  clomiphene, 332
  cysts/tumors, 266–267
  paclitaxel, 336
Overseas Educational Advisory
    Centers, 53
Ovulation, 81
Oxaloacetate, 154, 155, 167
Oxazepam, 309
Oxidative phosphorylation, 155
Oxygen. *See also* Nicotinamide
    adenine dinucleotide
    phosphate oxidase
  cardiac output, 345
  hemoglobin, 165
  methemoglobinemia, 165
  oxygen-hemoglobin dissociation
    curve, 369
  respiratory burst, 152
Oxytocin, 99

P

Pacemaker action potential, 344
Pacinian corpuscles, 91
Paclitaxel
  mechanism/clinical use/toxicity,
    336
Paget's disease of the bone, 169,
    232, 267, 284, 336, 362
Pain
  abdomen
    acute pancreatitis, 249
    Budd-Chiari syndrome, 247
    diabetic ketoacidosis, 263
    mifepristone, 332
    pancreatic adenocarcinoma, 250
    poliomyelitis, 254
    polyarteritis nodosa, 274

porphyrias, 165
    pregnancy-induced
      hypertension, 265
  algophobia, 131
  chest
    hyperthyroidism, 260
    panic disorder, 131
  flank
    pyelonephritis, 205
  joint
    systemic lupus erythematosus,
      257
  left lower quadrant
    diverticulitis, 246
  opioid analgesics, 313
  peptic ulcer disease, 245
  periarticular
    temporal arteritis, 274
  pericardial
    pericarditis, 273
  right upper quadrant
    Entamoeba histolytica, 193
  somatoform disorder, 130
  suprapubic
    urinary tract infections, 205
  tabes dorsalis, 256
  tumors, local effects of, 234
Palatine tonsil, 78
Pallor and aplastic anemia, 239
Palpitations and panic disorder, 131
Pancoast's tumor, 252, 255
Pancreas
  adenocarcinoma, 250
  carbohydrate digestion, 374
  cystic fibrosis, 146, 228
  embryology, 79
  endocrine cell types, 95
  enzymes, 373
  exocrine secretion, 373
  insulin, 161
  multiple endocrine neoplasias,
    260
  stimulation of pancreatic
    functions, 373
  Zollinger-Ellison syndrome, 264
Pancreatitis, 163, 249
Pancytopenia, 239
Panic disorder, 131
Papillary carcinoma, 261
Papillary necrosis, 278
Papillomaviruses, 199
Papovavirus, 195
Paraaminobenzoic acid (PABA),
    167, 295
Para-aminohippuric acid (PAH),
    357
Paracoccidioidomycosis, 191
Paracortex, 96
Parafollicular cells, 74, 362
Paragonimus, 301

Paragonimus westermani, 194, 195
Parainfluenza, 199
Paralysis/paresis
  Brown-Séquard syndrome, 109
  clostridia, 183
  Erb-Duchenne palsy, 111
  facial lesions, 109
  lower motor neuron, 109
  syphilis, 206
  upper motor neuron, 109
Paralytic ileus, 336
Paramesonephric duct, 80
Paramyxoviruses, 197, 199
Paranoid ideations, 128, 132
Parasitology. *See under* Microbiology
Parasympathetic nervous system
    (PNS), 91, 98
Parathion, 303
Parathyroid, 78, 216, 260
Parathyroid hormone (PTH), 237,
    252, 360–362
Paraurethral glands, 80
Parenchymal cells, 147
Parenchymal hematoma, 253
Paresthesias, 109, 168
Parietal cells, 370, 371
Parkinsonism
  amantadine, 299
  antimuscarinic drugs, 304
  basal ganglia, 100
  blood-brain barrier, 98
  deprenyl, 312
  drug reactions, 340
  levodopa, 307
  neurotransmitter changes with
    disease, 125
  pathology, 253
  pharmacology, 308
Parotid gland, 104, 370
Parotitis, 133, 199
Paroxetine, 311
Paroxysmal nocturnal
    hemoglobinuria (PNH), 214
Parvovirus, 195, 199
Passive *vs.* active immunity, 217
Pasteurella multocida, 186
Patau's syndrome, 226
Patent ductus arteriosus (PDA),
    224, 225, 313
Pathology. *See also under* Database
    of basic science review
    resources
  alcoholism, 280
  cardiovascular
    arteriosclerosis, 268
    atherosclerosis, 268
    Buerger's disease, 274
    cardiomyopathies, 270
    congestive heart failure, 272
    deep venous thrombosis, 272

Vikas Bhushan, MD

Tao Le, MD

Joshua Klein, PhD

Anil Shivaram, MD

Vikas Bhushan, MD

Dr. Bhushan is a world-renowned author, publisher, entrepreneur, and board-certified diagnostic radiologist who resides in Los Angeles, California. Dr. Bhushan conceived and authored the original *First Aid for the USMLE Step 1* in 1992, which, after 11 consecutive editions, has become the most popular medical review book in the world. Following this, he coauthored three additional *First Aid* books as well as developed the highly acclaimed 17-title *Underground Clinical Vignettes* series. He completed his training in diagnostic radiology at the University of California, Los Angeles. Dr. Bhushan has more than 13 years of entrepreneurial experience and started two successful software and publishing companies prior to cofounding Medsn. He has worked directly with dozens of medical school faculty, colleagues, and consultants and corresponded with thousands of medical students from around the world. Dr. Bhushan earned his bachelor's degree in biochemistry from the University of California, Berkeley, and his MD with thesis from the University of California, San Francisco.

Tao Le, MD

Dr. Le has led multiple medical education projects over the past seven years. As a medical student, he was editor-in-chief of the University of California, San Francisco *Synapse,* a university newspaper with a weekly circulation of 9000. Subsequently, he authored *First Aid for the Wards* and *First Aid for the Match* and led the most recent revision of *First Aid for the USMLE Step 2.* At Yale, he was a regular guest lecturer on the USMLE review courses and an adviser to the Yale University School of Medicine curriculum committee. Dr. Le earned his medical degree from the University of California, San Francisco in 1996 and completed his residency training and board certification in internal medicine at Yale–New Haven Hospital. Dr. Le subsequently went on to cofound Medsn and served as its Chief Medical Officer. He is currently pursuing research in asthma education as a fellow in allergy and clinical immunology at the Johns Hopkins Asthma and Allergy Center.

Joshua Klein, PhD

Dr. Klein is currently a sixth-year student in the MD/PhD program at Yale University School of Medicine. He is originally from Roslyn, New York, and went to college at the University of Pennsylvania, where he studied biology and music theory and graduated with a BA in 1997. He recently completed his PhD thesis, "Activity-Dependent Modulation of Neuronal Sodium Channel Expression," in Stephen Waxman's neurology lab at Yale. Earlier this year, Josh became engaged to Meredith, a third-year student at the University of Illinois College of Veterinary Medicine. They are planning their wedding for April 2005. This is Dr. Klein's fourth year working on *First Aid for the USMLE Step 1*. He can be contacted at joshua.p.klein@yale.edu.

Anil Shivaram, MD

Dr. Shivaram is currently a medicine intern at Mt. Auburn Hospital in Cambridge, MA after which he will become a first-year ophthalmology resident at Boston Medical Center (where he will finally be able to satisfy his curiosity regarding all things "eyeball"). He graduated from Yale University School of Medicine in 2003 with thesis research focused upon the migration of retinal microglia in inherited retinal degenerative disorders. Prior to a life in medicine, he completed his undergraduate studies at Columbia College of Columbia University in Sanskrit with further graduate studies at Oxford. Rounding himself out with a fellowship in medical ethics, he was recently described as "extremely busy" by Actiwatch criteria. While he may live in Boston, he still misses his family in Chicago and Los Angeles. When he is not on-call, post-call, short-call, or mini-call, he can be found cooking, cleaning, and generally pampering his seemingly overworked (but always self-proclaimed "amazing") girlfriend, Lisa. This is Dr. Shivaram's fourth year working for *First Aid for the USMLE Step 1*. Any questions about residency in Boston, medical school, ophthalmology, or something outside of medicine (please...), feel free to email him at anil_shivaram@hms.harvard.edu.

About the Authors

[Handwritten notes:] EL nido recort
894 - 5644
902 - 5962
Pos Palmas
637 - 42?
637 - 42
Princessa holid